GENDER, COMMUNICATIONS,
AND REPRODUCTIVE HEALTH
IN INTERNATIONAL DEVELOPMENT

McGill-Queen's/Brian Mulroney Institute of Government Studies
in Leadership, Public Policy, and Governance

Series editor: Donald E. Abelson

Titles in this series address critical issues facing Canada at home and abroad and the efforts policymakers at all levels of government have made to address a host of complex and multifaceted policy concerns. Books in this series receive financial support from the Brian Mulroney Institute of Government at St Francis Xavier University; in keeping with the institute's mandate, these studies explore how leaders involved in key policy initiatives arrived at their decisions and what lessons can be learned. Combining rigorous academic analysis with thoughtful recommendations, this series compels readers to think more critically about how and why elected officials make certain policy choices, and how, in concert with other stakeholders, they can better navigate an increasingly complicated and crowded marketplace of ideas.

6 Cyber-Threats to Canadian Democracy
  Edited by Holly Ann Garnett and Michael Pal

7 The Canadian Federal Election of 2021
  Edited by Jon H. Pammett and Christopher Dornan

8 CETA Implementation and Implications
  Unravelling the Puzzle
  Edited by Robert G. Finbow

9 Multilateral Sanctions Revisited
  Lessons Learned from Margaret Doxey
  Edited by Andrea Charron and Clara Portela

10 Booze, Cigarettes, and Constitutional Dust-Ups
   Canada's Quest for Interprovincial Free Trade
   Ryan Manucha

11 NORAD
   In Perpetuity and Beyond
   Andrea Charron and James Fergusson

12 Under the Weather
   Reimagining Mobility in the Climate Crisis
   Stephanie Sodero

13 Rethinking Decentralization
   Mapping the Meaning of Subsidiarity in Federal Political Culture
   Jacob Deem

14 Natural Allies
   Environment, Energy, and the History of US-Canada Relations
   Daniel Macfarlane

15 Gender, Communications, and Reproductive Health
   in International Development
   Carolina Matos

Gender, Communications, and Reproductive Health in International Development

CAROLINA MATOS

McGill-Queen's University Press
Montreal & Kingston · London · Chicago

© McGill-Queen's University Press 2023

ISBN 978-0-2280-1754-7 (cloth)
ISBN 978-0-2280-1755-4 (paper)
ISBN 978-0-2280-1809-4 (ePDF)
ISBN 978-0-2280-1810-0 (ePUB)

Legal deposit second quarter 2023
Bibliothèque nationale du Québec

Printed in Canada on acid-free paper that is 100% ancient forest free (100% post-consumer recycled), processed chlorine free

Library and Archives Canada Cataloguing in Publication

Title: Gender, communications, and reproductive health in international development / Carolina Matos.

Names: Matos, Carolina, 1973- author.

Series: McGill-Queen's/Brian Mulroney Institute of Government studies in leadership, public policy, and governance; 15.

Description: Series statement: McGill-Queen's/Brian Mulroney Institute of Government studies in leadership, public policy, and governance; 15 | Includes bibliographical references and index.

Identifiers: Canadiana (print) 20230166636 | Canadiana (ebook) 20230166644 | ISBN 9780228017554 (paper) | ISBN 9780228017547 (cloth) | ISBN 9780228018094 (ePDF) | ISBN 9780228018100 (ePUB)

Subjects: LCSH: Communication in reproductive health. | LCSH: Reproductive health in mass media. | LCSH: Reproductive health—Social aspects. | LCSH: Women—Health and hygiene—Social aspects. | LCSH: Women's rights. | LCSH: Non-governmental organizations. | LCSH: Feminists—Political activity.

Classification: LCC RA564.85 .M38 2023 | DDC 613/.0424—dc23

This book was typeset by Marquis Interscript in 10.5/13 Sabon.

Contents

Tables   vii

Acknowledgements   ix

Abbreviations   xiii

Introduction   3

1 Gender, Communications, and Women's Reproductive Rights in International Development: An Assessment   8

2 Transnational Feminism, the 'Female Body', and Global Gender Justice: Defining 'Sexual and Reproductive Health and Rights'   55

3 'Northern' and 'Southern' NGOs and Advocacy on 'Female Bodies' and Reproductive Health   64

4 Latin American Feminisms and the Struggle for Gender Equality and SRHR in Brazil and Beyond   75

5 Health Advocacy and Feminist Activism for SRHR in South Asia: The Indian Case   94
   Carolina Matos with Ambika Tandon

6 Development Communications and Advocacy for Women's Health and Rights: Why It Matters   105

7 Making Development Work for Women: Assessing Health Communications, Development Campaigns, and Entertainment-Education Approaches   113

8 NGOs, Advocacy Communications, and Feminist Digital Activism on Sexual and Reproductive Health and Rights   123

9 Content Analysis of Institutional Websites and NGO Communication Strategies: From Family Planning 2020 to Anis Brasil   135
Carolina Matos with Tatiane Leal

10 Deconstructing 'Gender Ideology' Myths and Digital Storytelling through Critical Discourse Analysis: A Case Study of NGOs' Social Media Engagement on Twitter and Facebook   174

11 The NGOs' Blog Posts and Digital Storytelling on SRHR: A Critical Examination   198
Carolina Matos with Sarah Molisso

12 Social Media and Advocacy Communications from South Asian NGOs Working on Sexuality and Reproductive Health   213
Carolina Matos with Ambika Tandon

13 Gender Development, Women's Reproductive Health, and Sexual Rights in Challenging Times: Communication Strategies Discussed and Concluding Remarks   225

Appendices

A List of Organisations   249

B NGOs by Region   251

C Budget Information for Twenty-Two NGOs   252

D NGOs and Type of Communications (Sample)   254

E Tables and References from the NGOs' Blogs   266

F South Asian NGOs' Social Media Engagement Figures   269

Notes   271

References   285

Index   307

Tables

9.1 Factors shaping NGO's SRHR communication strategies and advocacy   138
9.2 Forty-nine NGOs' web features   139–44
9.3 Budget information of ten largest organisations   146
9.4 Thirteen NGOs' web features and social media engagement   149–50
9.5 Six NGOs' web features and social media engagement   151
10.1 The top ten most active organisations on Twitter   177
10.2 The top ten most active organisations on Facebook   178

Acknowledgements

The research for this book emerged during the fieldwork conducted for my last manuscript, *Globalization, Gender Politics and the Media* (Lexington Books, 2016). I started then to examine the use of new technologies for mobilisation and the articulation of counter-discourses by feminist groups both in Latin America and across the world within the context of what I saw as a revival of transnational feminist activism and mobilisation globally. A lot of the material gathered for this previous research pointed to the importance of doing more work on how feminist and social movements, NGOs (non-profit organisations), and other third-sector actors within international development could make better use of media tools and practices and new technologies for advocacy around gender equality as well as on challenging areas such as sexuality and reproductive health. This was set within a paradoxical context for transnational feminist networks and movements, which, despite the recent growth in the last years and revival of feminism as a political global movement – as I argue here – were also subject to the growing pressures of populist, conservative, and other extremist movements throughout Eastern Europe to Latin America and the United States. These groups have also come to be represented politically by new players such as Trump in the US (2016 to 2020) and Bolsonaro in Brazil (2018–), attacking the 'equality agenda' and producing a series of setbacks across the world. These new political players have sought to undermine many of the underpinnings of Western liberal democracy, starting, in the last years, to present more significant challenges to the further advancement of progressive policies on women and minority rights, with the COVID-19 pandemic in March 2020 exacerbating some of these structural gender and social inequalities globally.

Many of the previous theoretical frameworks and much of the empirical work conducted in my last research led to this current study, which, in 2019, began to develop and take wider shape. This research project was supported by two small grants from the Global Challenges Research Fund (GCRF) scheme, covering the duration of this research from September 2018 until July 2021.[1] The core fieldwork for this research took place during the months of March and April of 2019, both in Brazil, during my stay at Instituto de Estudos Sociais e Politicos University of the State of Rio de Janeiro (IESP UERJ) as visiting professor, where I worked alongside two PhD students and another early career researcher in India through a partnership with the Centre for Internet and Society (CIS), and during the summer of 2019 in the UK. The second stage of the fieldwork occurred during the first term of 2020, from April to July, during the coronavirus pandemic, with the final research analysis stage and further data collection taking place during the summer of 2021.

The COVID-19 pandemic placed considerable pressure on the conclusion of this research due to my daily teaching commitments and childcare responsibilities, causing some delays in concluding the manuscript. However, an early version of the findings of this research was published in an online article by *Feminist Media Studies* (November 2020) and was made available in print in April 2022.[2] The entirety of the research was also presented in June 2021 at the London International Development Centre (LIDC) event for practitioners, known as 'De-Colonising Development', for its panel on gender and development as well as at IESP UERJ in June 2022.[3]

I am thus grateful to the Department of Sociology at City, University of London – where I was based before moving to the new Department of Media, Culture and the Creative Industries in August 2022, for having granted me sabbatical leave from January to May 2019 and, particularly, to Professors Rosalind Gill, Jean Chalaby, and Petros Iosifidis as well as to Dr Jenny My former head of department and chair of City's Network for Racial Justice. I would also like to thank PG City students and, in particular, those from the MA in International Communications and Development, whose energizing, thoughtful, and engaging debates during the seminars and lectures of the core module of the master's programme, as well as their research interests in the fields of gender development, health communications, NGOs, and the role of communications in social change, helped the intellectual thinking behind this project and to shape its core concerns.

I am also grateful for the support, guidance, mentorship, and collaboration provided by other researchers, development practitioners, and professors from outside City, both in the UK and abroad, including Visiting Professor of International Relations from King's College, Sir Myles Wickstead (KCMG CBE), for his kindness and encouragement; Professors Thomas Tufte, director of the Institute for Media and Creative Industries, Loughborough University; Professor Jairo Lugo-Ocando, director of the Executive and Graduate Education, Northwestern University of Qatar; Dr Linje Manyozo, senior lecturer in communication and development at the School of Media and Communications, RMIT University, Australia; Jan Nederveen Pieterse, Duncan and Suzanne Mellichamp Distinguished Professor of Global Studies and Sociology, University of Santa Barbara California, US; Professor of Media and Public Affairs, Silvio Waisbord, of George Washington University; and Shaku Banaji, LSE Professor in Communications, for her assistance with one of the early career researchers.

I would also like to thank the fifty-two NGOs and organisations that participated in this research and whose members gave up their time to be interviewed, either by answering the questionnaires or by providing in-depth interviews. I would particularly like to thank Erin Williams from the US's Global Fund for Women, the organisation Change, as well as Brazilian NGO Reprolatina and, in particular, Margarita Diaz and Francisco Cabral. I am further grateful for the research collaboration of IESP UERJ for inviting me to be a visiting researcher during the first stage of the fieldwork in 2019, and I am particularly grateful to Professor Joao Feres, then director of IESP UERJ, for the invitation. I would also like to thank Professor Ana Carolina Escosteguy, visiting professor of the Federal University of Rio Grande do Sul (UFRGS) for assisting with the early career researchers and inviting me to deliver a keynote speech at UFRGS in June 2022.

I am also grateful for other partnerships developed during the project, and which culminated in workshops in collaboration with Professors Thomas Tufte and Adilson Cabral from UFF. We developed two successful workshops – one in Brazil and the other in the UK – entitled 'Media, New Technologies and Development in Latin America: Political, Social and Economic Perspectives', bringing together a lot of scholars from the US, Europe, and Latin America working on development communications and democracy. Further presentations of early results of this research were also delivered in April 2019 at the International Relations Department at UERJ, following from the invitation made by Professor Hugo Suppo, whom I would also like to thank, as well as at the University of Coimbra, Portugal, in September 2019. Further, I would like to acknowledge the various discussions at these conferences and workshops, all of which contributed to deepening the theoretical frameworks and assisted in the development and the interpretation of the data gathered here. I am also thankful for the invitation to be an associate visiting professor at the School of Communication, University of Miami, US, in 2023 during the launch of this book.

I would also like to thank my editor at McGill's-Queen University Press, Richard Baggaley, for his understanding concerning the delays in finalising the manuscript as well as for reading and providing useful comments on the draft. I am particularly grateful for the support of Professor Rosalind Gill, co-director of the Gender and Sexualities Research Centre at City, University of London. A thank you also goes to the work done by the PhD research students during the first months of 2019, to Ambika Tandon from CIS, Alessandra Brigo, Aline Saytan, Tatiane Leal, as well as to Jamile Dalpiaz and to Sarah Molisso during the second phase of the project in 2020 and in its final stage in 2021. Finally, I would like to recognise the support given by my mother, Heliana, whose kindness and patience were always there, as well as by my closest friends and family, including my husband Norbert and my son Christian, all of whom had to be incredibly understanding of my use of weekends to finally complete this manuscript. It is to them that I dedicate this book.

Abbreviations

AADS	Acoes Afirmativas em Direito e Saude (Affirmative Action in Rights and Health)
AHI	Action Health Incorporated
AIDWA	All India Democratic Women's Association
APA	Asia Pacific Alliance
ASAP	Asia Safe Abortion Partnership
BPA	Beijing Platform for Action
CARE	Cooperative for Assistance and Relief Everywhere
CDA	critical discourse analysis
CEDAW	Convention on the Elimination of all Forms of Discrimination Against Women
CEPIA	Centro de Estudo, Pesquisa, Informacao e Acao (Centre of Studies and Research, Information and Action)
Cfemea	Centro Feminista de Estudos e Assessoria (Feminist Studies Centre and Consulting)
CHANGE	Centre for Health and Gender Equity
CHR	Commission on Human Rights
CLADEM	Latin American and Caribbean Committee for the Defence of the Rights of Women
CPD	Commission on Population and Development
CREA	Creating Resources for Empowerment in Action
CSE	comprehensive sexuality education
CSW	Commission on the Status of Women
C3	Centre for Catalysing Change
DFID	Department of International Development
EGDI	Expert Group on Development Issues (Sweden)
FGM	female genital mutilation

FHP	Family Health Programme
FWCW	Fourth World Conference on Women
GAD	gender and development
GBV	gender-based violence
GDP	gross domestic product
HDRS	human development reports
HERA	Health, Empowerment, Rights, and Accountability
IAW	International Alliance of Women
ICPD	International Conference for Population and Development
ICWRSA	International Campaign for Women's Rights to Safe Abortion (or Campaign)
IWHC	International Women's Health Coalition
MDGS	Millennium Development Goals
NGOS	non-profit organisations
NWICO	New World Information and Communication Order
Promsex	Centro de Promocion y Defensa de los Derechos Sexuales y Reprodutivos (Centre for the Promotion and Defence of Sexual and Reproductive Rights)
PRSP	Poverty Reduction Strategy Process
RESURJ	Realising Sexual and Reproductive Justice
SDGS	Sustainable Development Goals
SIDA	Swedish International Development Corporate Agency
SRHM	Sexual and Reproductive Health Matters (former RHM)
SRHR	Sexual and reproductive health and rights
SRI	Sexual Rights Initiative
STIS	Sexually Transmitted Infections
UN	United Nations
UNDP	United Nations Development Programme
UNESCO	United Nations Educational, Scientific and Cultural Organisation
UNFPA	United Nations Population Fund
UNICEF	United Nations Children's Fund
USAID	United States, Agency for International Development
WAD	Woman and Development
WAS	World Association for Sexual Health
WHO	World Health Organisation
WID	Women in Development
WLP	Women's Learning Partnership
WNU	Women's Network for Unity
WWHR	Women for Women's Human Rights

GENDER, COMMUNICATIONS,
AND REPRODUCTIVE HEALTH
IN INTERNATIONAL DEVELOPMENT

Introduction

The empirical research carried out by this Global Challenges Research Fund Project project, as well as the theoretical debates on gender and development, health communications, and NGOs' advocacy in the field of gender and sexual and reproductive health and rights (SRHR), are presented in the thirteen chapters of this book. The first chapter aims to critically assess the theories on gender and development at the turn of the twenty-first century, and the ways in which communications can be used for the advancement of gender equality on sexuality and reproductive health. It sets the core theoretical perspectives that are developed throughout this book, providing the frameworks within which to understand some of the discussions in the field of global health and development communications, as well as the advocacy and communication efforts of feminist and health NGOs working in the field across the world, both in the Global North and the Global South. These organisations work under challenging circumstances, which include a hostile geopolitical and economic climate as well as limitations on funding and other donor pressures on development programmes. They operate in a highly competitive, uncertain, and fragmented international development landscape (Gideon and Porter 2016), having had to respond to these challenges that have grown considerably in the last decade across different regions of the world (Petchesky 2003; Friedman 2003; Harcourt 2017).

Chapter 3, like chapter 2, further develops the theoretical debates explored previously and begins to include some of the empirical research and results of the in-depth interviews conducted with the gender experts and CEOs of the NGOs and other networks who participated in this research. While discussing the work of feminist and health NGOs, networks, and movements in the field, I adopt a *decolonisation* framework that seeks to avoid naivety and essentialising or simplifying the North/South divide – or the 'Northern' or 'Southern NGOs' (Narayanaswamy 2014) – and further call for the strengthening of partnerships between organisations in Latin America and those in the US, Europe, Latin America, and South Asia. I also argue for the need for further collaboration and new ideas and approaches from practitioners, organisations, and scholars with the purpose of advancing gender policies around sexuality and reproductive health so that there can be more transformative social change 'on the ground' for various groups of women and other vulnerable communities. This should be inserted within a framework that is truly forward-thinking, pro-feminist, anti-colonialist, and anti-imperialist and that favours equality and justice for all women irrespective of country of birth, socio-economic background, and status (McLaren 2017; Mohanty 2000; Fraser 2013). It further aims to look at *how* media and communications – from communication tools, practices, and strategies – can have a wider role in assisting social change for development (Wilkins 2016; Tufte 2012; Waisbord and Obregon 2012a).

The following chapters look at the concept of communications and why it matters. They also assess how communication has come to be more understood in terms of human rights as well as what we mean by communication for social change (CSC) and the role that this plays in development and in thinking about health and gender equality. They examine some of the research and theoretical debates on health communications, such as the use of some campaigns in the field of health, problematising the popularity of entertainment-education in the field as well as the growth of more human interest narratives and storytelling techniques (Lewis and Lewis 2015; Tufte 2012; Dutta 2011). As we shall see, despite the promises of wider participatory democracy provided by the online environment (Dahlgren 2009; Iosifidis, 2011; Della Porta 2012; Fotopoulou 2016a), communication is still controlled by powerful groups and is currently being disputed by various political actors across the world, from extreme right-wing movements linked to Trump, to other nationalistic groups in Europe, to other grassroots and professional organisations, including feminist ones.

Thus for those who master the *media logic* – from the adoption of communication strategies to the efficient use of online networks and social platforms – communication can go a long way. It can be a tool that, if used effectively, can help shape thinking, consequently influencing debate in the mediated and political (global) public sphere, resulting in (radical) social change, for the better or for the worse. The election of Trump in the US in 2016 and Bolsonaro in Brazil in 2018 are two concrete and recent examples of how the use of media played a prominent role in assisting in the inclusion of far-right populist politics and discourses within mainstream politics as well as in the mediated public sphere, with studies still assessing the extent of that influence (Arnaudo 2017).

I move on to examine the role of transnational feminist NGOs in development and their advocacy communication efforts and strategies, engaging with a discussion on the use of advocacy for sexual and reproductive health and rights (Wilkins 2016), and for women's rights more broadly. This is inserted within a context of rising feminist digital activism that has become more significant in the last decades and that has begun to receive more attention from social movements and other feminist scholars and communication scholars researching NGO journalism (McPherson 2015, 2017; Powers 2014, 2017). I then assess the results of the content analysis of the institutional websites of the fifty-two health and feminists NGOs, networks, and movements that participated in this research, among them organisations like Care International UK, CREA India, and SOS Corpo (Brazil) (see the methodology section of this book).

I then discuss the results of the critical discourse analysis (CDA) conducted on the data collected on the social media engagement of the organisations on Twitter and Facebook. This is contrasted to the other communication material collected from the organisations, which is examined further on in the book. This chapter also includes the results of the empirical work done on the communication narratives and practices of the organisations, such as the use of journalistic devices and 'fact checking' techniques, as well as the appeal to human interest stories, which have become popular with fundraising and other marketing practices employed by humanitarian organisations and others working in international development (Ascough 2018). This includes the use of communication practices such as digital storytelling, which were mentioned by many of the organisations interviewed here as communication practices that they have begun to use more frequently in their advocacy communication efforts relating to SRHR.

Finally, the *deconstruction* of language, discourses, and narratives around sexual and reproductive health and rights is something that some organisations and experts interviewed here emphasised as being an important aspect of the debate on advancing reproductive health and rights for women within the public sphere as a means of influencing public opinion, policies, and decision making in the field. They also stress the need to articulate new conversations around SRHR and gender equality within the necessary fields of gender and development and development communications as well as the need to connect more public health professionals with communication and development scholars and practitioners. This includes pursuing more *dialogue* with the affected communities, encouraging their wider participation and engagement with health messages and communications on sexuality and reproductive health mainly as a means of assessing what they would like to see more of from governments, NGOs, and other multilateral agencies regarding health promotion and communication campaigns for SRHS. I thus argue the need to *deconstruct* traditional language and assumptions around 'gender ideology' myths and discourses around SRHR, which have existed both inside and outside development discourse, further underscoring the need for NGOs to use communications more strategically, mingling offline with online and adopting different engagements and approaches to messages and content on sexuality and reproductive health.

In the concluding chapter, I propose an intellectual and epistemological framework, as well as communication strategies and practices, for organisations, practitioners, and other professionals working in the field with the purpose of advancing reproductive health and women's rights within international development. This framework needs to be centred within a *decolonising feminist* praxis, one that engages in a genuine *transformative dialogue,* one that is capable of thinking about sexuality and reproductive health, 'female bodies', as well as the role of women in societies, in developed and developing countries alike. It further pays attention to the differences and the particularities of national as well as local contexts and is sensitive to the current global challenges of our time. Thus communications, media content, and messages from the organisations on sexuality and reproductive health – as well as discourses and language relating to SRHR within the development industry – need to be better unpacked, discussed, and situated so that they can fully address the current global challenges. They need to have more capacity to be genuinely *transformative*, to be capable of contributing to combatting gender structural inequalities wherever these exist, and to to do so from a commitment to seeking equal opportunities, justice, rights, and dignity in life and well-being for all girls and women as well as for all other marginalised and disadvantaged minority groups.

I

Gender, Communications, and Women's Reproductive Rights in International Development

An Assessment

INTELLECTUAL FRAMEWORKS AND CURRENT CHALLENGES

It has become a well-known fact that the COVID-19 pandemic, which started in March 2020, has significantly reshaped the world, having placed even greater pressure on women's rights and having already exacerbated previous structural inequalities, from turning back the clock in gains on combatting poverty in developing countries to causing sharp increases in unemployment in developed countries amidst the expansion of a global recession. Research reports, such as the one released by King's College London in partnership with the Australian National University, commissioned by Oxfam (April 2020), underlines how the coronavirus pandemic could push 580 million people – or 8 per cent of the population – into poverty for the first time since the 1990s, having a further impact on everything from health care and education to maternal mortality. The authors argued for an expansion of social safety nets in developing countries as well as for a wider commitment from the international community in providing assistance.[1]

Organisations like the United Nations Population Fund (UNFPA) have also expressed concerns regarding the continuation of the commitment expressed by the international community to uphold gender equality, given that the COVID-19 pandemic will likely compromise the UN's 2030 deadline and its aim of achieving the Global Goals for Sustainable Development. The coronavirus pandemic could have a detrimental effect on some of these 2030 aims, from the elimination of preventable maternal deaths and the ending of the unmet need for family planning to the increase in unsafe abortion practices throughout the world, reversing some of the slow gains made in the last decades. This is at a time when achievements in the field of SRHR within international development, as well as the challenges and setbacks, have started to come more to the foreground in the last years. Morgan (in Grugel and Hammett 2016) underscored the year 2015 as important for SRHR, representing approximately the twenty-year anniversary of the 1994 ICPD Cairo conference, seen as a landmark for the attention placed on sexual and reproductive health and rights. Underlining how many women and girls still lack access to essential SRHR services in many countries, leading to unnecessary deaths, the Morgan (Matos 2016, 472) correctly underlined how improving women's health in the field 'is one of the most cost-effective development investments, decreasing maternal and child deaths, reducing poverty, improving economic growth, and encouraging gender equality' (DFID 2004; Stenberg et al. 2014 in Morgan 2016, 472).

Although maternal mortality rates fell by 49 per cent between 1990 and 2008 (Germain 2004), there are still differences between the richer and poorer nations, with the lifetime risk of maternal death in poorer countries being 1 in 480, compared to 1 in 4.3000 in more developed countries. Germain (2004) also underlines how the rate of maternal death has been seen as an indicator that separates a poor country from a more developed one. Nonetheless, this is likely to become more complex, given the concerns expressed by reproductive rights advocates that, in countries with restrictive abortion rights – such as the US following the overturning of the 1973 *Roe v. Wade* legislation in June 2022 – the risks of maternal deaths are much higher than in those that have decriminalized the practice, providing safe and legal services. According to the Centre for Reproductive Rights, 36 per cent of the world's population of women of reproductive age live in countries that allow abortion with restrictions only on the length of pregnancy, while another 39 per cent live in nations with strict standards (15 per cent of them do not permit pregnancy terminations at any time, while 22 per cent do so just to save the woman's life, and another 14 per cent do so to preserve her health).[2]

The impact of COVID-19 on turning back the clock on women's rights is not the only challenge to the advancement of gender equality policies in the field of SRHR, which, in the last few years, has seen an increase in vocal opposition around the world, from the US to Eastern

Europe and Latin America. Even before the rise of Trumpism (Cornwall, Correa, and Jolly 2008), the US had seen a lot of controversies and 'sex and cultural wars' being fought between progressives and conservative 'pro-life' groups, with innumerable examples of state-sanctioned policies that seek to curb women's rights and that have been largely supported by a renewal of the pro-family discourses propagated by populist far-right political and religious groups. On September 2021, the state of Texas introduced a law preventing abortions after the sixth week, something that was seen as a large step backwards by many American feminist advocates; however, it was not considered surprising given the increasingly hostile and contentious climate that has been established around sexuality and reproductive health in that country.[3] More shocking was the US Supreme Court's decision in June 2022 to overturn *Roe v. Wade*. Decisions like these, which have turned back the clock on women's rights, have not appeared in isolation, either in the US or in countries from the Global South. In fact, setbacks in legislation around sexuality and reproductive health and rights have been seen throughout different regions of the world.[4]

Thus the struggle to advance women's rights in the field of sexual and reproductive health within international development has been a complicated process that, among other things, has seen some significant advancements in the reduction of maternal deaths and the *decriminalization* of abortion, in the application of comprehensive sexual education in schools, and in the recognition of sexual identities in many developing countries. But, at the same time, it has placed in the foreground various moral, religious, and philosophical debates, including those dealing with cultural and social norms around definitions of female reproduction (Bordo 1992), women's bodies and sexuality, and the right to agency, as well as understandings of motherhood and of a woman's place in society. Feminists working in the fields of law, politics, anthropology, and public health have, since the 1970s, examined the debate on 'fetal versus women's rights' (Roth 2014; Heriot 1996; Petchesky 2003), with some denouncing what they see as the 'politization of pregnancy' (Roth 2014) and the essentialisation of the views surrounding 'personhood', which have also justified the 'monitoring of the unborn child' by the state (Heriot 1996, 187).

What is argued is that women's bodies are coerced and that their rights are undermined and pitted against those of the foetus. Establishing birth as the 'criteria of relevance', Warren (1989, 59 in Heriot 1996, 183) argues that 'it is impossible to treat fetuses in *utero* as if they were persons without treating women as if they were something less than people'. Also missing from the 'pro-life' arguments are a wider discussion of the economic and financial conditions of women, and the disruption that childcare can be in their lives (as well as in that of their partners) if these conditions consist, for instance, of financial hardship. SRHR concerns (and not just those of 'abortion') are thus closely interwoven with wider issues of poverty and deprivation as well as structural gender inequalities and economic development – issues that I examine throughout this book.

At the heart of all these debates are very specific beliefs, views, and assumptions around rigid and ahistorical gendered norms, including not only the status of women in societies but also the role played by men in fertility and childcare. This includes the 'appropriate place' that should be reserved for the *female body* within the family and the private sphere as well as the public space, including within the nation and the wider world (Yuval-Davis 2010; Friedman 2003; Butler 2019). It is precisely these ideas and beliefs that circulate in the public sphere and that end up becoming key challenges for health and feminist organisations, public health professionals, and NGO activists working in the field of sexuality and reproductive health across the world.

On another note, feminism as a political movement has seen a revival throughout the world, from transnational feminist advocacy networks to NGOs and other feminist grassroots groups. This has been more pronounced since the early 2000s onwards, with the entry of young feminist and other groups that have mobilised campaigns in favour of key issues, including combatting the gender pay gap in the workplace, sexual harassment and online misogyny, and other causes associated with the so-called 'new feminism' (Jonsson 2021). Feminism is also now more focused on individual forms of *empowerment*, careerism, individualism, and sexual pleasure. That said, the feminist movements of the last decades, particularly those associated with the 'third' and 'fourth' waves of feminism, have also contributed to further implementing and strengthening a variety of 'democratic' forms of engagement with various meanings and understandings of 'feminisms' (in the plural) (Alvarez 2014). This includes, among other things, the increase in concerns over race and ethnicity issues within feminism, with the feminist movement paying lip service to a wider commitment to 'democratising' the movement itself.

Despite the pessimism regarding the state of feminism as a political movement throughout the world, and its capacity to deliver de facto progressive change for multiple groups of women due to its numerous challenges – from operating within a marketized and neoliberal environment, to facing growing political opposition from conservative forces, to being attacked from sectors of the left for failing to fully *decolonise* and deliver justice to less privileged groups of working-class women, women of colour, or women from the Global South (i.e., the current attacks against the 'white [Northern] feminists')[5] (Jonsson 2021) – it is still possible to affirm that feminism continues to be a vibrant and influential political movement that has seen a significant revival as well as renewed interest in a whole range of gender issues, from online misogyny to sexual harassment and reproductive rights (Mendes, Ringrose, and Keller 2019; Fotopuolou 2016a; Dean and Aune 2015). This includes growing concerns with female and transgender rights, gender-based violence, the persistence of the gender pay gap in the workplace as well as gendered social norms in society and their continuous reproduction in the mainstream media despite 'postfeminist sensibilities and feminism being "undone"' (McRobbie 2009; Gill 2007b; Jonsson 2021).

Feminsim in the US and the UK has slowly started to take on board the criticisms of postcolonial scholars regarding the need to promote a more inclusive feminism, one that is attentive to anti-imperialism and concerned with decolonialism and with the 'normalisation' and dominance of 'white feminism' (Mohanty 2000; Spivak 1988; Jonsson 2021). It is thus being pressured to become more open to previously marginalised identities and to others from diverse backgrounds, ethnicities, and nationalities, many of whom are also increasingly engaging in global transnational network activities and seeking to unite in favour of greater solidarity and global gender justice for all groups of women. The increase in protests, demonstrations, and mobilisations throughout the world, in the last years in particular – from Eastern Europe, to Brazil, India, and the US – also show that feminism not only continues to be an influential political force and that it matters but that it has, in fact, been one of the most successful social movements of the past fifty years (Dean and Aune 2015).

In their article on the mapping of contemporary feminist activisms in Europe, written from a historical perspective, Dean and Aune (2015, 375) state that feminism continues to shape the continent politically, economically, and socially within a context in which feminism is changing rapidly within a global environment of economic crisis and austerity, emerging far-right politics, shifting geopolitical dynamics, and a backlash against women's rights. As Dean and Aune note, feminism as a transnational social movement has been widely examined (Hawkesworth 2006); however, within the context of globalization, in which problems and issues need to be addressed both locally and globally, feminism as a political force offers even more possibilities and is a force to be reckoned with. As Dean and Aune (2015, 376) further affirm, feminism transcends national borders and thus culminates in placing 'transnational solidarity at the heart of its wider political project' (Hawkesworth 2006).

There are abundant examples of the increase of feminist demonstrations and protests that have occurred in the last few years, from the worldwide #MeToo movement, which is popular in places like India, to further demonstrations of the persistence of domestic violence against women and feminicide, such as the Argentinian #NiUnaaMenos campaign.[6] Other rallies in favour of the decriminalization of abortion, for instance, have also taken place in developed and developing countries alike, from Ireland to Argentina. At the same time, discourses and rhetoric propagated by conservative and oppositional groups from the US to Latin America against the supposed imposition by governments, policy-makers, and gender advocates of 'gender ideology myths' have also grown in the last decades. Narratives around gender, sexuality, and reproductive health concerns and ideas have thus been framed around misinformation and 'common-sense' assumptions about reproduction, and motherhood as well as the feminist movement itself, with attacks that range from pigeon-holing feminists as being in 'favour of a culture of death' (Butler 2019) to accusations of attempting to enforce sex education in schools or arguing that reproduction health rights and concerns are solely about 'liberating abortion practices'.

As feminist scholars have pointed out, such discursive practices – which have occupied the public sphere more intensively in the last years – were initiated some time ago as part of a growing *countermovement* against the advancements in the gender equality agenda made by Western governments, multilateral agencies, and NGO advocates, which were secured globally through the UN-led conferences of the 1980s and throughout the 1990s (Friedman 2003; Machado 2018). This has forced many feminist groups, as well as NGO and public health advocates working in the field of SRHR, to be on the defensive and to respond to such accusations through new framing strategies and communication practices (Friedman 2003; Petchesky 2003; Harcourt 2017). Thus, the resistance here is not new and did not emerge only in the last years with the politics of far-right politicians such as Bolsonaro, Trump, and Viktor Orban, although it could be said that the political pressures have intensified in the last three decades.

Moreover, in an article written for Open Democracy in 2021, Reimeryte and Ferreira (2021) outline some of the sophisticated tactics that are employed by anti-abortion activists, from manipulation to the use of misleading terminology, further focusing on the activities of organisations that seek to persuade people who accidentally get pregnant not to gain access to abortion services (known as 'crisis pregnancy centres'). The authors point to a total of twenty-five hundred centres in the US alone that offer pregnancy tests and counselling coupled with anti-termination messages. Moreover, in 2020, Provost and Archer, in an article published on the Open Democracy website, reveal how, since 2008, US Christian right groups have been sponsoring 'pro-life' and other radical groups throughout Europe, pouring over $280 million in 'dark money' globally, and also engaging in similar practices throughout Latin America and Africa.

It is possible to trace some of the roots of this opposition to the discussions around reproductive bodies, motherhood, and women's bodies (from birth to menstruation) well back to the nineteenth century. Female reproduction already occupied the attention of the medical discourse and of other disciplines at that time (Martin 1987; Butler 1993; Foucault 1980), with these being inserted into discourses that were ultimately concerned with women's bodies and sexuality as well as with how to exercise control over these. In their discussion of the difficulties of addressing sexuality in development amidst the rise of 'sex wars' throughout the world, Cornwall, Correa, and Jolly (2008, 4) underline how historical studies pointed to the systems of control and punishment enacted against 'loose' female sexuality and homosexuality in Europe before the transition to modernity, including the role played by Roman Catholic inquisitions. The authors underscore parallels between the sex cultural wars of today with what was experienced in other historical realities.

Cornwall, Correa, and Jolly (2008, 4) further discuss how various 'globalization' theorists (i.e., Giddens 1991) identified shifts in gender and sex as part of the transformations that were occurring throughout the world. The core of their critique is that sexuality has been treated with a certain embarrassment in development, having been a 'frivolous add on' rather than having been connected to concerns around poverty and marginalisation (4–5). They further note that, within mainstream development agencies, sexuality has been traditionally dealt with as a health issue and treated with policies designed to prevent disease and to promote health, as was the case with the HIV/AIDS pandemic (5). This was to the detriment of emphasising concerns with the application of a more human rights approach to sexuality and development, one that could stress the rights of women and transgender people to lead pleasurable sex lives free of prejudice.[7] Thus the shift within development, mainly since the 1990s, away from the more narrow understanding of poverty as needing to be tackled through basic income, which had its roots in modernisation theory, towards a more sophisticated understanding of poverty as being connected to a 'web of disadvantages' (Chambers 2005) and a lack of opportunities and entitlements (Sen 1999). The latter view became more influential within the field, permitting wider discussions of oppression around sexuality and how this can contribute to intensifying poverty (Cornwall, Correa, and Jolly 2008).

Friedman (2003) examines in detail the advancement of policies on gender rights achieved by transnational feminist movements and NGOs during the 1990s, including at the 1992 UN conference on Environment and Development in Rio, Brazil, and the 1993 World Conference on Human Rights in Vienna, Austria, to the programs of action developed in the multilateral UN-led conferences of Cairo and Beijing. These achievements were seen as a direct result of the intense lobbying of transnational feminists and health advocates from NGOs across the world and other movements, including many from the Global South (Friedman 2003; Petchesky 2003; Harcourt 2009, 2017). Friedman (2003) underlines how feminists contributed to shaping the human rights discourse, moving it away from the previous commitment to individual rights and towards a wider notion of economic and collective justice.

In her discussion of women's health movements and the UN conferences, and the leadership role played by feminists from the Global South, Petchesky (2003) emphasises the pioneering role of Black feminists as advocates for SRHR, something that is often either ignored or downplayed. Authors writing about the impact of the ideas of postcolonial scholars and women of colour on feminism, particularly within the British context (Jonsson 2021), have noted how reproductive rights were an agenda espoused by Black feminists during the feminist liberation movements of the 1970s and were not exclusive of the demands made by liberal Western feminists. Petchesky (2003) also further notes how women in the North and the South made different use of the concepts of reproductive health and sexual rights in accordance with their circumstances.

As Friedman (2003) argues, throughout these years, feminist NGO and health advocates built on the experiences of lobbying, mobilizing, and making use of communications for advocacy. They would see successes in the last two conferences, which were seen as a significant turning point for NGOs working with gender equality (Alvarez 1998). It was during these last conferences, however, that an organised counter-movement represented by the New Right against the gender agenda, organised through conservative representatives in NGOs who attended Cairo in 1994, began to emerge, paving the way for the rise of the opposition to the equality agenda.[8] Despite the limitations imposed on the equality agenda, including on women's agency and the decriminalization of abortion, scholars and activists have been united in underlining that progress was undeniable during the 1990s (Friedman 2003; Correa and Petchesky 1994; Harcourt 2009). Women's health advocates managed to shift the very terminology in the field away from the early 'population control' discourse to the promotion of women's reproductive rights embedded within the human rights framework.

The rhetoric around women's reproductive health and sexuality thus moved away from the previous emphasis on fertility and 'population control' to incorporate a vision that equated women's autonomy and human rights with reproductive health (Garita in Harcourt et al. 2015, 269; Correa and Petchesky 1994; Lottes 2013). The Plan of Action of Cairo's 1994 International Conference on Population and Development (ICPD) was further praised for having used for the first time a definition of reproductive rights that included *family planning,* as one among broader elements of reproductive health (Harcourt 2009). In her book *Body Politics in Development,* Harcourt (2009, 45) provides a detailed outline of the strategies adopted by groups to advance the agenda, with health and women's movements merging to secure rights. New concepts, such as 'reproductive health', were combined with discussions on sexuality, empowerment, and cultural difference, all of which were seen as ground-breaking and that contributed to move the very playing field of development discourse (Harcourt 2009).

Despite the recognition of advancements, the ICPD legacy remains contested across the political spectrum. Some women's groups have criticised the 'Cairo consensus' as simply being an exercise in the co-optation of feminists that served to legitimise the 'old style population control' discourses on fertility control of poor women from the developed world (Hartmann 1994 and Spivak 1999, both in Petchesky 2003, 3). There has also been a clash in the last decades on the international stage between the 'population' and 'women's movement' debate when it comes to the applicability of reproductive health and choice for women. Freedman and Isaacs (1993) argue that there have been diverse approaches to the comprehension of population as a development issue. Theoretical perspectives on reproductive health, for instance, started to move the debate away from the merely Malthusian agenda of fertility or birth control, which had previously marked development programming approaches to poverty reduction in the 'Third World', particularly during the decades when modernisation was the guiding framework for development thinking.

However, the shift away from the notion of 'population control', a discourse embedded within the Eurocentric 'overpopulation' narrative, with its emphasis on the need to control fertility as a form of combatting poverty, in line with the Malthusian theory, to a notion of reproductive health and sexuality as being embedded in a human rights approach, has still not significantly changed the discourse in international development on women and SRHR. Instead, the latter has continued to reflect some of the biases of the modernisation framework as well as of the whole colonial and imperial legacy. These discourses are still widely supported by stereotypical notions of the femininity of the 'Other', coupled with outdated images of women from developing countries being in 'need of saving', disempowered and lacking in 'agency' (Wilkins 2016; Harcourt 2009; Matos 2016; Mohanty 2000). These discourses and practices have further culminated in the persistence of simplistic portrayals of women, and their reproductive health and rights, within population and family development programmes designed for developing countries (Wilkins 2016; Harcourt 2009, 2017).

Despite decades of criticisms from postcolonial scholars and other feminists from the Global South concerning the homogenizing tendencies within development discourses when it comes to talking about poverty and inequalities suffered by women and girls in developing countries (Mohanty 2000; Radcliffe 2015; Chowdhry 1995), the reality is that the experiences of women beyond the Global North continue to appear within the literature, as well as within the development industry and practices, in an ahistorical, fragmented, and distorted manner. It is the continuing perpetuation of such a legacy that has made the bridging of differences, with the intent of seeking unity, all the more difficult; however, this is a growing necessity given the need to tackle gender inequality as a global movement of transformative gender justice (Fraser 2013). Nonetheless, in the aftermath of the achievements obtained in advancing the feminist agenda globally during the last decades, including in the field of SRHR, a sense of frustration with the little progress made has resulted in renewed commitments and feminist engagement with the topic across countries from the Global South to the Global North.

In their discussion of the challenges faced by feminist health women's movements just ten years after Cairo and Beijing, Petchesky (in Correa, Germain, and Petchesky 2005, 110) identifies three major gaps: the failure to recognise legal abortion as a human right, the lack of mention of 'sexual rights' in documents, and the limited way in which it is defined, including the failure to take into account the impact on SRHR of larger macro-economic and political forces. Women who lived in the Global South, as well as migrant or indigenous women who lived in the developed countries, transgender, and queer activists, were for the most part not included in UN gender development debates. It was also further assumed that women in the developed North 'did not need developing' as they had 'money and access to rights ... which other groups of women in the rest of the world need[ed] to strive for' (Harcourt 2009, 30).

A well-known Brazilian feminist from the NGO CEPIA who was interviewed for this research talked about the impact that Cairo had on legislation in the field in Brazil:[9]

> I participated a lot as a part of an international group of feminists as well as being part of the Brazilian delegation. CEPIA had a fundamental role, having organised an event in Brazil in 1993 called 'Our Rights for Cairo 94' ... Then we organised together with Women Health Foundation a meeting of representatives of ninety countries and we produced a document ... Thus when we arrived at Cairo in terms of civil society this had been formed ... Cairo was fundamental for Brazil because after it the legislation on family planning was

proposed ... But it also influenced public policies, it influenced discussions on abortion in the sense that it put as a duty of the government to take on women who have had abortions in the sense of avoiding sequels, and also in the sense of offering safe abortion, including in the cases that the legislation permits.

Arguably, the expansion of the definitions of sexual and reproductive health and rights by the 1994 International Conference on Population and Development had an influence not only on the language used on issues regarding women's rights but also on the approaches to population programmes and wider reproductive health concerns that came afterwards. As Colle (2008, 131) notes, the Programme of Action for the ICPD reflected 'the convergence of many issues that had significance for a communication agenda', underlining as examples how men initially were not targeted by programmes for condom use whereas afterwards they started to be targeted also (Drennan 1998 in Colle 2008, 131).

In his discussion of population programmes and development communications, Colle (in Servaes 2008, 130) underlines how, for several decades, the programmes had been associated with family planning, making use of information, education, and communications in traditional ways, the aim of which was to influence people's contraceptive behaviour. The terms 'birth control' and 'family planning', for instance, were interchangeable, reflecting concerns with population growth and later with gender equality and human rights issues (Colle 2008). Underlining the importance of the role of the 1994 ICPD as having to contribute to 'broaden the scope of population programmes' (Colle 2008, 131), the WHO (1997, xi, in Colle 2008, 131) went on to define 'reproductive health'

> as the state of physical, mental, and social well-being and not merely the absence of disease or infirmity in all matters relating to the reproductive system. Reproductive health therefore implies that people are able to have a satisfying and safe sex life ... have the capacity to reproduce and the freedom to decide.

Many feminists, however, have lamented the lack of the structural transformation of the reality of more vulnerable women 'on the ground' as well as the excessive professionalization of feminist NGOs post-Cairo 1994, combined with what many saw as a reduction of women's rights to issues of safe abortion services. Wider macro-economic inequities, as well as different understandings of SRHR, were insufficiently problematised. Criticisms were further articulated around the tensions between individualistic liberal principles and the collective responsibilities of states (Correa and Petchesky 1996).

The lead of the UK's SheDecides feminist movement also criticised the predominance of the 'medical discourse' in the field, which left aside questions of women's agency:[10]

> I think another challenge that helps explain why we are stagnated is that, over time, the approach to SRHR has become quite *a medicalised one* ... What started off as a conversation around rights ... became a different kind of conversation. And we actually stopped seeing women's rights organisations in particular participating in SRHR spaces ... it ... became much more a question of quantitative targets ... 'what are the causes of maternal mortality, and what do we need to reduce it?' ... And so questions around agency ... seemed to disappear ... and now are being re-introduced ... [E]ven if you make certain technologies ... etc. available, if a woman still does not have the right to make that choice ... it does not matter that this technology is available ... If she does not have the agency to use that choice, if there is still stigma and misunderstanding around women's bodies ... and reproductive choices ... [A]t the root of this discussion of SRHR has to be the ability of women and girls to make these choices for themselves.

Thus the attacks on women's and reproductive rights intensified in the last years and have had a significant impact. From the early 2000s onwards, there has been a more visible and aggressive growth in movements of opposition to the expansion of the agenda on women's rights. The platform of the 'anti-gender ideology' agenda includes the opposition to feminism, LGBT rights, gay marriage, and trans and other minority rights. In the aftermath of the 2008 global financial recession, we have been seeing the growing stagnation of women's rights, with the rise of austerity and cuts to public services affecting less privileged groups, including women, while at the same time seeing the growth of far-right and populist political discourses throughout the world – discourses that stigmatise certain minority groups, including poorer or 'migrant' Third World women.

These reactions against the equality agenda can be identified as being part of a wider global geopolitical movement that has sought to challenge, somewhat successfully, the 'Western consensus' liberal democracy model that has prevailed almost as a given for the last few decades and very much so since the twentieth century. It exposed the weakness of the West's commitment to democracy and equal opportunities as well as to combatting structural inequalities, particularly those of class. Many have pointed to current developments, such as the actions of 'pro-life' US conservative groups, including the setbacks in reproduction health created by the Trump administration's application of the Global Gag Rule.[11] Like other governments in Eastern Europe, such as Hungary with Vicktor Orban and Brazil with Jair Bolsonaro, Trump's (2016–20) administration led a global campaign to promote family values and to reaffirm the privilege of the white male, further curtailing access to abortion as well as to LGBT rights.

These shifts in the 'political consensus', which many civil rights and other feminist groups took for granted, did not occur in a vacuum or emerge out of the blue. Feminist sociologists have long researched how gender operates within societal structures that reproduce inequalities through daily interactions, from cultural expectations concerning different groups to status differentiations between men and women (Ridgeway and Smith-Lovin 1999; Ridgeway and Correll 2004; Risman 2004). As Risman (2004, 432) underlines, not only do social structures shape individuals but they are also influenced by them: these social structures can 'enable or constrain social actions' (Fuchs 2003, 133). Influenced by Giddens's (1984) *structuration theory*, with its emphasis on the relationship between social structures and individuals, and how this has mutual impacts and can transform human action, this theory is an attempt to explain *how* social change can occur and how this process can be initiated by people through *transformative* action.

This is an acknowledgement that social change can occur in different ways and that it is not always for the better. These theoretical frameworks can help us think critically about *how* social change can take place, albeit gradually and almost invisibly, for better or for worse. Consequently, when the results finally manifest themselves more strongly, it can be too late. Among institutions and societies throughout the world this process usually occurs through the *reproduction* of the dominance of the status quo, manifested in the persistence of structural inequalities of class, gender, and race (and ethnicity). The reality is that these inequalities have in the last decades been largely reproduced and have become more entrenched – albeit with exceptions due to the resistance of more genuinely transformative forces working within societies' institutions – on a daily and consistent basis irrespective of the ideologies of the 'left/right' of the political spectrum. Thus change can be incredibly slow and is often disrupted due to the continuous reproduction of inequalities through everyday practices and interactions within social settings, institutions and the wider society.

The slow growth of counter-reactions over the last decades has occurred within various societal institutions throughout the world due to the reproduction and the maintenance of the values of the status quo as well as of the structural inequalities between groups within and between countries. This has occurred to the detriment of breaking with these conservative forces and, more broadly, with neoliberalism itself. The intensity of the reactions has, nonetheless, taken many by surprise. Attacks against scholars working on gender studies as well as on NGO activists seeking to advance women's rights have become more common, this being confirmed by some of the gender experts and CEOs interviewed for this research. Well-known and respected scholars like the American feminist theorist Judith Butler have also been the object of high-profile public attacks and have been victims of various hate campaigns.[12] Other challenges faced by many NGOs working in the North and South include censorship or attacks on their communication practices and online advocacy engagement around SRHR.

Examples of feminists and scholars who also came under attack included the blogger and professor Lola Aronovich, from the Federal University of Fortaleza, Brazil, as well as the anthropologist Debora Diniz, from the University of Brasilia, known internationally as an expert on reproductive rights and abortion. The latter left Brazil in 2018 after having received online attacks and death threats from Brazilian ultra-conservative groups amidst the election of Jair Bolsonaro for president in October of that year. Bolsonaro has been seen as offering a 'tropical version' of US Trumpism. Many of these Brazilian far-right groups have been accused of paying lip service to their US alt-right, pro-gun loving, uber macho counter-part groups, such as those led by the US influencer Jack Donovan, known for upholding masculinity as an aesthetics while forcing women to 'return' to their supposedly traditional reproductive role.

The head of the health commission of the International Alliance of Women (IAW),[13] interviewed for this research, provided a very detailed account of the coordinated network of individuals and organisations who are currently posing serious risks to the advancement of SRHR throughout the world:

> Those opposed to the gains of the 1990s extended in turn their powerful alliances ... The AGENDA EUROPE[14] is a powerful enemy of SRHR ... According to the European Parliamentary Forum Population and Development, it is a 'reactionary and expansive network' ... If the network attains its set goals [the] decade-long progress of SRHR would be annihilated. The manifesto of the movement claims to restore a 'natural right' disturbed by the sexual revolution. The separation of the sexual act from its primary destination, the procreation, was to be cancelled ... Countries with a record of 'no interference by traditionalists and by religious creeds' have better advanced ... In Europe, Sweden and the Netherlands are part of an eight-country initiative to sign up for a fundraising to counter D. Trump's anti-abortion move ... Africa offers only a few positive examples, I'd quote Malawi for child marriage and sexual education, and Burkina Faso for FGM/C ... In South America: Uruguay, Argentina, Chile have advanced ... Less advancement, even loss of acquired rights, are known from Poland, Hungary, Slovakia, Lithuania.

The urgency of the topic has already begun to mobilise different NGO activists and feminists working in the field across the world. In November 2018, groups of NGO advocates working with reproductive health, from organisations like the International Planned Parenthood Federation to Amnesty International and the World Association of Health, held a workshop at The Hague entitled 'Effective SRHR Messaging in Changing Times'. This workshop was organised by the Dutch NGO Share-Net Netherlands Community of Practice (CoP),[15] and it focused on the retreat of civil society groups in Eastern as well as in Central Europe. The 'Effective SRHR Messaging in Changing Times' workshop seminar nonetheless sought to engage NGO organisations and advocates working in the field with a few pertinent questions, having provided some suggestions for consideration, such as the need for a wider engagement with affected communities. It was suggested that the NGOs should seek to find out more about how these communities form their ideas on gender equality and on more contested topics such as abortion. The workshop underlined the need to 'reframe' language so as to create greater impact and to reach out to wider publics, thus better communicating with communities.

The last few years have seen a growth in the mobilisation of various feminist groups against the persistence of practices that continue to control sexuality and gendered norms and, thus, to deny women's agency, autonomy, and control over their own bodies. A series of protests that have taken place throughout the world in the last few years have occurred in parallel with the increasing opposition to the 'gender ideology agenda', in response to counterattacks and as a way of upholding past conquests as well as the small victories for women's rights. Many across the Global North and South have taken to the streets in anger at the slow advancement of the equality agenda, following from the disappointment with the lack of sufficient progress, mostly 'on the ground'. Amnesty International went so far as to proclaim 2018 as the year of 'resistance' for women globally: from India to the US many women's groups took to the streets to demonstrate against various issues concerning the body, from sexual violence and harassment – epitomized in movements such as the #MeToo campaign – to abortion rights. Others demanded less restrictive laws in countries like Argentina and Ireland, with the former, after much heated debate, seeing success in the formal approval of new legislation in December 2020.[16]

In all these campaigns communications had a fundamental role to play in raising awareness, mobilizing transnational feminist networks and NGOs, and attempting to intensify the reach and impact of the agenda on women's reproductive health and rights. It further sought to unite diverse groups and activists from around the world, seeking to find points of empathy and solidarity and, at the same time, reviving some of the past transnational feminist activism associated with the 1990s. Various of these women's groups and NGOs have also played leading roles in many demonstrations, contributing to frame the debate on gender across key areas, thus contributing to 'setting the agenda' on public policies in the field in the years to come. They managed to make some progress in agendas such as women's discrimination in the workplace (symbolised in ground-breaking documents like the Convention on the Elimination of Discrimination Against Women [CEDAW], adopted in 1979) as well as interweaving the concerns of gender with the environment, sustainable development, and reproductive health and sexuality in multilateral and national documents and legislations.

I am thus interested in how communication can be used strategically by NGOs and organisations working in the field of SRHR to improve messaging, content, and discourses on the topic within this current highly complex, challenging political and socio-economic post-pandemic environment. I argue that it is precisely around issues affecting the body, sexual harassment, violence, and reproductive rights that feminists can begin to transcend differences of class and ethnicity (McCann and Nicholas 2019), seeking to find common footing and uniting around causes in the quest for meaningful social transformative change for different groups of women across the world.

Questions asked here include: How can communications and media be used more strategically and in the pursuit of social change? How can they be used to undermine societal prejudices and, instead, to promote more empathy, assisting in the improvement of debate in the public sphere on reproductive rights? Developing from this is the question of *how* discourses around women's advancement have been challenged in the last years by conservative groups, particularly regarding the notion that 'gender' is a form of *social construction*. Arguments espoused here include defending the abandonment of the term 'gender' in favour of biological sex categorisation, which emphasises the existence of two sexes and the idea that men and women's gender roles should be fixed. Thus, the previous *constructivist* approach to gender, presumed to be a consensus, began to be slowly undermined in the public sphere by counter-discourses articulated by these oppositional groups, which contributed to impede further progress on women's rights.

Given the divisions between groups of women and the persistence of the exclusion of poorer women, women of colour, and those from the Global South from mainstream society and from the political arena of governance – as well as from within the feminist movement itself – how is it possible to pursue transformative dialogue capable of transcending the barriers of difference, further seeking equality in order to deliver real change for women 'on the ground'? How can resistance to discourses of reproductive health, sexuality, and women's bodily autonomy be better fought in the public sphere? How can we further connect women's groups and NGOs from the North with those from the South in the pursuit of globally advancing gender equality and reproductive health for sustainable development? These are just some of the questions that I explore here, some of which are hard to provide with full answers. Based on the results of this research, I attempt to articulate a theoretical platform for wider *gender global justice*, emphasising key communication strategies and processes for advancing communication practices and discourses by NGOs on SRHR. These are examined in the concluding chapter.

First, though, it is important to state that any discussion of the role of communications for social change needs to be realistically assessed. The reality is that communication practices remain dominated by the West, and it is still the case that the more powerful nations, and their media groups and communications, control the representations, discourses, and images of women in developing countries. Despite the changes in the last decades within the wider feminist movement when it comes to recognising intersectionality and acknowledging the diversity of the experiences of oppression suffered by different groups of women, from working-class to minorities, as Gill (2007a) states, much of feminist scholarship is still accused of reinforcing a hegemonic colonial view of the world. In the last decade specifically, among British feminists but also in the US, there have been some attempts to engage in uncomfortable conversations and theoretical debates around postcoloniality and imperialism (Jonsson 2021). These have followed from the criticisms made by postcolonial feminist scholars and other women of colour (Yuval-Davis 1997, 2010; see also Minh-ha 1991; Mirza 1997; Ang 2001 [all in Gill 2007a, 27]). 'White feminism' has been accused of having been ignorant of the ways in which race and gender structures intersect, and how these are experienced differently by women (Jonsson 2021). Many representations, discourses, and media images of women from the Global South, be they in the general media or in development campaigns and communications, continue to carry (sometimes implicitly) patterns of the current colonial legacy that have begun to be more challenged within Western institutions, the academy, and the feminist movement.

Despite the criticisms of modernisation theory within international development from postcolonial scholars and feminist from the Global South, the reality is that the more dominant and powerful voices still come from the North, from those players who continue to speak in the name of the powerless, including women, who continue to struggle to exercise their agency (Steeves 2003; Spivak 1988; Wilkins 2016). Communications approaches in development discourse and practice have only tended to reinforce these hegemonic forces (Melkote and Steeves 2001), despite the criticisms and the 'fall from grace' of the so-called 'grand theories of development'. Modernisation theory can thus be seen, by default, as continuing to be the dominant theoretical framework for a lot of thinking on international development – as well as on the role of media and communications within it – in areas ranging from health to gender equality.

Under the continued influence of modernisation theory and its 'technological deterministic' view of the role of technologies in helping the developed world 'catch up' with the North, there has been a growth of research within development studies and other fields that seeks to examine the role of information, communication, and new technologies (ICTs) in development. As I discuss, there has also been a shift towards more *participatory-led* forms of communications, particularly since the 1990s, with discussions on how popular communication approaches used in development campaigns – such as *entertainment-education* in health advocacy campaigns – can contribute to social change across development problems, from poverty, to education, to health (Tufte 2012; Lewis and Lewis 2015; Dutta 2011; Serveas 2008; Manyozo 2012a; Wilkins 2016). Since the 990s, there has been a proliferation of studies on how online technologies and communications can provide wider spaces for transnational feminism and mobilisation, and how these can be used to advance women's rights. Feminist research from across the humanities and social sciences has also been critical of the role played by communications and new technologies as necessarily enabling social change and promoting progress for women, underlining how often online tools can be used to reproduce offline structural inequalities and reinforce the status quo (Fotopoulou 2016b; Wajcman 2000; Plant 1995; Grint and Gill 1995).

Therefore, I have decided to focus on examining the various uses of communications by health and feminist NGOs and networks, including online platforms. However, I do not restrict my discussion to how these are used for SRHR advocacy. There is a growing literature on how NGOs and civic and human rights organisations are using online communications, particularly social media, for advocacy around a series of humanitarian causes. This has occurred within the context of research on NGO communications and journalism, and how, in recent years, these have emerged as important communication (and political) players, capable of competing with the mainstream media for sectors of the public as well as helping to shape public opinion in the mediated political public sphere around a series of causes, from HIV/AIDS to climate change (Thrall, Stecula, and Sweet 2014; McPherson 2015, 2017; Powers 2014, 2017).

It is within such contexts that much of the sexuality of women from developing countries continues to be stereotypically understood, defined, talked about, and discussed within and across international development. This has resulted in an urgent need to transcend colonial patterns of representation, discourse, and imagery when it comes to women's bodies and issues around reproduction, motherhood, and maternity (Harcourt 2009: Wilkins 2016; Matos 2016). It could be said that the fact that these stereotypes and ideas have continued to prevail, with women's voices still being marginalised, has indirectly culminated in discussions on sexuality and on women's reproductive health not being fully addressed within international development (Cornwall, Correa, and Jolly 2008; Harcourt 2009, 2017). Given the fragility around these commitments, this has made it easier for the few advancements in women's reproductive rights, among others, to come under scrutiny and to be vulnerable to attacks by oppositional groups, resulting in the reproduction of discrimination towards less privileged groups of women and other minorities and sexual identities.

I argue elsewhere about the need to further strengthen the bridges between different feminist movements and women's groups on a transnational level, moving beyond the persistence of ingrained narratives of 'Otherness' and making further points of connection between the North and the South in development discourse, thinking, and practice. Despite acknowledging the difficulties in pursing these avenues of female solidarity that cut across borders, and within the difficulties created by socio-economic differences and backgrounds, I believe that SRHR is among one of the few areas within the women's movement where such bonds could be pursued. Some gender experts interviewed for this research have also defended the need to overcome these differences and to continue to build more bridges between different groups. The programme director for Sexual and Reproductive Rights at the US's Global Fund Women also stressed the importance of improving communications between feminist organisations,[17] further stating that the current 'voices that are pushing for gender equality are coming from the South'.

Given the various studies that have shown that, due to differences (including class and ethnicity) that often function as barriers to collaboration, women do not easily unite in a 'sisterhood' of solidarity and cooperation. Thus the assertion that, through certain issues – such as women's bodies and reproductive health – opportunities and spaces for diverse groups of women to get together might exist can sound at first like wishful thinking. If I acknowledge that there is a sense and a feeling that, around certain issues, women *do* unite – and in a context within which the need to dismantle bridges is becoming all the more necessary given the complexities of the current global challenges and the various threats to our livelihoods – this acknowledgement must be taken with a pinch of salt. We must recognise the difficulties of transcending the challenges and divisions that still exist within the feminism movement as well as within the international development sphere.

A revival of transnational feminist support, mobilisation, and solidarity – embedded in discursive practices that aim to recapture language and discourse around women's bodies, sexuality, and reproductive health, has definitely occurred and has begun to take shape throughout the world. The post-pandemic context, and the exacerbation of the structural inequalities that already existed, further demand a renewal of energy and the re-establishment and fortification of transnational feminist links around the world. These will continue to be upheld across different levels and institutions to advance global gender justice, whether in developed or developing countries.

My epistemological stance is rooted in pragmatism insofar as it reflects a genuine commitment to furthering social change and seeking more equality for those who have not yet benefitted from the promises of democratisation. For this reason, my research has engaged with organisations working with gender equality and reproductive health from across the world, although there are also specific case studies of countries from the Global South, including two of the most populated and larger emerging democracies in the world – India and Brazil. These, despite their differences, share many similarities when it comes to social structural inequalities, gender discrimination, poverty, and extreme right-wing politics (Modi in India and Bolsonaro in Brazil). Both countries have also had strong social movements, including feminist NGOs and networks that have helped shape thinking on gender equality policies from a feminist transnational perspective, either internationally through lobbying or mobilizing within the UN circuit as well as nationally through other local and grassroots initiatives (Narayanaswamy 2014, 2017; Alvarez 1998, 2009).

These countries also share similar democratic paradoxes of having high gender, health, and social inequalities while also being home to vibrant feminist movements and NGOs that work under challenging circumstances, co-existing alongside highly conservative and hierarchical cultures that have assigned women a submissive place. The different priorities and understandings of sexuality and reproductive health, and how these are discussed in the public sphere in each country, is also of particular interest. This taps into the argument that the debate here runs much deeper than a mere 'defence of abortion' by feminists who 'cultivate a culture of death'; rather, it is one that is rooted in understanding the complexities of sexuality and reproductive health, and their connection to poverty and inequalities, such as the importance of safety networks and welfare systems for more vulnerable groups of women and girls.

India is an interesting case for studies that seek to examine the role of communications in development with regard to SRHR. Traditionally, the country is seen as liberal in its approach to SRHR, but the reality on the ground remains one of sharp structural inequalities, particularly when it comes to the experiences of less privileged groups of women in its rural areas. When it comes to SRHR, India has managed to achieve a sharp reduction of 77 per cent in maternal mortality, going from 556 per 100,000 births in 1990 to 130 in 2016, thus managing to move closer to reaching the Sustainable Development Goal (SDG) target of below 70 by 2030. Although it should be noted that the pandemic has put some pressure on the nation's achieving this.[18]

India has also had an early focus on family planning and population control, having legalized abortion in 1971. In the last decades it has fully adopted neoliberalism, seeing an increase in the divide in its health service between the richer segments of the population, who can afford to pay for private health care, and the poorer segments, who are left with an under-funded state health system.[19] India also figures prominently in debates about the 'digital divide'. Although only 26 per cent of the population have access to the internet, and many working-class women use new technologies for practical purposes, the opportunities that these technologies are providing Indian women to fight gender injustice is beginning to be examined by journalists and scholars. India has over 460 million internet users and is home to the second largest online market, being ranked only behind China.

A similar situation exists in Brazil, where the under-funded SUS (Sistema Unico de Saude) health system, modelled on the UK's NHS and other European public health systems, attends to less privileged groups in contrast to private health care, which is used mainly by middle- and upper-class groups. Like India as well as other Latin American countries, Brazil, which is a highly patriarchal and misogynist society, also has many vibrant feminists and NGO groups who have influenced debates on women's rights and on reproductive health transnationally as well as at the local level. It is also one of the world's largest emerging democracies and, in the last decades, has sought to strengthen liberal democracy and economic neoliberalism. It has also seen the rise of far-right movements (like the Bolsonarismo political movement) that have been influenced by global 'populist' politics as well as by national specifications, including the historical legacy and baggage of the right-wing military dictatorship in Brazil of the 1960s and 1970s.

Speaking within the South Asian context, the senior director of the NGO Human Rights Law Network, where she heads the Women's Justice Initiative, underlined the various challenges faced by organisations working to advance sexual and reproductive rights:[20]

> I would say India has just taken the first few steps ... because look at Bangladesh, they have made such great strides when it comes to maternal deaths. India has made some progress, women have been standing up and demanding services, and there is a debate about 'health for all' ... I think there are very few feminist organisations – see the feminist movement in India has been very elitist. I don't think it is percolated to the grassroots. How many feminist organisations stand up and hold the government accountable for a woman's death on the hospitable table? None. How many have stood up to say that abortion services are the right of a woman? ... I've always been a person working in the grassroots, and I don't see any of that dialogue ringing in Delhi ... We work right with the grassroots and ensure that there is a discourse in those spaces. Movements haven't picked up these cases though ... whatever has happened is not enough to bring any change.

This problem is not restricted to South Asia. The director of advocacy of the International Planned Parenthood Federation (IPPF) also underscored how essential it is for NGOs working in the sector to reach out to the most marginalised communities across the world:[21]

> Safe abortion is an area which is neglected, and it carries so many ideological issues. But also, SRHR is not one thing, SRHR is several themes that have been defined by the Guttmacher and

Lancet Commission ... the new definition of SRHR ... it includes infertility and a few things. We have defined what we're talking about and definitely from that big range of issues, safe abortion probably is the most neglected, but I think that beyond the themes is that we need to look at people. We need to reach the women who are marginalised, who are indigenous and live very far from health services ... who have a different sexual orientation and gender identity, who are too young to make a decision.

It is crucial to assess the stagnation affecting the furthering of women's rights in the field of SRHR within this complex myriad of socio-political and cultural challenges. The failure of liberal Western governments to provide responses to the economic crises, and the growing uncertainties in social and political life, has without a doubt paved the way for the rise of cynicism, disillusionment with democratic politics, and a sense of disenfranchisement for many of the population, culminating in the endorsement of nationalist parties and right-wing extremist movements, from the US to Brazil, Hungry, and Italy. At the same time, the last decade has been hailed by scholars, journalists, and critics as the 'decade of the protest:'[22] movements against global inequalities, capitalism, austerity, and climate change have been seen in countries from Belgium to Lithuania, from the US Occupy Wall Street protests to the Arab Spring uprising.

Many argue over a deep and existential Western crisis that has produced a sharp sense of angst within the status quo. Where progressive change could have appeared as perhaps the obvious first alternative there emerged instead the rise of new authoritarian movements and a regrouping of right-wing groups in new packages, shapes, and forms. These had spread roots against the advancement of gender policies in reproductive health and in other areas since the UN-led conferences of the 1980s and 1990s (Friedman 2003). However, it was only following the 2008 economic global recession that attacks on human rights principles, including gender and minority rights, became more evident throughout the world.

The need to provide more and better information, knowledge, and communications on SRHR, and engaging in strategies to deconstruct myths and misinformation on SRHR through discourses, narratives, language, images, and representations, has been underscored by various gender experts and communication professionals from the organisations interviewed here. They further point to the current challenging context for NGOs working in the field. In her discussion of the activities of the transnational women's movements at the UN conferences of the 1990s, and the lobby around the inclusion of women's rights language in official documents, Friedman (2003) underlines how different frames for women's rights had already begun to compete. Resorting to 'framing' theory, and making use of idea of 'framing contests', Friedman (2003, 351) argues that:

> 'frame' and action 'repertoires' are the strategic processes through which movement participants develop and execute shared understandings ... Frames refer to a 'pattern in participants' beliefs about the causes of and solutions to contested issues', or the collective understandings that ... bind together ... participants (Clark et al. 1998, 5; Snow and Bedford 1992) ... Putting issues on the agenda is one marker of success that provokes countermovement (Meyer and Staggenborg 1996, 17); having done so movements may become engaged in 'framing contests' ... [T]he countermovement coalition led by the Vatican responded to the success of women's rights advocates' 'gendering the agenda' by establishing a frame of 'women's rights as threat to family, nation and god' to protect religious or traditional constructions of gender relations.

These dominant 'frames' and discourses around gender ideology myths continue to proliferate in the mediated political public sphere in both national and international contexts. These discourses around the centrality of the family, and the position of women in society primarily as 'mothers' dedicated to the private sphere, as well as the need to control women's bodies and their sexuality (or 'sexual liberation and promiscuity tendencies', in Foucauldian terms), have been rearticulated by these groups in recent years through new communication practices and discourses. These have often been articulated as economic concerns (e.g., that certain groups are 'being privileged' over others), although paradoxically the discourse that prevails is the social and cultural one (e.g., 'feminists teaching sex education to kids'), whereas the economic interest is often downplayed or obscured. It is nonetheless the key concern here given the interest of these groups in strengthening economic neoliberalism and capitalism. To do this, they create fear and uphold the 'nuclear family' as a vital discourse of influence that then becomes central to the debate. However, this discourse has taken on a *popular* form, hiding its true economic interest and instead masquerading as a 'legitimate concern' of the 'disenfranchised working classes and underprivileged communities' who have been 'hard done by' on the part of cosmopolitan global elites and others preoccupied only with 'identity politics', minority rights, and sexual identities (i.e., the so-called 'woke crowd').

Thus, far from being simply about 'moral' or 'Christian religious concerns', these narratives are being appropriated by groups embedded in all the nooks and crannies of capitalism and neoliberal economic politics, and they are fighting against the 'threats' posed in the last decades by the Western democratisation project itself and by social democracy. Confusion around terminology on SRHR is thus encouraged, including misinformation and/or prejudice around the topic of reproductive health. These are part of a whole arsenal of manipulative efforts and tactics deployed by conservative groups throughout the world who seek to roll back rights and, in doing so, to gain the support of segments of the population.

There is a need for new conversations, thinking, and empirical research on gender equality and SRHR. And engaging with the important role that communications has within the public sphere is vital to all the fields involved, from public health, gender, and development to health and development communications professionals and scholars. It is particularly pertinent in the post-pandemic context. It is crucial to start to examine the role that communications can have in constructing/deconstructing these misguided and manipulative discourses around sexuality, women's bodies, and reproductive health. Thus, one of my core aims is to examine *how* such discursive practices, articulated by vested interest groups, are being propagated in the mediated and political global public/private sphere. I also assess how these are contributing to further undermining public policies on gender equality and reproductive rights globally, thus contributing to the stagnation of women's rights globally.

RESEARCH RATIONALE AND METHODOLOGY

This book adopts a critical view of the role of communications for social change within development. It assesses the ways in which various health and feminist NGOs working with SRHR, located in countries in both the Global North and the Global South, from small to large organisations, can make better use of a variety of communication methods, practices, and strategies, as well as communication technologies, mingling online and offline media tools in their advocacy efforts around gender equality and reproductive health. Given the complexity of the subject matter and the problems that exist around communications on health, particularly when it comes to women's rights and reproductive health, this study engages in cross-disciplinary research and draws its theoretical frameworks from various disciplines, from gender and media studies to communications, sociology, and development studies.

This research aims to contribute to the theoretical debates on gender equality and reproductive health in development by arguing that a connection exists between the persistence of certain types of discourses on women's bodies (Harcourt 2009; Wilkins 2016; Matos 2016), particularly in developing countries from the Global South, and practices in international development that are failing to engage in a more holistic approach to SRHR, grounded in a more in-depth understanding that ceases to reinforce stereotypes and instead attempts to address structural inequalities of gender and health with the intention of boosting women's rights. It further aims to contribute to discussions on the role of advocacy communications and NGOs for social change (McPherson 2015; Powers 2014) as well as for feminist perspectives on health communications, feminist activism, and advocacy around SRHR (Harcourt 2009, 2017; Alvarez 2009; Wilkins 2016).

I also seek to contribute to the work of scholars within the field of gender, health, and development communications (Obregon and Waisbord 2012; Wilkins and Mody 2001, 2016; Tufte 2012; Dutta 2011; Lewis and Lewis 2015), advancing discussions on the role of feminist NGOs in the Global South and their wider role within international development and, in particular, in the field of SRHR (Alvarez 1998, 2009; Harcourt 2009, 2017; Cornwall, Correa, and Jolly 2008; Gideon and Porter 2016). With my current focus on the advocacy communication efforts of NGOs located across the world, from Europe to the US, Latin America, and South Asia, I seek to contribute to the literature on transnational feminist activism, organisation, and mobilisation, which, in the last decades, has attracted a lot of research in the fields of sociology and political science (Hawkesworth 2006, 2018; Alvarez 1998, 2009; Gajjala and Mamidipudi 1999; Gajjala 2003; Harcourt 2013; Keck and Sikkink 1998; Fotopoulou 2016a and 2016b).

My current research further expands on my previous work concerning democratisation and the combatting of structural inequalities, and the ways in which media and communications can be used for assistance in development and for social change, particularly in developing countries but also in the Global North. It builds on my earlier work on how contemporary feminist movements in Latin American and Brazil, in negotiation with other transnational global and feminist movements, have made use of online technologies to articulate counter-discourses and to pressure for change (Matos 2016, 2017). Here I concentrate on the role of NGOs working in the areas of health and gender and their use of strategic communications for SRHR advocacy, enacted locally but also pursued through transnational forms of activism and engagement and in a process of dialogue with other countries of the South and North.

I use a mixed-methods approach, combining mainly qualitative methodology with some quantitative methods to assess the ways in which NGOs working with women's health have made strategic use of communications to advocate for reproductive health and justice. A total of fifty-two health and feminist NGOs working in the field across the world were selected from a larger sample to participate in this research.[23] I conducted a one-month process of evaluation of the organisations, from an initial list of over one hundred, finally reducing this to a total of fifty-two health and feminist NGOs, networks, and movements located in the US, Europe (UK, Belgium, and Switzerland), Latin America (Brazil, Argentina, Peru, and Uruguay), and Asia (India and Philippines). Of these, a total of nine were from Asia, eleven were from Europe, nineteen from Latin America, nine from the US, and a further four were not specified and were classified as 'international' due to the fact that the organisations were present in more than one country and could be defined as being 'international networks'.

In-depth interviews with gender experts from the organisations as well as the application of a survey-style questionnaire to the communication professionals was combined with a content analysis of the institutional websites of the fifty-two NGOs. This included a critical discourse analysis (CDA) of their engagement on social media platforms, in particular on Twitter and Facebook (Fairclough 1998; Van Dijk 2016; Wodak and Meyer 2016; Gill 2018). Further CDA was also conducted on a selection of blogs from a sample of the NGOs. The content analysis of the institutional websites of the organisations included within this sample a total of fifteen websites from

NGOs that were examined in isolation as nobody was available for interviews. Of the original fifty-two NGOs, twenty-one had some form of blog on their website. A total of nine South Asian organisations were also the focus of a critical discourse analysis of their social media engagement.[24]

A total of fifty-eight interviewees, including gender experts and CEOs from these organisations, as well as communication leads and directors, also took part in this research. The interviews were conducted by me as well as by two research assistants, with Alessandra Brigo conducting most of those in Brazil and Ambika Tandon those in India. I conducted a total of twenty interviews internationally, particularly in Europe, the UK, and the US, while Sarah Molisso took on another two interviews. The survey-style questionnaires were applied to the communications directors of these organisations with the aim of assessing their advocacy work and the ways in which online and offline communication strategies were used for SRHR advocacy communications. Some interviews were conducted face to face and some via email, while others responded via the questionnaire or opted to do both. Another seven people, mainly gender experts and others from various human rights and civic organisations who had done work on SRHR and gender equality, were also interviewed. However, the organisations to which they are currently affiliated were not included as part of the institutional website sample list, and they gave interviews solely as experts.[25]

I argue that the expanding literature from communications scholars on NGOs communications and journalism makes it clear that there is still not enough knowledge about *how* civic and human rights organisations are making use of communications and information technologies, from the adoption of journalistic practices to the use of social media in their advocacy efforts around various causes (Powers 2014, 2017; McPherson 2015, 2017; Waisbord 2015). Over the last few years, within international development, politics, and international relations there has been a growing debate over the capacity of NGOs working in development or humanitarian causes to actually make a difference and to contribute to advancing change (Bebbington, Hickey and Mitlin, 2008; Thrall, Stecula, and Sweet 2014), a discussion also pursued by Powers (2014, 2017). Some of the classic definitions of what constitutes an 'international NGO' (Yanacopulos 2016, 49) state that these are organisations that function as intermediaries between concerned Northern publics and the beneficiaries of development work, usually located in the Global South, indicating a core/periphery, South/North division. However, the reality of globalization and the complexities of a world in which inequalities have become part of the lived experiences of countries in both the North and the South has meant that this division has become less clear cut.

In the introductory chapter in the *Journal of Communication*, 'Communications, Social Movements and Collective Action: Toward a New Research Agenda in Communications for Development and Social Change', Obregon and Tufte (2017, 638–9) argue for more research on how development institutions work with NGOs, the private sector, and governments in their pursuit of communications for development and social change. They also outline the similarities, not the antagonisms, that can exist in communications 'coming from the top' and the one 'coming from the bottom' (i.e., community-led). Despite the differences in the organisations' approaches (i.e., the more activist-led versus the institutionally conventional) to communications for development and social change, as well as the positions that they occupy within society, Obregon and Tufte (640) further problematise this top/bottom division, arguing that there can be little difference in the mobilisation of actors from both sides (64). They state that movements within development led from 'above' can also make use of communications to mobilise stakeholders towards a concrete goal. An example is the case of the Global Polio Eradication Initiative, which included public-private partnerships led by governments and partners such as the World Health Organisation, the Bill Gates Foundation, the US Center for Disease Control and Prevention (CDC), and UNICEF.[26]

This research is concerned with *how* the use of communications by NGOs who work in the field of SRHR can contribute to creating wider awareness and mobilisation and, most important, how they can engage in wider in-depth dialogue and debate on the topic in the public sphere, with a view to dismantling misinformation, prejudices, and resistances as well as seeking to deepen knowledge, understanding, and information on sexuality, reproductive health, and women's bodies and rights. It's aim is to examine how this could be further strengthened and where the exchange of knowledge and advocacy around issues of sexual and reproductive health and rights can – and should – be improved, particularly when it comes to reaching out and influencing target audiences, from the media and policy-decision arena to citizens and other affected communities.

Many of the gender experts and NGO directors interviewed confirmed that SRHR is still widely misunderstood by the public and that there is a need to invest in communications for advocacy to move the discussion forward, deconstructing the idea of a supposed 'gender ideology' and returning to debates on *why* sexual rights and health matter and are part of a human rights framework, and why these are essential to women's basic rights. Aware of the complexity of researching this topic from a global perspective and of the challenges of conducting cross-national, multidisciplinary research, I strive to insert some flexibility into the structured interviews, particularly with regard to the standard set of questions designed for the communication professionals and gender experts.

Sensitive to the diversity of local contexts and the approaches to the topic in different countries, to the achievements and barriers as well as to the political pressures around SRHR, both the question sheet for the in-depth interviews and the survey-style questionnaire provided scope for the interviewer to apply some flexibility. The standard set of questions initially designed for the gender experts and CEOs of the organisations was done in a way that permitted adaptability to the local contexts, their specific histories and challenges, while also covering a range of topics around women's rights and SRHR, from the achievements in the field in the aftermath of the 1994 ICPD conference, to specific questions on the ambiguities around terminology, to further questions on advocacy communications.

With the assistance of one of the early career research assistants, Jamile Dalpiaz, a thematic analysis was developed to help sort out the data obtained from the interviews with the gender experts and CEOs. This was developed into what we identified as the main themes, which we considered the most important and which we explored with all the gender experts interviewed. The six themes selected are: (1) *achievements relating to SRHR at the ICPD Cairo conference*; (2) *the role of NGOs in advancing sexuality and reproductive health*; (3) *SRHR terminology and use*; (4) *investments in communications*; (5) *online communications use*; and (6) *future challenges for SRHR*. Words and phrases were selected from the interviews and then coded according to the core themes that ran through the responses. All research material, data collected, codebook, questionnaires, and consent forms were uploaded to a Google Drive so that the project could be shared by all members, and this facilitated the work of the early career researchers who joined at different stages of the project.

The design of the communications survey-style questionnaire that was applied to the media professionals of the organisations mingled directly with indirect questions and also provided the interviewee with optional answers. These were provided with space to write more details on their communication strategies, campaigns, and activities. The communication professionals were also asked to evaluate how they made use of communications for advocacy in their attempts to influence a diversity of publics, including being asked to assess the differences and impact of online and offline communications on their target publics. Contrary to the in-depth interviews with the gender experts, which were done either face-to face or via Skype, the communications questionnaires were sent to the head of communications of the organisations, and they were then given a time for answering them.

The communications questionnaire also sought to look at how NGOs use digital communication technologies in a range of ways, including how they combine these with their offline traditional media activities, such as their development of press releases or contacts with the mainstream media. They were also asked to think about how they use their online communication tools and interactive features on their websites for advocacy communications on sexuality and reproductive health. There were specific questions related to funding, money, and the need for further investments (or not) in their communication activities. The core objectives here were to examine the nature of the communication and information flows being carried out by these organisations to assess the ways in which media, as well as online tools, could be better used to the advantage of NGOs in their advocacy communication efforts. The research questions here were: (1) How can health and feminist NGOs and networks make better use of communications for SRHR advocacy? (2) How do these communication strategies and practices reflect the daily advocacy efforts and activities of these organisations? (3) What are the discursive communication strategies used, and in what way can these have a wider impact? And (4) How have offline (and online) communication efforts assisted these organisations in achieving their goals, and what are some of the future challenges for SRHR advocacy communications?

First, the core data for this research were collected during its initial stage, which was conducted during fieldwork I carried out in Brazil when I was on sabbatical (January to May 2019) and was a visiting academic at IESP UERJ in Rio de Janeiro. The first stage of the data collection was from March to June 2019, whereas the second stage occurred post-COVID-19, from April to August 2020, and was carried out in the UK. This included the writing up stage and the initial findings being submitted to a journal in the field.

During the first stage of the fieldwork, three PhD research students worked alongside me at IESP UERJ during different stages of the esearch, while another student research assistant based at the Centre for Internet and Society (CSI) in India, Ambika Tandon, assisted me in the initial gathering of the data, analysis of the websites and blogs, and the conducting of the interviews in India in 2019. During the April-August 2020 period, at the height of the start of the coronavirus pandemic, another PhD research assistant from City, Sarah Molisso, aided in making sense of the data, conducting a few final online interviews, and carrying out some discourse analysis of the NGOs' blog posts collected between 2019 and 2020. Finally, another early career researcher in the UK, Jamile Dalpiaz, assisted in the last months of the project in 2021 before the completion of this manuscript in October of the same year.[27]

The first stage of this project consisted of an initial mapping of the NGOs and organisations who work with gender equality, particularly with SRHR, in order to build a representative sample that could do justice to the diversity of the organisations represented by civil society actors and by third-sector actors who are working in the field of development and seeking to improve policy in gender equality and reproductive health through a series of diverse approaches and strategies, dealing with different levels of donor funding, support, and resources as well as policy influence. This is in a context in which many of these organisations work under challenging circumstances and within an environment that lacks funding for health NGOs seeking to advance women's rights and agency with regard to reproductive health (Gideon and Porter 2016).

To better reflect the organisations that work in the field, this study seeks to include health and feminist NGOs, networks, and movements working in both the North and the South – these may be either large organisations or more grassroots feminist movements, but all of them have managed to influence debates, thinking, and policies on reproductive health. These organisations are based in different geographical locations and have different epistemological understandings of SRHR, according to their culture and socio-political contexts, although all of those that participated place sexual and reproductive health within the human rights framework (Cornwall and Nyamu-Musembi 2006; Kindornay, Ron, and Carpenter 2012).

The criteria for selecting the organisations that are included here took into consideration a range of factors, such as their policy work, political impact and clout (i.e., what they have managed to achieve through legislation, policy, and/or political standing in their countries), as well as media influence, engagement with the targeted publics, and their approach to the use of communications for advocacy on women's health. All organisations selected are doing work on gender equality more broadly, with some including SRHR as part of their work and others focusing exclusively on reproductive health. Moreover, not all these organisations can be classified as being exclusively 'feminist' or as necessarily an 'NGO'. Some may be placed more within the medical research field, while others may be classified as being a 'feminist network'.

The final sample for the NGOs was chosen from the research and put into selected phrases on Google. These were: 'NGOs sexual and reproductive rights', 'feminist NGOs and reproductive rights', and 'feminist NGOs, gender equality, and human rights'. The identity of the organisation, its mission or vision statement, history and goals, was also examined, including the impact and relevance of its work in the field. This list included NGOs who work both 'on the ground' and at the grassroots level as well as more professionalized and larger NGOs. Examples of some of the NGOs included range from more medical-focused organisations like Ibis Reproductive Health, to the global development Care International UK, to the more feminist Latin American NGOs and networks like Anis in Brazil. Organisations like Amnesty International and Care International, which do not focus primarily on gender equality, were nonetheless included since they conduct some relevant work in the field and are influential within international development.

The NGOs selected included large organisations with a more research- and health-focused approach as well as mid-range and small grassroots feminist networks that define themselves as 'activists' and that work more on the advocacy of single issues (such as the defence of abortion, contraceptives, or family planning), many of which are largely composed of a few volunteers or a small group of employees. These have different resources and money at their disposal, including for both online and offline media and communications activities, and this has implications for the type of advocacy communication activities with which they engage.

Recently, the growth and diversity of the organisations that compose the third sector, and their placement somewhere between civil society and the market, has been the subject of much debate and research in the fields of politics, international relations, and international development (Bebbington 2007; Yanacopulos 2016). Despite some limitations, and the fact that some organisations overlap in what they offer (e.g., being a service-orientation NGO with a participatory framework), McPhail (2009, 67–9) provides a useful distinction between the different types of NGOs, grouping them together in four key categories. These are: the *charitable-orientation* organisations, with their top-down effort and insufficient use of participation; the *service-led* organisations, which offer provision in health, family planning, or education, with programmes often designed by the NGOs themselves; the *participatory-orientation* organisations, in which local people are included in projects; and the *empowerment-orientation* organisations, in which local groups work on issues that affect the poor. Most of the organisations that participated in this research could be classified as being either of the service or participatory-orientation type, with a few exceptions being some of the local feminist grassroots movements and networks, which can also be categorised as a type of 'empowerment' NGO. Many were single-issue based, focusing on particular areas, such as family planning and contraception, while others engaged with SRHR within their wider work on gender equality (i.e., gender-based violence and women's economic empowerment).

I found myself having to overcome the challenges of going over the vast range of information, data, and research material put out by these fifty-two health and feminist NGOs and networks. I had to make my way through the abundant data, images, discourses, and debates on SRHR that they produced. The enormous challenges of doing this cannot be dismissed. Here I would like to borrow from an expression used by Sonia Alvarez (2009, 178) concerning the 'vast constellation of knowledge products generated by NGOs', which she uses to describe the richness of the work carried out by these feminist organisations within the context of her critical examination of the paradoxes created by the whole 'NGO-ization' process that took place throughout the 1980s and 1990s as they gained influence at the UN-level (Friedman 2003).

Here the use of the term 'NGO-ization' refers to the process of how wider funding was provided to these organisations by the UN and other multilateral agencies following from the successes achieved at the international conferences of the 1990s. This term is used to criticise the co-optation of previously 'radical' or grassroots feminist groups into the mainstream by packaging ideas on gender equality, sexuality, and reproductive health into more 'acceptable' discourses on women's rights grounded in notions of 'individual empowerment' and choice rather than in the right to agency – for instance, the right to reproductive justice as well as to quality state-funded health and other medical services (Harcourt 2009; Narayanaswamy 2014, 2017).

The advocacy communication efforts of the NGOs on sexuality and reproductive health, at least some of the initiatives, could be seen as being part of their strategies of 'self-branding', of acquiring and strengthening their respectability, credibility, and clout with members of the public and decision-making elites. This, however, should not function to dismiss their efforts, as it is often the case that a blurring of the boundaries between the use of media and communications for advocacy on specific campaigns and programmes in the field can be the result both of a genuine commitment to advance social change and an indirect attempt to enhance the organisation's image ('its branding') and profile. Therefore, some scholars (Enghel and Noske-Turner 2018) argue that, within international development, there is frequently a dilemma between 'appearing to do good or looking good'.

I have thus adopted the view that these practices are not necessarily that far apart from each other and that there is often overlap. Frequently it is in the organisation's interest to enhance its own profile through the advocacy of certain development programme campaigns in the field, many of which are not totally dissociated from concerns with using media and communications for the advancement of SRHR at the policy level. Thus, out of the fifty-two organisations examined here, there were clear differences in positionality, funding, and resources as well as various forms of communication practices and strategies, including advocacy communications and specific action on SRHR. Some organisations, for instance, made use of more activist discourses, while others supported themselves more on the basis of research-driven arguments, including reports, facts, and statistics.

As I show here, the frequent use of more *facts-based* arguments and reports for advocacy – as well as the evocation of emotion and human interest – has become a much more common communication and marketing practice used by NGOs within humanitarian and international development (Ascough 2018). As I argue, there is still a frequent blurring of the lines between more militant activist styles of advocacy communications and the more rational, factual, 'objective', and professional informational-led type, which are more rooted in journalistic jargons and their practices. Emotional appeals, human interest stories, and digital storytelling have also become popular communications devices widely deployed in fundraising campaigns by charities and humanitarian organisations working in international development, and they have produced mixed results and debates on how individual personal interest stories can often *depoliticise* complex structural development issues. If designed well, and if they are embedded in participatory frameworks, these personal stories of 'suffering' and hardship can contribute to creating wider empathy, compassion, and engagement from the public for that particular cause (Ascough 2018; Hemer and Tufte 2016). This is because many throughout the world are not immersed in 'compassion fatigue' (Chouliaraki 2006) and, instead, are genuinely moved by structural inequalities, poverty, and famine, and by various social injustices.

Moreover, advocacy communication activities around SRHR have sought to make use of language, narratives, discourses, and various communication strategies with the intention of *persuading* groups of people around a particular cause to influence policy. Often it is the case, as this research shows, that the 'objective' and the 'subjective' are blurred, with emotional testimonies frequently being layered on top of 'fact-checking' initiatives and other statistical data and information. Wilkins (2014, 57) states that 'advocacy' entails the engagement of forms of public communication 'in support of a particular political cause', with the intention of gathering social support for policy change by focusing on some strategic programmes.

Thus, in order to dive into this 'communication overload' and to make proper sense of the richness of the 'vast constellation of knowledge' (Alvarez 2009) presented before me, I decided to design a codebook to make sense of the data and the communication work that these organisations and networks put out. The latter enabled the early career researchers and me to add the data collected for the project during the course of its two years duration. The design of this codebook was influenced by political communication typologies, including the one provided by Foot and Schneider (2006) and further developed by Stein (2009), as well as Auger's (2013) work on NGOs' use of Twitter and Facebook. Stein (2009, 755) uses a typology that includes categories such as presenting information and promoting interaction, including through hyperlinks, which are frequently used in political communication campaigns to mobilise supporters or promote the image of a candidate.

This work also considers ethical considerations associated with conducting research on data gathered from the internet, according to the ethical guidelines provided by the Association of Internet Researchers (2019). For the analysis of the institutional websites, I combined both content analysis and discourse analysis, having developed categories for the codebook to ensure reliability as well as to make better sense of the data. To assess the communication approaches of these organisations, the qualitative content analysis sought to examine the type of features included on the organisations' websites, from the hyperlinks of podcasts to videos, press releases, and reports to blogs.

I apply here also a *feminist intersectional epistemological* lens to my methodological approach. Quoting Oakley's (1981) classic text on the contribution of feminist thinking to methodology, 'Interviewing Women: A Contradiction in Terms', Michailidou (2018, 20–1) discusses the criticism of the previously dominant positivist paradigm of sociological research and the shift towards the interpretivist methodological frameworks and qualitative tradition that has marked not only feminist sociology but also media and cultural studies scholarship. It has also become somewhat the dominant methodological tradition. I am interested here specifically in Michailidou's (2018, 23) discussion of Haraway's (1991) relational concept of *agency*, particularly in relation to how the research process can be transformative for both the 'knower and the known'. This is what I seek to do here by engaging with NGOs from across the world, with the research process and collection of data being an enriching process for all parties involved. Thus knowledge gained from the NGOs was transferred to the researcher while at the same time, I assisted the organisations in their strategic thinking on communications, gender equality, and SRHR.

As Michailidou (2018, 23) notes, Haraway (1991) redefined 'objectivity' and, in her discussion of the 'epistemology of situated knowledge', argued in favour of the subject of knowledge being 'conceptualized as shaped by the space and time coordinates as much as the object of knowledge. The acceptance ... of embodiment and ... social positioning of the "interested" agent not only signifies that he or she is conceptualized as a member of an ... epistemic community ... but has also implications for the power relationship between subject and object'.

I thus sought to combine qualitative methods with some quantitative methodology concerns. I start by using qualitative social media data analysis to examine public posts made by the organisations. The media content, videos, campaigns, and social media posts are all part of the public domain and have no privacy requirements. The campaigns that are discussed were referred to by the interviewees or included in the questionnaire sheet, with the links provided. There are no direct quotes taken from the videos, each of which is provided with its title, a description, and an analysis of its content, with user anonymity being protected. The blog posts that are mostly discussed were also referenced, with the names of the authors included.

I was not interested in conducting a merely quantitative study, which would have mainly sought to measure the frequency of social media use. Such a study would tell me little about exactly *how* these organisations are using communications for SRHR advocacy, such as, for example, the strategies used to mobilise, influence, and shape policy as well as to create awareness. It would have been mainly concerned with measuring the intensity of the communication material put out by the organisations during a specific period. This type of work would have been more suitable for studies concerned with assessing the efficacy of media content and posts in achieving specific goals and targeting certain audiences, mostly with the intention of evaluating how such approaches were successful in securing funding and resources from private and public bodies, including donations from the public, or how this had an impact on policy-makers. These do not constitute the core concerns of this study.

Quantification was used in a limited manner to capture the frequency of certain messages, but this was done with the purpose of aligning the data to the qualitative interpretation of the content collected. Thus, the quantification of the sampled data had as its main purpose *identifying recurring trends* and sorting out patterns of communication activities and forms of engagement. Non-frequency content analysis was combined with quantitative concerns regarding the *quantity* and diversity of communicative content posted by the organisations on social media and their use of different communication tools (offline and online) for advocacy on their institutional websites (George 2009; McMillan 2009; Krippendorff and Bock 2009). Quantitative content analysis was used to count the number of stories posted during the period of analysis and to assist in sorting out content (words, messages, texts, and phrases) and how it is used for different types of communications. The purpose of this was to understand how different media content and communications can be appropriated either for advocacy purposes, or to persuade people to endorse a particular cause (inserted within a category that I classify as being part of 'emotion[s]'), or to provide knowledge, information, and facts on sexual and reproductive health and rights (the emphasis being on rationality, or 'reason').

Strategies were further developed to improve the reliability of the qualitative material, creating the means to document its analysis using the codebook. The discourse analysis of the social media content tended to draw on what Lindekilde (2014, 18), quoting Dahler-Larsen (2012), classifies as 'displays', which can be understood as being a 'condensed, visual depiction of qualitative data, which facilitates analysis and helps detect patterns/trends/themes'. This can, for instance, include the presentation of the results of a discourse analysis in display format (e.g., matrix display, such as tables with cross tabulations of codes). In my research this resulted in the application of thematic analysis to some of the data, such as the interviews, while the CDA of the media content of the NGOs (such as that of the blogs) included the use of a codebook with categories created to make better sense of the qualitative material collected. The aim is to identify patterns as well as recurring themes and trends, to permit comparisons between organisations.

As argued previously, a lot of the literature on NGO journalism underlines how the communication strategies of civic, human rights, and other NGOs in many ways matches the communication practices and professional journalism style of the mainstream media and other news organisations in their publicity endeavours (Waisbord 2001; 2015; McPherson 2017; Powers 2014, 2017; Keck and Sikkink 1998; Thrall, Stecula, and Sweet 2014). To discuss how the NGOs apply their SRHR framework to their advocacy communication practices, I develop Powers' (2014) discussion on the components that shape civic and humanitarian NGOs' publicity and communication strategies, outlining some of the factors that affect their organisational dynamics, from the feminist approaches to SRHR to the type of publics targeted, the resources used, and communication strategies. All these factors shape the information and communications on SRHR put forward by these organisations, as well as their intended outcomes and the challenges that they face.

The use of critical discourse analysis emerged as the natural and preferred method for the investigation of the communicative content espoused by the organisations, be it through their websites, on social media, or on their blog posts. It goes without saying that the relationship of language to power is essential here (Jaworski and Coupland 2014). As Fairclough (2001) argues, 'discourse' can be understood as *social practice* and is explained by the way social agents act in the world. The analyst needs to look outside of the physicality of the text to understand how people use texts and discourses in everyday practices, and how this is connected to power dynamics as well as to how they make meaning from them (Wodak and Meyer 2016).

In her discussion of the variety of discourse analysis approaches, which have been drawn from the fields of critical linguistics, social semiotics, and critical language studies (Hodge and Kress 1988 and Fairclough 1989 in Gill 2000, 3), Gill (2000, 2018) notes how all of these reject the realist position that language is something merely neutral, simply reflecting reality. In their examination of how discourse has been studied within the social sciences, Wodak and Meyer (2016, 4) further explain that discourse can mean 'anything from a historical movement ... a policy, a political strategy, narratives in a restricted or broad sense of the term ... to language per se'. This includes the notion of certain *types* of discourse, including racist and gendered discourses. Discursive practices in societies can thus function to reproduce power relationships and, historically, such practices have been embedded in systems of knowledge that uphold the status quo (Foucault 1972).

Ideology then is the *site of struggle* for power and authority (Bourdieu 1991, in Jaworski and Coupland 2014). Particularly within the context of the CDA tradition (Van Dijk 2016; Wodak and Meyer 2016; Gill 2000, 2018; Jorgensen and Philips 2002; Fairclough 1998), a key concern has been with the deconstruction of ideologies. This is often done through 'the systematic ... investigation of semiotic data (written, spoken or visual)' (Wodak and Meyer 2016, 4). I attempt to do something similar, concentrating on examining how some of the communication material collected here has explicitly attempted to deconstruct discourses, misinformation, and narratives that uphold misinformation and 'gender ideology' discourses around women's sexuality or wider reproductive health rights. Battles around SRHR and women's rights ultimately involve disputes over meaning.

It is precisely within the realm of discourse that we can find clashes between groups regarding ideas around motherhood as well as who has control over a woman's body. Here lie the tensions between liberalism's emphasis on individual rights and the collective responsibilities of the state and government, represented in the access to quality public health services and the obligation of the state to ensure these rights. Thus, when it comes to the field of women's rights and reproductive health in gender and development, I argue that part of the cultural and social resistance and constraints around SRHR are interwoven with philosophical, moral, ideological, and political struggles over competing discourses, definitions, and meanings concerning women's bodies, reproduction, and fertility as well as parenting, childcare, and the role of fathers.

Thus, when I refer to 'gender myths' around SRHR, these include common-sense assumptions and discourses, such as the notion that 'sexual and reproductive health and rights is all about abortion', to more controversial accusations, such as 'feminists promote a culture of death.' As I show, many organisations engaged in advocacy communications on reproductive health rights often do so from a position of defensiveness, having to point out 'the facts' and the 'truth' about the need to decriminalise abortion due to public health concerns. Thus, the circulation of these discourses within the mediated public sphere ends up contributing to creating anxiety around the 'breaking down of families', culminating in having an impact on the perpetuation of forms of discrimination and the marginalisation of less privileged groups of women and other sexual identities. As I explore here, a lot of the battles fought today in the field are embedded in prejudices, misinformation, and lack of an appropriate understanding of what constitutes sexuality and reproductive health. Here communications has played, and can play, a better and more influential role in deconstructing such narratives and, instead, improving information, communications, and debate on health communications around SRHR.

My purpose is not simply to 'play' with discourse and language in my discussion of sexual and reproductive health: I would also like to make use of some of the criticisms of CDA's moral and ethical dimensions (Graham 2018). Examining the limits of CDA in his discussion of Van Dijk's (1993) work on racism and its focus on how discourses are reproduced rather than on how to alter racist discourse itself, Graham (2018, 194) maintains that we need to 'change social systemic discourse, including elite media and other institutional discourse (Scene)' as well as 'the cognitive systems of Agents who are framed as discourse 'recipients'. This is because discourses in isolation cannot change institutional structures and their inequalities. Despite acknowledging these limits, Graham defends the validity and merits of CDA against accusations of its being *unscientific*, acknowledging its primary concern with ethics and with building equitable spaces for equality and democracy. As he further states, CDA 'aims to transform action and values such that the social system becomes increasingly equal', and this has much more to do 'with law than with grammar' (202).

I use the foregoing conceptual frameworks to analyse and discuss the social world, reinforcing how it needs to be fully embedded within social and political practices and placed firmly within empirical reality. All of them have been useful for examining the competing discourses in the public sphere around SRHR and how organisations working in the Global North and in the Global South are using advocacy communications within a highly complex and challenging global environment. I further conceptualise my understanding of 'communications' as being above all a *dialogical* process, rooted in participatory dimensions and supported within a human rights framework. I am thus critical of the behaviourist models traditionally associated with the health communication messages of development campaigns promoted in developing countries within the logics of the modernisation framework (Waisbord and Obregon 2012a; Tufte 2012; Manyozo 2012b; Dutta 2011).

A core question is *what type of communication* are we talking about? All these conceptual frameworks led me to design a codebook that seeks to capture all the types of communication content, messages, and information used by the organisations for advocacy on reproductive health, both online and offline. The codebook is divided into nine key parts represented by separate sheets in an Excel Spreadsheet file. The first and the second sheets include the mapping out of the organisations, from their location to the type and issue focus (i.e., their mission statement), the language used (English, Spanish, or Portuguese), their defining features and design, and how they use media and present themselves to the public. This includes other information, such as the names of their experts and the budgets with which they work (see appendices). To make better sense of the *type of communications* and information put out by the NGOs on their institutional websites, I developed certain categories based on the dominant features usually encountered on online platforms, including the words 'Facebook', 'Twitter', 'YouTube', 'Emails', 'Instagram', 'video', 'podcasts', 'blog', 'e-learning link', 'discussion forums', 'LinkedIn', and any other unique link.

The third sheet of the codebook was developed to capture the type of communication strategies used by the organisations. To do this, I developed five core categories under which to include the communicative material: *fundraising, advocacy, community engagement, mobilisation,* and *information*. Under each category, four to seven items were included. These were policy reports, press releases, media articles, publications, facts and figures, CEO speeches, and archives (for *information*); information (emotion), campaigns, events, discussion forums, membership, volunteering, and newsletter (for *advocacy*); emails, discussion forums, contact organisation, member profiles, local events, workshops and training, and international agenda (for *community engagement*); donations, funding, partners, and lobbying politicians (for *fundraising and resources*); and online petitions, action alerts, protests, and organisation of campaigns (for *mobilisation*).

Community engagement refers to the *type* of dialogue and flow of communications that takes place between the organisation and its targeted publics, while *mobilisation* is associated with activism, protest, campaigns, and events. Part of this process evidently involves different forms of engagement with community members. The same can be said of *advocacy* and *information,* as facts, policy reports, statistics, and more 'objective' and scientific material can be placed under the latter as well as under the former. Advocacy is associated more with an appeal to emotions, passion, and persuasion and, in contrast to information, is seen as more 'subjective' and opinion-led, being open to dispute and contestation. It can be difficult to fully distinguish between these categories as they are often blurred, and certain content can easily be placed under both. Nonetheless, it is precisely in the realm of this type of ambiguity that confusion can be created, for facts and statistics can be disputed within competing discourses by different groups of people and interests with diverse forms of access to societal power structures. Moreover, such categories can also be used to undermine certain facts on the grounds that they may be deemed too 'subjective', their 'truth claims' being open to dispute and attack.

The fourth sheet of the codebook looks at the 'effects' of online communications and is part of the gathering of data from organisations on how they assess digital communications in relation to offline media. This was included as part of a question in the questionnaire for the communication heads. I attempted to assess the *type of communications* online (under any of the five categories, such as advocacy) according to the 'effect' (very effective, somewhat, not effective, or more effective than offline lobbying and/or successful online campaigns). Most organisations answered this question by focusing on their advocacy communications efforts (e.g., listing successful online campaigns), but they also mentioned examples of strategies for community engagement and mobilisation. Most claimed that their online communications were 'very effective' or 'somewhat effective'. The fifth sheet was on *online communication aims*, which was part of a question also included in the survey and that offered the following options from which to choose ('networking and connections', 'influence policymaking', 'influence politicians', 'the media', 'public opinion', 'all the above', or 'other').

The coding for the Twitter and Facebook feeds include a division of the communication material between 'emotion' and 'reason', which are further combined with the five categories mentioned above as well as with the item 'lobbying'. I was ultimately concerned with examining *how* communication strategies and goals translate into everyday policy and advocacy practices. Waisbord (2015) views the very act of policy advocacy as, in essence, an *exercise in communications*, demanding both persuasion *and* participation, such as the mobilisation of citizens to influence policy-makers to concentrate on certain policies. As he further notes, this 'entails the mobilisation of various publics who engage and persuade other actors ... to support their causes through a range of communication acts, such as information sharing, dialogue, public deliberation, street actions, consultation, and media tactics' (150).

Communications can and should be more embedded in the policy advocacy process of the whole organisation, from their design to the ways in which they can generate more impact, and how best they can be enacted using a diverse range of channels both at the global and local levels. At the same time, the limits of communication processes in enacting social change need to be factored into the whole equation and must include not just those associated with new communication technologies, with commercialization or the 'digital divide' but, rather, those associated with the knowledge that communications cannot work in isolation and need instead to be inserted within the specific historical contexts of the societies in which they are immersed. In other words, they must be fully connected to their economic, social, cultural, and political realities.

It is important to assess *how* these communication strategies could be better exploited and appropriated by these same organisations to enhance their causes, many of which are currently misunderstood, and to which there is still a lot of misinformation (and prejudice and stigmatisation) attached. Thus, the strategies of *constructing/deconstructing discourses* around SRHR used by health and feminist NGOs in their advocacy communication efforts are of crucial interest to me. This is particularly the case given the fact that the need to deconstruct discourses, language, and narratives around sexual and reproductive health and rights has been emphasised by a number of the experts interviewed here as being crucial in the debate on advancing equality for women's rights globally. This is why we need to articulate new conversations and narratives around sexual and reproductive health and rights. These are issues that I turn to next.

2

Transnational Feminism, the 'Female Body', and Global Gender Justice

Defining 'Sexual and Reproductive Health and Rights'

Within the dominant modernisation framework, mainstream development theory conceptualised development as economic growth, neglecting women altogether during the 1950s until finally incorporating them in response to criticism. However, despite decades of various feminist scholars, postcolonial scholars, and others from the development communications field (Cornwall, Correa, and Jolly 2008; Harcourt 2009, 2017; Wilkins 2016) pointing out the shortcomings of mainstream development theory, particularly regarding the persistence of colonial and patriarchal patterns of thinking, the reality is that development as it is currently practised still pays lip service to the modernisation framework and can be seen as largely embedded within neoliberal economics and market dynamics.

Debates within gender and development have been influenced by the different 'feminist waves', from liberal feminism, associated mostly with the Women in Development (WID) framework, to radical, Marxist, and postcolonial versions, which affected the thinking around Woman and Development (WAD) and, particularly, gender and development (GAD) (Sen 1999; Chua et al. 2000). This included the discussions on the shift from the word 'woman' to the word 'gender' (Sardenberg 2007). Feminist theorists within international development thus contributed to thinking on policy, with debates moving away from earlier calls to simply include women in development interventions, as was the case with WID (Parpart et al. 2000; Rai 2011; Mohanty 2000), to the examination of *how* women were included and the power dynamics at play, as was the case with GAD. Development programmes applied to developing countries during the early years of the modernisation period were accused of having been ineffective at providing transformative gender justice to more vulnerable groups of women.

Many of the development campaigns dedicated to women in development from the early modernisation period of the 1950s and 1970s were mostly focused on health and family planning practices and were constructed within social marketing imperatives and behaviourist communication models. Many of these were also criticised (Dutta 2011; Obregon and Waisbord 2012a). Feminist scholars working in international development have, in the last few years, begun to examine more critically the notion of 'women's agency' and 'empowerment' within the field in theory and practice (Cornwall and Rivas 2015). As the crux of the argument goes, not only do 'women' from developing countries still lack legitimate 'agency', but they also continue to be stereotyped within the discourses that speak of female *reproductive bodies* in the Global South. Debates have moved on to cultural and social factors that affected development as well as to analyses of discourses and representations of 'women from developing countries' and how these are defined (e.g., the criticisms of Mohanty [2000] regarding the homogenization of the 'Third World woman' within development).

What is thus still argued is that, when 'women' are included, this usually continues to be problematic or insufficient, mainly articulated within neoliberal discourses of 'empowerment' associated with individual success and inserted within the dicta of capitalist frameworks. This is particularly the case for women from the Global South (Wilkins 2016; Harcourt 2017; Matos 2016; Cornwall and Rivas 2015). These discursive practices do little to fully combat structural inequalities for all groups of women 'on the ground', including in the area of women's health (Giden and Porter 2016). The last decades have also seen the development of more holistic understandings of poverty and inequalities, and how this affects women and girls from developing countries beyond the previous North/South *core/periphery* dichotomy of the modernisation framework. Throughout Western institutions, this has culminated in debates on the need to *decolonise* knowledge, expertise, and thinking, from academia to the international development industry itself, relating to practices and discourses, power dynamics, and relationships between different players – that is, the 'Northern' versus 'Southern' NGOs (Narayanaswamy 2014) – as well as the to role of women and other vulnerable groups.

In response to the criticisms of the modernisation framework and its view of development, the 1990s saw the increasing popularity of the commitment to participatory approaches in development, including wider concerns with the role of culture in shaping development. This included a movement away from a mere focus on understanding development as economic growth and productivity, one disassociated from the impact of social factors and from more complex understandings of inequalities and poverty within development (Nederveen Pieterse 2010; Kotahri and Minogue 2002; Sen 1999; Cornwall, Correa, and Jolly 2008; Chambers 2005; Kabeer 2015). Moreover, the emphasis on the social and on the need to construct more participatory-led programmes built within a language of human rights and gender mainstreaming (Walby 2000) began to take place alongside the rise, since the 1980s, of neoliberal economics, which significantly affected development thinking as well as donor funding (Wilkins 2016; Green 2002). It contested that it is often the case that women largely constitute the poorer segments of society in developing countries. This led to gender gaining central stage within social development programmes, alongside 'vulnerable groups', such as children and minorities (Green 2002, 60). This, in turn, led to the problematic view of equating poverty and underdevelopment with women, contributing to the tendency to *universalize* the diversity of the experiences of women from developing countries, including situating them in an ahistorical period devoid of time and space, thus as eternally oppressed and as the 'victims of patriarchy' in their own cultures and in 'need of saving' (Mohanty 2000).

Poverty thus acquired a 'feminine' face – with the term 'feminization of poverty' (Chant 2011) becoming a popular expression within debates on gender and development – that stands in contrast to the 'masculine' domain of 'hard' economic development, which has continued to define international development practice. Poverty began to be viewed not just in terms of basic income, or in numerical or quantitative terms, but also more qualitatively, in terms of notions of entitlement, empowerment, and capabilities (Sen 1999). Within this view, to be fully 'empowered',[1] humans need to have access to a range of rights, from political and cultural rights to economic opportunities and security as well as being able to access quality education and health services. As Green (2002, 61) argues, the classification of groups as 'vulnerable' has led, paradoxically, to the 'marginalisation of social development within development agencies and discourse', leading it to be viewed as secondary to trade, economics, and governance. Similarly, other scholars, like Harcourt (2009, 29), underline how gender 'has remained the soft issue of development' as opposed to macro development, including the restructuring of markets.

Poverty issues, social and gender issues, as well as health inequalities intersect in reproductive health. Far from being an issue that is restricted to 'social engineering' within programmes dedicated to social development (Nederveen Pieterse 2010), I argue that the focus on advancing sexuality and reproductive health is tied to any given country's democratic project of deepening women's rights and furthering their economic status and productivity. In other words, other social aspects of development should not be seen as secondary to the supposedly 'more important' emphasis on economic development. The 2030 Agenda for Sustainable Development pledged commitments to reproductive health and universal health access, also asking member states to commit to the Sustainable Development Goal (SDG) target 3.7. The latter underscored the need 'to ensure universal access to sexual and reproductive health care services, from family planning, information and education, and the integration of reproductive health into national strategies', including target 5.6, which guaranteed 'universal access to sexual and reproductive health and reproductive rights as agreed in accordance with the ICPD Programme of Action.'

As I argue, the renewed interest in sexuality and reproductive health and rights is taking place precisely within a complex set of dynamics that includes the recognition that not enough has advanced in the last decades, despite commitments made at the Beijing and Cairo conferences and at the UN assemblies of the 1980s and 1990s. The 2018 report of the Guttmacher-Lancet Commission, *Accelerate Progress: Sexual and Reproductive Health Rights for All*,[2] points out that the gains of the past decades have been inequitable among and within countries. Services have fallen in quality and people have insufficient access to SRHR services. As the report (2018, 2642) states, improvement in people's well-being depends on individuals 'being able to make decisions', such as 'the right to control one's own body, define one's sexuality ... and receive confidential and high-quality services'. The report also defends a more holistic approach to SRHR, one that can tackle neglected issues, from adolescent sexuality to gender-based violence, abortion, diversity in sexual orientations, and gender identities. As it affirms, 'progress in SRHR requires confrontation of the barriers embedded in laws, policies, the economy and in social norms and values – especially gender inequality – that prevent people from achieving sexual and reproductive health' (2018, 2642).

Various authors working in the field of health and gender have also criticised the growth of the impact of 'marketization' on development programming and practice, speaking further of the existence of a 'democratic deficit' in terms of women's health in international development. These authors advocate for a wider role for NGOs in influencing decisions in the field (Gideon and Porter 2016). This includes, I would add, the difficulties in gaining access to quality and accurate information on women's reproductive health.

Discussions around SRHR have shifted in the last years towards not only the *rights of the female body* but also towards the notion of reproductive justice (Garita 2015; Lottes 2013; Morgan 2016; Parker 2009). As Freedman and Isaacs (1993, 19) argue, reproductive health needs to be addressed 'in the way women experience it, not as a series of isolated biomedical phenomena, but as an integral part of everyday life'. Scholars working on gender, sexuality, and development within the human rights framework have for some time underlined how sexual and reproductive health and rights are closely interwoven with debates on poverty. As Cornwall, Correa, and Jolly (2008, 29) state, Chamber's 'Web of Poverty's Disadvantages' discusses the intersection between sexuality, poverty, and development within the specific context of the deprivations suffered by urban poor LGBTs in the Philippines. It is quite illuminating in the ways in which it connects social, cultural, political, and economic pressures in the creation of a 'web of disadvantages'. This 'web' includes everything from the mere access to institutions, to physical well being, to support provided by social relations, to lack of education and access to adequate information on health.

Moreover, Cornwall, Correa, and Jolly (2008) point out that development had taken on board a largely essentialist view of sexuality, and they argue instead for the need to adopt a more constructivist approach – one capable of recognising greater variations in sexualities across cultures. Writing in the introduction to Cornwall, Correa and Jolly's *Development with a Body: Sexuality, Human Rights and Development* more than a decade ago, the then UN special rapporteur on the rights to the highest attainable standard of health, Paul Hunt, argued that SRHR had an important role to play in 'the struggle against intolerance, gender inequality, HIV/Aids and global poverty' (Cornwall, Correa, Jolly 2008, xi). I believe that this remains true within the current post-pandemic context.

Debates on sexuality are thus far from new. Anxiety over sexual pleasure has been a topic of much discussion among social scientists, with the work of Foucault on the history of sexuality being particularly important and having an influence on various studies across different disciplines, from gender and sexuality studies, to feminism, to the media and development studies. In the first volume of *The History of Sexuality*, Foucault (1980) provides a rich overview of the emergence of the proliferation of discourses around sex within Western culture during the eighteenth and nineteenth centuries. From that time, sex started to be 'policed' and confined to certain spaces deemed appropriate for discussion. Anxieties around the discussion of sexuality and pleasure within the public sphere have continued well into the twenty-first century in developed and developing countries alike. Sexuality, and particularly the female body, has been the subject of heated debate, from arguments on biological distinctions between the sexes to the shift towards the current consensus to conceptualise gender and sexuality within a constructivist approach (Parker 2009; Lottes 2013).

There has been a growing literature on bodies within development, with an increasing call for an acknowledgement of reproductive rights and sexuality within debates on women's agency, gender equality, and health (Petchescky 2003; Cornwall, Correa, and Jolly 2008 cited in Harcourt 2017, 191). Such work aims to make visible the diversity of gendered experiences and the connection of sexuality and reproductive health to the legacies of racism and colonialism, patriarchy, fundamentalism, and militarism (Wilkins 2016; Harcourt 2009, 2017). The *rights of the body* – including the struggle against the patriarchal control of it within the framework of affirmation of the right of choice – are thus closely intertwined with the process of decolonisation. As Vargas (2017, 303–4) states, 'body politics emerges both as an intersection and as a convergence of ideas, histories, concepts and embodies lives. Today the notion of body politics has broadened ... to which different movements and feminisms add their own experience and meaning ... and ... highlight the need to deconstruct, decolonize and depatriarchalize them.'

Writing about medical metaphors for women's bodies in her discussion of the impact of culture on science, Martin (1987) examines from a historical perspective the thinking around women's and men's bodies, such as how scientific ideas and the medical discourse were infused by cultural assumptions and by particular understandings of women's menopause and bodily fluids. These were seen as unclean and as waste that needed to be discharged. Despite the early claims that both women's and men's bodies were similar, as stated in the literature from ancient Greece until the late eighteenth century (30), the reality is that women's genitals were perceived as being inside the body, as opposed to those of men, signalling the idea that female bodies were somehow *lacking* in contrast to male bodies.

By the early nineteenth century, the notion that women's and men's bodies were similar came under attack. Writers underlined the biological distinctions made between the sexes based on ideas about society and the 'natural order of nature', according to which hierarchies between men and women were articulated under the notion of 'body heat'. Men were seen as dominating the public world due to their 'greater perfection' as well as to their 'excess heat' (Martin 1987, 31–2). Men could sweat to remove impurities whereas females menstruated to remove imperfections, menstrual blood being seen as unclean (32). Here, one sees the roots of men's and women's social roles as 'grounded in nature' and dictated by their bodies.

Within the context of international development, Correa and Jolly (2008) note how, from the eighteenth century onwards, sexuality began to occupy a controversial political terrain, with science having contributed to underpinning this essentialist idea of sex. They further state that it was only in the last decades that scholars from different disciplines (22), from social anthropology to feminist and queer theorists, including scholars like Plummer (2000), Weeks (1985, 2003), Parker and Ganon (1994), and Parker and Aggleton (1999) among others (all cited in Cornwall, Correa, and Jolly 2008), challenged this essentialist approach through their constructive theories around sexuality. Sexual identities were thus seen as being constructed *culturally*, with sex practices being embedded in power dynamics within institutional and social discourses. Bodies and 'sex' were also seen as being reproduced by social meanings (Cornwall, Correa, and Jolly 2008, 24), with fixed ideas about men's and women's sexuality (e.g., that men should be macho and take risks).

In her discussion of *female embodiment*, Harcourt (2009, 20–1) borrows from a Foucauldian understanding of bodies and power as well as from Haraway's *A Cyborg Manifesto* (1992) to argue how *biopolitical strategies* – from population statistics to medical records and ideal bodies – categorise modern bodies within development. Bodies were thus seen as interwoven with the social and economic and were not identified as being 'objects' but, rather, 'subjects'

(Harcourt 2009, 25). Bodies should thus be seen as sites where the interplay between power, knowledge, and resistance is played out. Body politics challenges the very notion of maternity itself as the ultimate experience of embodiment (Harcourt 2017, 2009). From this perspective, bodies should be seen as being 'sites of contestation in a series of economic, political, sexual and intellectual struggles' (Harcourt 2009, 24). Making use of Foucault's concept of *biopolitics,* Harcourt suggests that new technologies can open 'up the possibilities of questioning the body in new ways', further seeing 'the new communication and bio technologies as fresh sources of power' that can be harnessed by feminists (22).

The reality is that, more than ever, bodies are now at the centre of political agendas and societal debates across the world in what seems to be a continuation of previous historical discussions on sexuality, pleasure, and the role of the body. Writing in the context of the 1990s, Correa and Petchesky (1996, 169) had already underscored how fundamentalist religious movements, form Roman Catholicism to Protestantism and Islam, were showing signs of growth throughout much of the world. They viewed women as *instruments of reproduction,* a vision that goes against 'any notion of reproductive rights'. Many feminists from the Global South have discussed the relationship between women's bodies, patriarchy, and European colonialism, making a link between the former exploited colonial countries and images displaying the exotic hyper-sexualised bodies of the 'Other' (Radcliffe 2015; Mohanty 2000; Rai 2011; Matos 2016). Scholars have noted how assumptions about women influenced the type of discourses articulated within the development field, including communications practices that represented women from less powerful countries and that further shaped Western literature, policy, and the media (Wilkins 2016; Matos 2016; Harcourt 2009, 2017).

Wilkins (2016) points to the 'objectification' of women that still occurs within development discourse and that has parallels with the commodification of women present within popular culture. This functions as a form of constraint over women's sexuality and bodies, culminating in placing the value of women (particularly from the Global South but also in the West) solely, or mostly, on their reproductive function or their capacity for it. The issue of fertility thus emerges as a form of *control,* of either women's sexuality and social status within her society or as a restraint on her political power and capacity for resistance. It is precisely in understanding sexuality from a constructivist and holistic perspective that we find the potential to change rigid definitions and positionalities, to create more equal and diverse lifestyles for all groups and sexual identities.

Sexuality then ceases to be seen as a problem (related to 'population control', for instance) and instead emerges as a 'source of affirmation of pleasure'. This, however, does not exclude the fact that many women are forced into sex due to poverty and economic dependency (Cornwall, Correa, and Jolly 2008, 37). Cornwall, Correa, and Jolly conclude that essentialist views of sex leave little room for seeing sexuality as connected with social change, democracy, and human rights, thus compromising the very notion that 'development' is synonymous with the improvement of human subjectivities (23).

The next chapter thus moves on to further debate the ambiguities, contradictions, and complexities surrounding the discussion of feminist and health NGOs working on SRHR, from both the North and the South, in international development. It then explores some of the interviews with the gender experts from the organisations that participated in this research, examining their views on sexuality and reproductive health as well as how these organisations conducted their advocacy activities, seeking to advance thinking on the topic to influence policy in the field. This is done not just within the context of the Global South but also within the advocacy practices conducted by organisations working on SRHR across the world.

3

'Northern' and 'Southern' NGOs and Advocacy on 'Female Bodies' and Reproductive Health

In the last decades, particularly since the 1990s, third-sector and non-governmental organisations (NGOs) have assumed a key role as important political players in international development (Alvarez 1998, 2009; Narayanaswamy 2014, 2017; Baltiwala 2007) or as 'agents of development' (Desai and Potter, 2014; McPhail 2009). This has been done during the increasing marketization of the sector due to the impact of neoliberal market politics – to the detriment of the classic role of the state as the main agent in the development process (Wilkins 2016; Desai and Potter 2014). NGOs have been hailed as important players in shaping and defining debate in the public sphere, in bringing issues to the 'attention of audiences' in a highly saturated and mediated global environment (Thrall, Stecula, and Sweet 2014; Powers 2014, 2017), thus competing with the mainstream media in influencing the public on important social causes (McPherson 2015, 2017).

With the expansion of the NGO sector throughout the world since the 1990s (McPhail 2009), another discussion that has emerged within development studies as well as within politics and international relations concerns the role that is played by these organisations in actually delivering change. Also discussed is how to situate them (between the market or civil society); their accountability and transparency; their relationships with governments, donors, and other actors; as well as their capacity to make a difference (Bebbington, Hickey, and Mitlin 2008). Scholars also underline the importance of NGOs within the international sphere and as part of transnational civil society and social movements (Kavada 2014; Bebbington 2004; Yanacopulous 2016).

NGOs have taken the space once previously occupied by the state in many areas, from poverty reduction programming to women's welfare, following from cuts in state public spending and the rise of austerity policies throughout many countries in the world. Developing countries have taken the brunt of the impact of structural adjustments programmes and reforms throughout the 1980s and 1990s, sold as a 'recipe' for the development of many nations of the Global South and seen as a kind of 'passport' for their insertion within the neoliberal global market economy. Moreover, one of the key characteristics of transnational advocacy networks, as Keck and Sikkink (1998, 3) state, is their creative use and deployment of information to reach certain goals as well as their use of sophisticated political campaign strategies. A key strength is their ability to use information strategically to persuade people and to gain leverage over more powerful organisations and governments. They 'frame' issues in a way that can contribute to changing the very nature of the debate as well as targeting audiences and bringing attention to these topics in order to encourage action and mobilisation. Quoting Silverstone (2007) and Cottle and Nolan (2007), Powers (2014, 104) underlines how 'NGOs have been hailed for doing more than influencing elite decision-making', having the role of 'connecting individuals and groups ... encouraging solidarity across national boundaries and creating the basis for a more cosmopolitan civic order'.

Authors have noted a tendency for the vast literature on NGOs within the social sciences either to be overly critical of NGOs or to be naively or 'excessively optimistic' (Bebbington, Hickey, and Mitlin 2008 quoted in Narayanaswamy 2014, 577). Others problematises the role of 'Southern women's NGOs' in development, including the Northern/Southern NGO division and how the latter is situated in relation to the former (Narayanaswamy 2014). Moreover, the term 'NGO' is seen as lacking in definitional clarity. Quoting the work of Alvarez (2009) on 'NGO-ization', Narayanaswamy (2017, 89) contends that 'non-governmental organisation' is a term 'indiscriminately deployed in development discourse to refer to any social actor not clearly situated within the realm of the state or the market', being used to describe anything 'from peasant collectives ... to research oriented policy think tanks'. The use of the expression 'Northern NGO' also unites all organisations of the North into one group of a supposedly resource-rich, professionalized, and powerful body, belonging to a global network of organisations to which their 'Southern counter-parts' are subordinate, appearing as mere appendices to the more powerful Northern players.

Narayanaswamy (2014, 576) notes that the phrase 'Southern women's NGOs' continues to define 'Southern women' as a category of supposedly 'politicized agents who share trajectories of historical and contemporary oppression'. Borrowing from Cornwall and Brock (2005), Narayanaswamy further states that 'Southern women's NGOs' has been a weakly defined concept, becoming almost like a 'buzzword' in development, like the terms 'women's empowerment' and 'agency', which have been overused and thus deprived of their initial radical edge. These 'Southern NGOs' are then dependent on funding, donation, and support from their more powerful Northern partners.

I argue, however, that NGO efforts pertaining to advocacy around SRHR have been inserted into larger struggles over *meanings*, including different understandings and approaches to reproductive health, many of which are built within a human rights and public health framework that is not always necessarily 'activist' driven. It is also possible to state that NGOs working on SRHR operate differently than do other civic or human rights organisations, which are more explicitly militant, when it comes to advocacy and activism (a discussion that I pursue in more detail later). Many engage in advocacy from a less explicitly political position; however, others are more grounded in research and technical expertise, and do not always shy away from engaging with feminist perspectives in addressing reproductive health.

Many of the gender experts from the interviews conducted here underscored an important role for NGOs working in the field in shaping debate and advocating for change. According to the International Alliance of Women (IAW) co-coordinator of the WP project and convenor of the IAW Commission on Health,[1] the role of NGOs in local and international contexts is to advance progressive politics:

> The role of progressive NGOs in both contexts was essential. My example from the local context was, and still is, a close cooperation with an NGO in Burkina Faso working for the abandonment of FGM/C and for better access of women and adolescents to contraception. My examples from the international scene are statements we drafted at sessions of UN agencies located in Geneva and New York, then asked like-minded NGOs to endorse. An example is the debate at WHO and the HRC [Human Rights Council], on the effect of family planning on maternal mortality. An African member-organisation of IAW

[International Alliance of Women] provided an analysis which we used as a basis for a one-page oral intervention.

According to the director of policy research from the US Center for Health and Gender Equality (CHANGE),[2] it is crucial for NGOs to develop partnerships and a range of networks in order to be able to push for change in the field:

> Two things: one thing is that partnership is critical to our work, it is how we work. CHANGE is not an organisation that is sitting in Washington DC and deciding how US policy should be for women and girls. Our whole work is based on the voices of the public and girls and the impact of US policy. From our perspective, our fact-finding work, we meet with a large sample of civil society, women's organisations, rights organisations ... that is ... where our work comes from. Our reporting on the Global Gag Rule, we have a great analysis of the impact of the loss of funding. But that said, most of our work is *quality*, and is taken from countries that are impacted by US government funding.

In her discussion of her work on funding NGOs, the program director of sexual and reproductive justice from the US's Global Fund for Women noted the complexities of the advocacy work that is done by those working in the field.[3] She discussed how advocacy is approached differently according to the specific interests of the NGOs as well as their overall structure, underlining how some organisations can contribute to maintain the status quo:

> I think there is a difference between an NGO and a movement. I think that women's movements globally comprise ... a network of people who are concerned with different ... social issues and who come together to make transformative social change. Some of it happens through networking, some with NGOs ... so the whole spectrum of a women's movement is very different from large international development organisations or NGOs who are focused on service delivery or who are focused on women's practical needs. Practical needs are very important. I think what is also important to recognise is that strategic interests of women, in being control of decision making, shifting the power is important. For me, the work that I have done in terms

of funding women's advocacy organisations and women's movements is that they are utilizing information that they receive, working with women on the ground, and then they are trying to get governments accountable ... That is a key distinction. You may be an NGO but not be a feminist NGO, or an advocacy NGO. And some NGOs may be replicating or continuing to maintain the status quo in some way.

The co-founder of the organisation Women Help Women,[4] a telemedicine service for abortion and contraception that has worked in community projects in Asia, Africa, Europe, and Latin America, stated that her organisation is a 'loud advocate' for the state's role in abortion care. In her interview she focused on discussing the situation of Europe, comparing Poland and Brazil:

I want to say that our organisation, despite a movement of groups that are working with this self-management option, is a very loud advocate for state responsibility to provide abortion care. By no means this is an ideal agenda. We base this advocacy in human rights and on the state's responsibility to provide abortion care, including clinical care, but at the same time we advocate for all forms of safe abortion ... It is the idea behind this that we can self-manage, we can do it ... but there should not be any legal or other regulatory obstacles for reaching the actual potential of these [birth control] pills. And that is what we have been seeing everywhere, including in Brazil, [which] has been routinely over-regulated with licences with various obstacles to access it [i.e., abortion], and also of course criminal laws on abortion, which bottom line prevents people from having safe abortions when they need them.

In her critical examination of different case studies of gender and population programmes in international development in *Communicating Gender and Advocating Accountability in Global Development,* Wilkins (2016, 34–5) notes how these created roles for women in terms of their potential fertility. She further states that there was insufficient recognition of gendered power dynamics within development programmes. These programmes' discourses and language on SRHR reflected assumptions about gender, rights, and health, encouraging the idea that targeted publics will respond appropriately given the right type of communication campaign. Traditionally, population programmes have been justified in terms of their perceived benefits, tending to see women in terms of their breeding potential (or their 'reproductive function'). Discussing population development programme interventions in Egypt, Wilkins (2016, 172) states that the reproductive rights model values women's choice and emphasises individual selection, thus functioning to undermine structural concerns, including the problem of availability of health services.

Maternal health programmes have thus frequently stressed the role of women as individuals who can make choices, such as when and how to marry (Wilkins 2016). This has tended to ignore the power dynamics of family relationships as well as the structures of health resources made available to them, making it difficult for these development programmes to be truly gender transformative. The responsibility for their problems is placed exclusively on girls and women as individuals, with interventions being viewed as only needing to target women in order to promote individual behavioural change (172). Absent from such narratives are wider concerns with tackling structural inequalities as well as the impact of neoliberal policies on health systems across the world at a time of cuts to public health services.

Thus part of the debate on 'sexuality and reproductive health' is not just the public health argument on how important SRHR is, or whether it should be grounded in feminist arguments around women's autonomy. As I point out in previous chapters, the examination of the terminology around SRHR has been of crucial importance since the International Conference for Population and Development and the move towards placing reproductive health within a human rights framework. Discussions in this area explore a range of issues, from the definition of concepts and use of language when we speak about 'sexuality', including what we mean by the term 'sexual and reproductive health and rights', to wider understandings regarding the role of women as mothers, the choices they make regarding reproduction, and the role of men and external forces and actors in assisting or constraining women's agency.

The regional communication adviser for Latin America and the Caribbean for the United Nations Population Fund pointed out how the debate around terminology has been crucial at the UN,[5] affirming that it is important for those working in the field to revisit language and to deconstruct the misconceptions regarding sexuality and reproductive health that circulate in the political and mediated public sphere:

We have done a lot of work with the UN system; we were able to provide an update on the human rights and sexual orientation and gender identity documentation that is the framework of the work of the UN. In order to agree with that language, it requires a lot of effort that takes years ... We work on every committee and session to secure the right language in that case, in terms of human rights, sexual identity, and orientation in terms of the global level ... Now in the region, for example, recently last year we worked together with the UN system in order to have a document explaining the concept, what is 'human rights', 'sexual orientation' ... what is the meaning ... and how can we convey that approach and resolution to the governments, and from that we can develop a series of messages ... So when we see this opposition taking place in different ... shapes and contexts in different countries, we have a common language that helps us approach the government ... to help them craft the right message and statements, that can help them be proactive and up to date ... We need to go back to understand the meaning of words ... in order to understand the message that is being used by right-wing groups, and then we need to go back to understand the language, and in order to do that, we need [to] do an exercise in deconstructing that message ... and then we need to reconstruct it in order to construct a message that is understood by the public ... We need to understand, what are the semantics, every single meaning of the words that are being used today ... We need to decodify these words ... and then we need to build again on our strategy and improve ... We need to take those messages, deconstruct, repackage it, and go back to governments and the champions of rights.

The CEO of the Brazilian NGO Reprolatina also underlined the problem of acknowledging how we use the concept of 'sexual health' to the detriment of 'sexual rights',[6] reflecting the earlier discussions on the difficulty of addressing sexuality within development:

Sexual and reproductive rights are human rights ... Why is there still ... confusion [over this]? Because people don't know. I think there are ... few people who understand ... that ... a sexual right ... [is] different from ... [a] reproductive right. And this is in institutions. I was also a WHO consultant for many years. I got tired of fighting with WHO because WHO is still working in reproductive health. The concept of 'sexual health' does not exist within WHO. They work on reproductive health ... Sexual rights, they don't embody. See official WHO documents. And, like it or not, WHO influences policy ... So it's complicated.

The vice-president for research at Ibis Reproductive Health is one of many voices that have argued in favour of shifting the debate towards the notion of reproductive justice:[7]

I think that there are several different ways that we can think about the evolution of the SRHR agenda since 1994. I think certainly ICPD was a moment where a feminist perspective was brought to the table and concerns about equity and coercion were highlighted, and I think that, following from the idea, there were some changes in the way family planning talked about the goals of family planning, and you know, trying to link family planning programmes with women's empowerment ... I think there was certainly a rhetorical shift. I am not sure, though, that looking at family planning programmes today we can say that there was all that much of a programmatic shift, certainly family planning programmes continue to, in essence, mark their successes by the number Iusers ... One of the things that I think has happened over the course of the last ten years or so is thinking about reproductive justice instead of focusing on the human rights framework, incorporating more of a reflective justice framework that enables us to think of wanted fertility, wanted use of family planning, that people should essentially choose whether and when to have children and to have the infrastructure and things that they need to have this. And what is exciting about that framework is that it takes into consideration the whole person and helps to contextualise the different scenarios in which women are choosing when and how many children to have.

These debates continue to divide and overwhelm those working in the field, creating barriers for advocacy as well as for discussions of SRHR within the public sphere. The coordinator from the South Asian NGO Asia Safe Abortion Partnership (ASAP) India underscored the political barriers that many civil society players still face when discussing the topic.[8] She fears that the spaces in which these discussions are taking place today might be contracting instead of expanding. This is particularly so around understandings of what exactly constitutes 'sexuality' and debates on the role of the 'family':

> We had the whole struggle with the MDGs focusing on maternal health instead of anything else, then you got the SDGs that have so many indicators and so many things to be done that SRH got completely lost ... To start with, to have a conversation around family planning when all of us are trying to depoliticise and say that family is whatever you want to be family, not a heterosexual couple with children. They're still calling it family planning, not contraception ... There's no conversation around failure of contraception because those are not who the funders want to have ... The politics is present in everything. Civil society is not funded or vocal enough ... ICPD was this brilliant moment, I don't know if we are going to have that kind of moment anytime soon. Because even if you go to these so-called civil society spaces, for example the Asia-Pacific Conference on Sexual Health and Reproductive Rights, that was originally a forum where civil society could meet and talk about ... holding their governments accountable for implementation of ICPD. Now if you go to these conferences it'll be held at a posh conference centre, half the participants will be from UNFPA. It is not what it was set out to be – so I think those spaces are getting lost.

Thus the advancements secured in UN-led international conferences, such as the 1994 ICPD, and the discussions that followed, are still taken as a starting point to reassess what has been achieved and what still remains to be tackled in the field of SRHR. The former president of the US NGO Centre for Health and Gender Equity stated that the achievements made at the UN-led conferences meant that organisations working in the field could pressure more governments and make them more accountable.[9] Part of the commitment of liberal democracies is precisely the provision of quality public services to citizens, ensuring that health systems can continue to deliver services from safe abortion to maternity services, anti-natal delivery and post-partum care, breast cancer treatment and treatment for sexual health problems, including sexually transmitted infections and treatment for infertility (Colle 2008; Richardson and Birn 2011). As she affirmed:

I think one of the biggest achievements has been, when it comes to SRHR and achievements, since Beijing ... there are more than forty countries who have legalised their abortion laws ... We have regional agreements that we made over the years, not only in sexual and reproductive health and rights and access to services but also on LGBT rights, sexual orientation and gender identity, HIV, women, and girls. I think we can really look to concrete points where we have made an impact. Exactly that is how we were able to get the US government to adopt the term 'sexual and reproductive health and rights'. Because we were able to present to them 'look at all these different agreements, different forums were SRHR is acknowledged' ... And being able to come to them and with that 'look the rest of the world is moving along' and the United States government needs to do [so] also ... I think one thing is, I mentioned this in the previous interview on communications, is the fact that the Trump administration is rolling back the language, framework, and rights on SRHR ... The fact that they are undoing that is bringing the attention of people, who are more outraged and saying, 'What do you mean we cannot talk about gender?' 'What do you mean that we cannot talk about sexual and reproductive rights?' ... Suddenly people are seeing that they are retreating on something that most people did not know we had made progress on.

There are thus various social and cultural barriers, as well as political and economic challenges, that contribute to perpetuating structural gender and health inequalities throughout many regions of the world, impeding the advancement of basic women's rights regarding the provision of better sexual and reproductive health services 'on the ground' in accordance with women's realities and the struggles of economic hardships that they face.. It thus comes as no surprise that women's reproductive bodies continue to be conceptualised within development discourse and practice in a stereotypical and simplistic manner. This is in despite of the diversity of women's experiences and the criticisms of the homogenization of the bodies of women from developing countries (Mohanty 2000). There are also the problems around understandings of sexuality in development and the acknowledgement of the importance of improving SRHR outcomes as part of wider strategies to combat global poverty. Such improvements seek wider global gender justice for all women in a postcolonial world. These 'female bodies' are still seen as *lacking* and are easily subject to control and surveillance by families, friends, the state, and other external forces. These practices continue to reinforce patriarchal (and colonial) views of women from developing countries, further perpetuating the marginalisation and oppression of bodies and sexualities, be it by the state or religious groups, across the Global South and beyond.

The programme director of SRHR at the US's Global Fund Women emphasised the importance of enabling the agency of women from the Global South so that they can work on advancing their own rights, thus moving towards solving their own problems, including tackling structural inequalities in the field and reaching out to the most marginalised:[10]

> We are a Global North organisation focused solely on supporting Global South activists. We have also supported and ... build national-level and regional-level women's funds, so by levering funding moving to women's funds globally has been an important strategy ... Women in the Global South need to have absolute control over resources, and not just be the ones receiving grants. By supporting women's funds to get off the ground, and to be sister organisations to us, is a very important strategy that we are using in terms of grant making and funding. And trying to leverage other donors, to be in an initiative to lever other dollars, as we may not have the money ourselves ... It is critical, we need to focus on those most marginalised, and then we look at those who are not. Women who are on the fringes, as it will not work otherwise.

These are numerous roadblocks to pursuing wider progress on equality for women's rights at the global level, particularly in the field of sexuality and reproductive health. I turn now to the specific case of transnational feminisms and activism around gender equality and SRHR in Brazil and in Latin America in general. This is a region that has vibrant feminist movements and NGOs that have helped shape some of these debates internationally while, at the same time, it restricts abortion for nearly 90 per cent of women and is home to a deeply rooted patriarchal and misogynistic culture.

4

Latin American Feminisms and the Struggle for Gender Equality and SRHR in Brazil and Beyond

There has been considerable debate among feminist scholars in the social sciences and humanities regarding the emergence of Latin American feminist movements and the influence of 'second wave' feminism on their formation, not to mention the role that these feminist groups played in the struggle against the right-wing military dictatorships of the 1960s and 1970s as well as their role in reconstructing their nation-states from the 1980s onwards (Sternbach et al. 1992; Waylen 1996; Maier and Lebon 2010; Sardenberg 2007; Alvarez 2014). Nonetheless, the vibrant Latin American feminist pursuit of the emancipation of women has co-existed with widely held Northern assumptions that women in Latin America do not like or understand feminism and are happy to be oppressed (Sternbach et al. 1992).

Since its origins, feminism in Latin America and its struggles against patriarchy have intersected with struggles against state authoritarianism and colonialism (Sternbach et al. 1992). As various scholars like Sternbach et al. (1992, 397) argue, despite the diversity that exists between the countries in the region, Latin American feminisms have a distinctive characteristic that sets them apart from other feminist movements across the world, particularly regarding their origins and emergence during the dictatorship period. This has given the feminist struggle in Latin America a particular characteristic and distinctive look, mainly that of being a movement whose aim is to tackle state authoritarianism within the public sphere as well as patriarchy within the private sphere.

As feminist scholars like Alvarez (2014) note, as do the gender experts and others from organisations in Latin America interviewed for this research, much of the Latin American left saw the feminist movement when it emerged during the dictatorship period as being composed mainly of petit-bourgeoisie and middle-class feminists, largely disassociated from the more important socialist class struggles against capitalism, which was seen as the ultimate oppressor of women. However, feminism ceased being seen as a 'dirty word' or as something restricted to small, privileged groups of women (Sternbach et al 1992; Waylen 1993). At first, feminist movements in Latin America were supported mainly by women involved with leftist politics. However, over the last decade the movement has significantly evolved and shaped itself into what is now the contemporary Latin American feminist movement: a vibrant, plural, and creative force, a multi-racial and multifaceted movement that is also socially and politically heterogenous as well as class and race conscious (Sternbach et al. 1992; Vargas 2017; Maier and Lebon 2010; Matos 2016).[1]

In the last decades Latin American feminisms have widely acknowledged the importance of identity politics, the role of intersectionality, and the multiple layers of oppression suffered by working-class and less privileged groups of women. Various authors (Alvarez 2014; Sternbach et al. 1992) have been quick to point out the association between the interests of feminists and those of working-class women and more vulnerable groups – those groups that are mainly affected when it comes to sexual and reproductive health and rights. This fact contradicts the early assumptions that Latin American women were not 'feminist' enough or were unaware of their own oppression.

Thus from the previous marginalisation of feminism during the 1980s, the 1990s would see feminism very much enter the mainstream, propelled by the success of the UN Decade of Women as well as in response to the transnational feminist lobbying that occurred during these years (Friedman 2003). The gender-equality agenda reached the global centre stage, with governments and nations adopting gender mainstreaming in their programmes, putting out legislation and expressing concerns with women's rights. As Alvarez (2014, 1998) argues, feminism was taken on board across the political spectrum, from the left to the right. Throughout much of the world, following from the success of the international conferences of the 1980s and 1990s, centre-right politicians, corporate groups, and the media all jumped on the 'bandwagon' of gender equality.

Alvarez (2014, 1998) identifies this process as being interwoven with the rise of neoliberalism and the insertion of development within the market forces. It is within this zeitgeist that the process of the

NGO-ization (Alvarez 2009) of feminism movements, particularly those in Latin America, took place. Alvarez (1998, 2014) underscores the paradoxical role that feminist NGOs played here, with various grassroots feminists being 'co-opted' by neoliberalism, thus diminishing their previous 'radical credentials' and contributing to the creation of new forms of power inequalities and divisions between 'card-carrying feminists' and those working with affected local communities.

This period marked the initial phase of the transformation of many feminist NGOS. The argument is that this 'co-optation' and division within feminist NGOS, involving more middle-class career-minded feminists working around the UN circuit, created a sense of disconnect with other NGOs who represented more local or working-class groups (Narayanaswamy 2014, 2017; Mitra 2011). Narayanaswamy (2017) examines this debate within the South Asian feminist context and the NGO-ization process, criticising the dominance of the interests of middle-class Indian feminists in the country's NGOs. Nonetheless, the last decades have seen the emergence of alternative forms of transnational feminist activism, mobilising, and engagement, with the realisation of the conferences of the World Social Forum (WSF) being an example (Alvarez 2009; Harcourt 2009, 2017).

Research also shows how various health and feminists NGOs from the Global South, not only throughout Latin America but also in Asia, played an important role in advocating for reproductive health (Richardson and Birn 2011; Alvarez 1998, 2009; Narayanaswamy 2014, 2017). Richardson and Birn (2011, 190) acknowledge the essential role of women's health organisations and NGOs in advancing reproductive health rights in Latin America:, stating that 'NGO service providers, such as *Orientame* and *Profamilia Colombia* ... which work alongside advocacy and research organisations, have helped to make sure that sexual and reproductive health issues are raised'. Latin American NGOs are thus seen as having had a role in impeding setbacks as well as in seeking justice through courts and other human right bodies. Countries like Mexico, Argentina, Chile, and Peru even submitted reports to the UN on reproductive health (Richardson and Birn 2011, 191). However, the reality is that sexuality and reproductive rights have not always played a major role within the feminist movement in this region, even with progressive actors on the left.

The CEO of the Peruvian organisation Promsex,[2] a very active and influential Latin American organisation working in the field, underscored its use of communications to raise debate and awareness. She outlined some of the difficulties faced, including the lack of integration between decisions made in international spaces and what happens 'on the ground'. She also emphasised the persistence of the division between the NGOs of the North and those of the South:

> Feminist organisations have been very active in international negotiation spaces because, in many cases, feminists have been able to integrate official delegations. This has not necessarily translated into greater compliance by the state or substantive improvements in terms of surrender of accounts in national spaces ... Thus even though the international participation of feminist NGOs has shown good results in terms of commitments, there has not necessarily been a connection with the national scenes. This explains why many times the states make very advances statements with very little correlation with what happens in the countries. The other very serious problem is that the high professionalization has made it very difficult to transfer skills, because many times the number of representatives cannot be expanded ... I believe that NGOs have an important role and are until now the most validated group to represent the voice of women. I think that, in terms of innovations, the feminist NGOs of the South have managed to position themselves; however, there is also a kind of North-South separation, which does not seem to add up, much less to achieve a more global positioning.

The director of research policy at CHANGE also outlined some of the work carried out by the organisation across the Global South, including in Latin America:

> CHANGE [was] created in 1994 in direct response to the ICPD conference, and CHANGE believes that one of its greatest contributions to the global women's movement is holding the US government accountable ... Since the beginning ... CHANGE has been doing advocacy, doing evidence-based programming, rights-based programmes, focusing on young girls and women particularly in sub-Saharan Africa ... Yes, as an organisation from the US, our work had a previous presence in Latin America in previous administrations. And there was more US money going to Latin America, and so many of these countries, US-based granted countries, our focus has been where the money

has gone – so far sub-Saharan Africa. As for Zika, as it was in Latin America and around the world, as this was a big part of our work, and we were working with Debora Diniz in Brazil. And some of the interesting conversations that came out of that ... [were about] the work among SRHR reproductive health organisations, and those women['s] organisations [concerned with] ... living with disabilities who were instrumental in shaping conversations on access to health services and rights-based programming around pregnancy, childbirth, and child bearing.

As in many other parts of the world, contemporary feminisms in Latin America have experienced a period of intense change and revival. Movements have changed their composition, and new players, such as younger groups of women from more diverse backgrounds, have joined and are participating and calling the shots at centre stage.[3] In keeping with the widespread use of communications and new technologies by feminists groups throughout the world – which many have argued is a defining feature of the recent 'third' and 'fourth' waves of feminism – Latin American feminist groups have taken to digital communications as a form of engaging politically, creating awareness and advocacy around a variety of causes, from climate change to poverty reduction (Matos 2017; Ferreira 2015; Gomes and Sorj 2014; Natansohn, 2013; Vargas 2010).

Race has also played an important part in the development of Latin American feminisms (Alvarez 2017; Vargas 2017), moving from what was initially seen as a separate movement with different interests from those of white 'middle class' feminists to finally being incorporated into the plurality of feminists' struggles. A key feature of the contemporary Latin American feminist movement has been the political debate around the theory of coloniality, developed by Anibal Qujano (Vargas 2017, 296). The decolonial framework, as Vargas argues, sought to modify the contemporary patterns of power, introducing a 'racial dimension to the understanding of past and present colonial socio-economic and political processes in the construction of the state' (297).

Moreover, writing within the context of an assessment of Latin American development programmes in the field on gender equality, Sardenberg (2007) underscores the separation that sometimes exists between the terms 'gender' and 'feminism' within the area – a separation that has been influenced by the 'co-optation' of the 'gender agenda' by the political mainstream. This has affected programmes by depriving them of a feminist critical perspective, resulting in a division between 'doing gender' and 'doing feminism' in certain policy-thinking around gender programmes in Latin America. Sardenberg cites the rise of technical 'gender experts' and a few examples of programmes in Brazil and Colombia that were shut down when power relations and domestic violence came up against the more 'apolitical' and technical use of 'gender' within the programmes.

Contemporary Latin American feminisms – from the grassroots movements to the more technical/apolitical spaces where 'gender' and 'women's issues' play out (e.g., in some of the women's health NGOs) – have incorporated multiple possibilities, opening various avenues for understanding these current feminist movements as being, as Alvarez (2014) puts it, 'discursive camps of action'. This term allows for a wider understanding of these movements and their ongoing processes of democratisation and expansion as well as their contradictions and the extent to which they have been 'co-opted', thus creating possibilities for more fluidity and dynamism as well as encompassing more pluralistic approaches to feminism. These can be more inclusive of early signs and manifestations of feminism that could, in principle, be deemed as too timid, technical, and not sufficiently political but that, in the long run, through dialogue, discussion, and debate, can take on a deeper purpose, with more political commitments and strategies for mobilisation and the improvement of women's lives.

What is problematic, though, and what we should avoid doing, is pushing aside forms of feminism that we consider 'weaker' when we encounter a context in which a stronger sense of feminism and empowerment is yet to emerge but is slowly taking shape. It is crucial not to forget the importance to the feminist movement of shifting from the term 'woman' to the term 'gender'. This has opened various possibilities for the discussion of multiple sexual identities and genders, with feminism no longer being restricted by the binary biological distinction that prevailed for many centuries and that was associated with the medical and scientific discourse. This has forced institutions and policy-makers, and others in the public sphere and political life, to seriously address the impact of power and other forms of oppression and inequalities on the making of people's gender, opening a whole field for solid empirical research deserving of funding and continuous debate. It has forced us to recognise how inequalities are produced, and how these can affect women's lives. Many can suffer from multiple forms of marginalisation yet still, should circumstances permit, encounter the means to engage in a gradual process of 'enlightenment', cultivating a stronger sense of self-respect and feminist engagement.

Thus various groups of women from Argentina to Brazil have started to demand control over their bodies and their sexuality and are seeking to influence policy-making and new legislation on reproductive rights, including on abortion. These groups have engaged in political debate and advocacy against the persistence of control over women's bodies, which is expressed largely in everyday discourses and practices but also through restrictive legislation. The use of communications and new technologies by various social movements and feminist groups throughout Latin America has permitted more communication and advocacy around SRHR between groups, with the younger generation frequently gaining access to information on reproductive health on social media directly through NGOs and blogs as well as through *WhatsApp*. I discuss this further later, as well as in a separate article on the results of the focus groups that I conducted in partnership with the Brazilian NGO Reprolatina.

Latin America has seen some advancements, albeit very insufficient, from the increase in educational levels to the growth of the participation of women in politics and in public life. There has been a decline in the culture of sexism because of the pressures for change and wider political democratisation that has occurred throughout the region over the last three decades. Structural adjustment programmes, which were applied throughout Latin America during the 1990s, have had various effects on the health systems of these nations as governments have been pressured to lower public costs. This has produced mixed results when it came to SRHR (Richardson and Birn 2011, 186).

Latin America is known to have the second highest rates of adolescent motherhood after sub-Saharan Africa, with 30 to 50 per cent of sexually active women aged fifteen to twenty-four not using any contraceptive method (Richardson and Birn 2011). Maternal mortality rates have nonetheless been declining continuously since the 1980s, dropping by 40 per cent in the Caribbean and 70 per cent in the Andean region. Latin America also has the lowest infant mortality among the developing regions, and fertility rates have fallen significantly in South America, Mexico, and Costa Rica (Kulezycki 2011, 199). As the Centre of Reproductive Rights states, however, many countries have problems of access to proper maternal health services as well as to comprehensive sexuality education.

Abortion is illegal for over 90 per cent of the women in Latin America; however, the practice is widespread, with clandestine abortions leading to more than one thousand deaths and 500,000 hospitalizations per year. Yet it has recently become safer due to the increased availability of contraceptive pills, including the growth of the use of misoprostol.[4] Statistics have frequently underlined how groups of privileged women from the upper classes have abortions in private illegal clinics in countries like Brazil, while those from poorer and more working-class backgrounds often risk their lives having unsafe abortion procedures (Diniz and Medeiros 2010).

Countries in Latin America have traditionally navigated between double standards when it comes to sexuality and morality. Many nations have been known for the dominance of strong gendered norms and for the persistence of chauvinistic attitudes, beliefs, and views concerning women's bodies and sexuality. The region has frequently defied superficial depictions of it being 'sexually liberal', 'easy going', or 'religiously and culturally tolerant', registering instead the co-existence of restrictive abortion legislations alongside a history of deeply ingrained misogyny. It also has one of the world's highest rates of female homicide and gender-based violence. According to the *Mapa da Violencia* (Map of Violence), published by the Latin American Faculty of Social Science in 2015, the feminicide rate in Brazil is 4.8 homicides per 100,000 women, giving this country the fifth highest rate in the world.[5] The Gender Equality Observatory for the Economic Commission for Latin America and the Caribbean also notes that fifteen countries in Latin America and the Caribbean registered at least 3,282 victims of femicide in 2018.

Various scholars working on Latin America (Machado 2018; Miguel, Biroli, and Mariano 2017; Miskolci and Campana 2017) as well as feminists working in the North (Butler 2019) have begun to conduct more research on feminism, sexuality, and religion, which is still an under-researched area within feminist research. Discussions include the impact of religion on ideas of womanhood and maternity, sexuality and the female body, and women's role in society as well as how these can have an impact on resistance to the advancement of women's rights. This involves not only influencing public discourses on women's rights more broadly but also, specifically, the problematic field of sexuality and reproductive health. As Miguel, Biroli, and Mariano (2017) show, despite the timid support of Brazil's MPs for reproductive health rights across the political spectrum, the conservative 'pro-life' discourse and the 'rights of the foetus' have been largely upheld by the extreme right in Brazil.

Miguel, Biroli, and Mariano (2017) researched the discourses on sexual and reproductive health and rights in the Brazilian Congress from 1991 to 2014. They attempted to examine how the debate was shaped and discussed in the public sphere as well as how it influenced public opinion and the impact it had on policy discussion relating to abortion. Although the topic occupied a lot of space in the 1990s, it was mainly from the early 2000s – particularly from 2010 – that conservative groups began to unite more strongly and to emerge as powerful forces in the Brazilian Parliament against reproductive health policies and any attempt to decriminalise abortion, working instead to make the law more restrictive (Miguel, Biroli, and Mariano 2017; Machado 2018; Miskolci and Campana 2017). This period would also see an expansion in the attacks framed around 'pro-life' discourses, including the targeting of politicians who defended the practice of legal abortion, even in exceptional circumstances where the law permits it, such as when not performing one would pose a health risk. This was seen as a response to the advances made by left-wing governments throughout the region (Miskolci and Campana 2017), particularly up to the mid-2000s, from Lula in Brazil to Nestor Kirchner in Argentina, Jose Mijuca in Uruguay, and Evo Morales in Bolivia.

Miguel, Biroli, and Mariano (2017) argue that the right of a woman to terminate her pregnancy became an important debate in Brazil from the end of the re-democratisation period onwards. However, they also note a retreat from across the political spectrum, as well as from some of the progressive sectors, when it came to defending a woman's right to abortion, be it through the discourse of support of the right to bodily autonomy and agency or on the grounds of public health. In their detailed account of the diversity of discourses articulated by politicians in Parliament during the period examined (1991–2014), from the 'right to life' to 'social injustice', the authors underscore the complexities of this debate, showing that it is not simply divided across the centre right/left political spectrum as it does not have unanimous support even among the left. Miguel, Biroli, and Mariano (2017) reveal how 'right to life' was the argument that appeared most frequently in the MPs' statements, receiving a score of 30.8 per cent, followed closely by 'no argument' (17.9 per cent), 'religious dogma' (11.5 per cent), and 'public health' (10.3 per cent). The arguments that could be more associated with a progressive stance, such as 'individual liberty' and 'bodily autonomy', only received 3.8 per cent and 0.4 per cent, respectively.

Some of the gender experts interviewed here underlined the Latin American left's lack of commitment to advancing the agenda on sexuality and reproductive health, which is in line with some of Miguel, Biroli, and Mariano's (2017) findings regarding the Brazilian Congress's undermining of the public health discourses around women's bodily autonomy. The coordinator of the research programmes of the Uruguayan NGO Mujer y Salud stated that a core problem for the advancement of SRHR in the region has been the lack of support from progressive politics. Uruguay is an interesting example, as it is considered one of the most liberal countries in Latin America and was among the first to legalise divorce, while Chile – where abortion was made illegal during the Pinochet dictatorship – has the lowest maternal mortality ratio and has been an early adopter of family planning (Kulezycki 2011, 209–11).

The coordinator and the executive director of Mujer y Salud both talked about the growing opposition to SRHR, further criticising the timidity of the Latin American left:[6]

> Well, yes, we have, let's see ... those conservative forces be[ing] reactive at the beginning of the century ... and for the first time, in 2014, we have an evangelical bench, and Uruguay, a secular state, one of the first secular states in all of Latin America ... Uruguay for these groups ... is a bad example because it has the law on legal abortion services, same-sex/gender marriage, marijuana, trans law and assisted reproduction ... Therefore they are targeting a whole battery that they reproduce in other countries, the campaigns against sex education, which they call as if they are carrying out an initiative to renew the abortion law in 2013 and they lost ... However, the left is usually very conservative ... And it is also an agenda that the left never fought, but always negotiated ... If you see it, all the leftist parties that assumed power in the last decade and a half, all their leaders are conservative: Daniel Ortega, in Nicaragua; Cháves, in Venezuela; from Ecuador, Carrera; Evo Morales himself, in Bolivia; well, Lula, who negotiated with all the affection with his allies to have ... governability; Cristina, Tabaré Vázquez himself in Uruguay. All the left leaders who came to power in the last

decade and a half, on the sexual and reproductive rights agenda, were extremely conservative ... And the left does not position those issues in a convincing way, as a new horizon of social structure or way of being among people ... Yes, those of us who are working on sexual and reproductive rights ... are really fighting all the time against the judicialization of the law ... And sexual and reproductive rights ... [have] only been defended by some feminist organisations ... I believe that we have to work much more ... in understanding that sexual and reproductive rights are understood on a daily basis, what it means for boys and girls ... If we demarcate within the social movement those who work on sexual [rights] ... we are a minority within the ... movement ... we are a minority within the progressive movement itself.

Moreover, the distinction between biology and gender is again being deplored by many conservative groups in their attempts to denounce the agenda on women's rights, from advocacy to policy-making and the work of NGOs in the field. These are all seen as being part of a 'gender ideology', which attempts to equate the struggle for the advancement of gender rights with other grand 'ideologies', from communism to Nazism (Butler 2019; Machado 2017; Miskolci and Campana 2017). As many have argued, countries that have criminalised abortion, or that have attacked comprehensive sexuality education in schools and have sought to make taboo discussions around sexual pleasure and reproduction, have often done so on the grounds of morality, religious opposition, or fears of 'disrupting traditional family values'. They have not sought to promote in-depth discussion of these topics from a public health, moral, or even philosophical perspective. For example, instead of advocating for more condom use or the provision of instructions on the use of contraceptives – or even the assessment of the choices concerning fertility treatments and how these are affected by financial constraints – some of these groups opt rather to encourage chastity and abstinence. This breeds hypocrisy and functions as a form of control over people's private lives. It also ignores how social and cultural constraints, as well as economic hardship and lack of access to health services, can lead many disadvantaged young girls from working-class backgrounds or rural communities to opt for extreme measures to terminate unwanted pregnancies, often utilizing unsafe medical procedures.

Miskolci and Campana (2017) provide a detailed overview of the origins of the 'gender ideology' discourse within the Roman Catholic Church and how it has proliferated throughout Latin America. They trace the origins of these debates to the writings of the previous pope, Joseph Ratzinger, who in 1997 wrote that 'there is a distinction made between the biological phenomena of sexuality from its historical forms to which "gender" is designated, but the intended revolution against the historical forms of sexuality culminates in a revolution against the biological assumption' (Ratzinger qtd in Miskolci and Campana 2017, 726). Miskolci and Campana argue that the 'gender ideology' agenda has been raised as a form of resistance to the advancements in SRHR seen throughout many countries in the world, from those in Europe to those in Latin America (778).

Miskolci and Campana (2017) further unpack the complex and often paradoxical role that religion has played in Latin America. The Roman Catholic Church, for instance, joined social movements and others in the fight against right-wing dictatorships in countries like Brazil, upholding the flag of 'social justice', despite having previously espoused support for some of these regimes. The adoption of this progressive stance, however, did not extend to feminist movements and LGBT rights (Miskolci and Campana 2017, 733). In the case of Latin America, a turning point was the increase of the offensive against women's rights, particularly from the 2010s, which took place in parallel with the launch of the Argentinian Jorge Scala's book *La ideologia del genero: O el genero como herramienta de poder* (The ideology of gender: Or gender as a tool of power). This book had a significant impact in the country and throughout Latin America. In it Scala defines 'gender ideology' as being a 'discursive-political instrument of alienation with global dimensions' – one that 'seeks to establish a totalitarian model with the intention of imposing a new anthropology' that could lead to the destruction of society (Scala qtd in Miskolci and Campana 2017, 725).

Despite the democratisation process of the last decades in many of the Latin American countries, in nations like Brazil the legacy of authoritarianism, and its intersection with women's oppression, has persisted. This has developed in new contemporary forms, actions, tactics, and discourses that have sought to essentialise women's experiences not just in the Brazilian Parliament but also throughout the country's institutions and wider society. Women are being brought back to the private sphere of the family, and to the *naturalization* of their biological function. This has been expressed most notably in the *bolsonaristas'* ideology and in the new type of military government installed through direct democracy in 2018 in a highly questionable presidential election facilitated by the proliferation of misinformation on political opponents as well as 'fake news' (Arnaudo 2017), including in the field of sexuality and reproductive health, with sectors of the left, among others, being accused of promiscuity.

The communications adviser of Latin America for UNFPA discussed the problems of the gender ideology discourse in Latin America in 2018, underlining how these debates have defined the careers of politicians, as was the case with Bolsonaro in Brazil:

> There is a lot of misinformation on social media ... this is the type of environment that is being used by different people ... People really get scared and do not understand the conversation. We put together a tool that helps us to listen carefully to all social media channels ... With specific words, 'gender ideology', 'abortion,' 'teenage pregnancy,' we have basically twenty-four words to listen to what is the meaning when we talk about 'abortion', and how ... the general public is using that word, abortion is *tabu* ... it is against the church ... Then we realized that the conversation in every country is ... based on who is using that word, we understand that politicians use the word 'gender ideology', that means that there is a huge conversation around that, but at the same time, who is in the middle of that? ... After that exercise we learned that there are some opinion leaders who can put something in social media and then the different other groups will start debating ... When we realized we can map different actors and institutions in one side, and leaders on another ... based on what is happening in Guatemala, in Colombia, Peru, and everything is shaped by the political situation ... So, we can go back to the case of Brazil, and how that conversation was shaped ... Those topics that were used as the political campaign for president, these were abortion ... 'gender ideology', all those terminologies were used to bring political groups together, and then they were able to mobilise citizens themselves to secure votes. That helps us understand that every single word that is interesting in [the] reproductive health and rights area is being used as decision-making power for governments and for people to advance

positions ... You know Brazil, Bolsonaro and the conservative groups were supportive of that campaign, using the words that we have seen used in the US. The big discussion is about gender, so every political movement in Latin America totally uses the word 'gender' ... and 'reproductive health and rights'. That is in the middle of the political discussion in every single country.

When it comes to policies around gender, particularly in the field of sexuality and reproductive health, the Bolsonaro government, like Trump's in the US, largely voted in alignment with countries that oppose SRHR at the international level and at the UN Council on Human Rights Convention. Elected as president of Brazil in 2018, Bolsonaro has instituted a series of measures intended to roll back women's rights and reverse many of the conquests of the last three decades following from the re-democratisation phase. He has attacked the rights of workers, Indigenous groups, LGBT people, and women, culminating in instituting various measures and policies that radically oppose previous advancements in gender and human rights agendas.

Brazil is also one of the countries in the region with the most restrictive laws, with abortion being allowed only in cases of rape, risk of death for pregnant women, or risk of abnormality of the foetus. In March 2019, representatives of the Brazilian Foreign Office at the UN were sought out by US governmental officials who wanted to persuade the Brazilian government to veto references to SRHR themes, reflecting a sharp change in direction from the country's stance during the administrations of Cardoso, Lula, and Dilma and their work on advancing women's rights and reducing poverty.[7]

Various NGOs, human rights advocates, and others working in the field of SRHR face a series of threats to their advocacy work on gender equality and reproductive health in many regions of the world as well as in Latin America. In Brazil, the rise to power of extreme conservative groups, supported by evangelical movements, culminated in the exile of the country's first openly homosexual MP, Jean Wylles, in 2019. Such pressures are not recent. Throughout the 1990s other countries in Latin America, like Chile and Colombia, were already seeing the rise of a growing opposition, with illegal abortion clinics suffering from crackdowns and repression (Richardson and Birn 2011).

Some of the gender experts interviewed here emphasised the importance of acknowledging the role played by religion in the oppositional discourses around SRHR and in the difficulties encountered when trying to adopt a more constructivist, critical, and historical approach to the notion of sexuality as well as a more holistic understanding of women's bodies. This was the case for the secretary of the Brazilian NGO Movimento Nacional das Cidadãs Positivas:

> I don't know if it's just religion, I think it has to do with the concept with which we learned, with the way we learned sexuality, the way we still work on sexuality within families. I think there are several factors and religion is one of them. But prejudice, stigmas of populations, I think it's growing. Maybe it's not just connected to religion ... There is a whole belief in what is ugly and what is beautiful, in short, what is normal, what is not. I think this is still very strong in people, including young people.

It is important to note that religion is not the only factor at play here and that not all religious groups are necessarily opposed to women's rights and the advancement of the SRHR agenda. Arguably, it has been religious evangelical groups that have been the most vocal opponents of reproductive health rights in the country. The last decade has also seen a significant growth in the political influence of these groups within the Brazilian Congress and in wider society. Statistics point to an increase in evangelical groups throughout Latin America to the detriment of the Roman Catholic faith. Recent research (Sotelo and Arocena 2021) further reveals how the rise of the evangelical church in Latin America has culminated in significant cultural change in the last decades, resulting in the growth of the number of evangelical politicians in the Brazilian Congress and the Bolsonaro political movement.

The coordinator of Catholics for the Right to Decide in Brazil recognised the challenges facing NGOs working in the field and advocated for gender and minority rights. However, she also noted that there have been some considerable advancements:[8]

> We do not work directly with the population, what we do is advocacy, not just with the parliamentarians but also with civil society and religious leaders. We have a proposal of dialogue which thinks the question of violence and how religion ends up perpetuating forms of violence against women ... I think that

we managed to implement various public policies in different countries. I remember that, although abortion has not been legalised everywhere, progress has been made in public policies, in the implementation of the distribution of inputs, [and in] information on health. The area of sexual health has advanced enormously in terms of policy as well. Brazil became a reference in the treatment of HIV/AIDS worldwide ... a significant advancement in public policies, not only in the implementation of health but also in terms of guidance and clarification to the population.

Some of the feminist and health activists from organisations in Latin America, such as the former coordinator of the Colombian NGO La Mesa por la Vida de Las Mujeres (and current secretary of Las Mujeres de Medellin),[9] underlined how feminists have managed to intelligently adapt themselves to the structures of the state. She argued that conservative forces have struggled to undermine the advances in women's rights:

I believe that it is undeniable that more effective, tougher response movements against conservative mobilisation are taking place and that they modify, in some senses, points on the agenda, especially on public policy issues. Well, they are living, they are managing to permeate, but I still would not say that the forces are equivalent, because I believe that the work that feminists have done ... in relation to all incidence, will lead to different levels and areas ... What the Cairo action plan means is to organize the women's agenda ... And proof of that success is the imitation in the way in which [as] feminists we have done things. Because I believe that feminists, especially those who opted for institutional views, understood very well how the institutional framework of the state will work and managed to implement gender mechanisms ... It has not been so easy to reverse what had been built. I think that already, for us, it is almost like an immediate minimum in the discourse of sexual and reproductive rights and that La Mesa activists, like me, are young (even if they don't seem like it). Well, La Mesa is twenty-one years old, but there are activists from La Mesa who were part of those processes, and who likewise brought us to the Colombian reality and to Colombian activism.

Moreover, a well-known Brazilian feminist from CEPIA pointed to the bottom-up work that the NGO does with young people and the importance of listening and learning from them:

> I think it is very important to build arguments, building knowledge on the subject is fundamental. CEPIA advocates to debate with the judiciary ... to have ... legitimacy and recognition. I think it's important to count on young people ... young people are bombarded by a culture against diversity and human rights. CEPIA is involved in working with young people in public schools, seminars ... listening to them ... Not from top to bottom ... We have a downloadable app, 'Partiu Papo Reto', made by young people. You will dialogue with the STF [Supreme Federal Justice court in Brazil] and ... work with vulnerable youth from the periphery, bringing them skills ... so that they can be authors of change. Another thing is the realization that the university, but the NGO as well, carries out research that allows a greater foundation of knowledge for an advocacy action. The other is the construction of solidarity, in a plural society ... starting from their diversities, [we] must know how to create bridges and act politically with the strategic capacity that overlooks what makes us different.

The role of Latin America as one of the leaders in the field, despite the numerous difficulties faced by the organisations, was stressed by many of the experts interviewed here. This was the case of the Reprolatina CEO, who outlined some core breakthroughs that she saw in the region:

> Historically, contraception was not a right. Birth control was done very much based on women's bodies ... And I'm talking about the beginning of the 90s ... so, 1995 we go to Beijing, nobody talked about freedom of choice ... But the concept of freedom of choice, in which the woman is the subject and not the object, of family planning programs, I think this was an advancement ... In Latin America, Brazil is very [much a] leader, because the feminist groups here were very strong. They had a lot of influence, for example, in the Women's Health Program, at the Ministry of Health. It had a great influence ... [on] feminist groups at the time. So, we have enormous progress ...

although in recent years we have had other setbacks ... Because all these changes are influenced by political changes. During Dilma's government, when she made an alliance with the evangelical bench, we started to lose, we started to notice the setback ... But we have advanced a lot in this area of contraception, in public policies throughout Latin America ... Everyone was very aware that they had to retreat in Cairo to be able to advance. It was accepted that we should leave the phrase 'sexual and sexual health' within reproductive health, which is ridiculous, for reproduction is within sexuality, but the sexual is not within reproduction. But it was a way to remove that word 'sexual', so that we could ... get this agreement ... this was a very conscious thing ... Latin America well accepts the concept of 'sexual and reproductive health'. There has also been ... progress in policies for comprehensive education in sexuality.

Others interviewed here were less optimistic – for example, the professor of the Federal University of the State of Rio de Janeiro (UNIRIO) and member of the Comite de America Latina y el Caribe para la Defensa de los Drechos de las Mujeres (CLADEM):[10]

I think there is a manipulation of these terms and I think we created certain terms ... We coined certain terms that were strategic for advancing political strategy, but they do not necessarily reach the population and I don't think it's a question of class. When we also keep repeating our left-wing discourse, which uses certain jargon, this drives away a good part of the population ... If we form a group of women not to talk about obstetric violence but, instead, to talk about childbirth experiences, we will certainly find reports of obstetric violence and we would have an opportunity to dialogue with women about it, without necessarily using these terms. I think conservatives end up winning because they manage to manipulate these terms that we used and that have now become a bit demonized.

However, the 'gender ideology' discourse has not managed to influence the entire debate in the public sphere, and it is important not to overstate its impact. Opinion polls conducted throughout Latin America in the last decades have revealed a growth in public recognition that pressing issues such as SRHR need to be better addressed, including debate on the decriminalisation of the abortion law. The 2011 FLACSO cross-national study of public opinion on abortion, which captured opinions in countries like Brazil, Chile, Mexico, and Nicaragua, revealed that the characterization of the abortion debate as polarised between two contrasting views was simplistic, with many favouring more liberal legislation and supporting legalising abortion under certain circumstances as well as seeing the need for a more participatory debate on the topic in their respective countries (Richardson and Birn 2011).

More recent statistics show similar results. Recent research by Ipsos, which surveyed global attitudes towards abortion, shows that seven in ten adults in twenty-seven countries support a woman's right to choose, indicating a growth in defence of legalisation in Latin American countries (79 per cent in Argentina, 64 per cent in Brazil, 73 per cent in Chile, and 59 per cent in Mexico).[11] In the next chapter I discuss how sexual and reproductive health is being understood by health and feminist NGOs working within the South Asian context.

5

Health Advocacy and Feminist Activism for SRHR in South Asia

The Indian Case

Carolina Matos with Ambika Tandon

As one of the largest and most unequal democracies in the world, with high levels of social inequalities and problems of access to quality health services, India shares many similarities with other countries from the Global South, such as Brazil, as well as some important differences when it comes to the nature of the debate around sexual and reproductive health and rights, how it has been constructed within the public sphere, and the specific cultural and historical contexts that define it, including how it has been shaped politically. Discussions around reproductive health and rights in India have included concerns over the controversial tradition of privileging the birth of boys over that of girls, a debate that is different from the 'pro-life' and 'gender ideology' discourses propagated by the religious and conservative groups examined earlier. However, issues of religion, morality, and tradition are also at play here. There are also similarities concerning the discrimination against women and girls, and the attempts to control their bodies and agency. This adds yet another layer to the complexities of analysing the advancement of sexuality and reproductive health in India, including the debate on abortion, further indicating that SRHR should be approached differently depending on local contexts and their cultural and historical specificities.

Similar to countries like Brazil, however, gender inequalities run deep in India and are closely interwoven with the persistence of cultural attitudes and the reproduction of patriarchal ideas about womanhood, maternity, and women's place in society. Both countries have high rates of violence against women as well as low representation of women in politics. India also fairs poorly on women's representation, with the Global Gender Gap Index 2021, revealed by the World Economic Forum, placing the country 140th among a list of 156 nations. India emerges as the third worst performer in South Asia, ahead only of Pakistan and Afghanistan.[1] Violence against women is seen as a very serious problem, with India having high rates of both feminicide and female infanticide.

Numerous scholars have underlined how gender inequality has persisted across various dimensions in India and how, ultimately, it has its roots in a deep-seated patriarchy that constructs gender roles for women and subjects them to gendered norms (Ghosh 2018). UNICEF India underscores how there continues to be a contrast between global Indian women who have a powerful voice and the majority of Indian women and girls who still do not fully exercise their rights.[2] Women are seen to fare poorly on key indicators of human development – from literacy and life expectancy to mortality rates (Ghosh 2018).[3] India's GDP has grown in the last years but the reduction of gender inequalities has remained stubbornly disappointing. Since the liberalisation of the economy in the early 1990s, India's GDP has grown by about 6 per cent, with education of women rising and fertility rates falling. The labour force participation (LFPR) for women has fallen from 42.7 per cent in 2004–05 to 23.3 per cent in 2017–18,[4] placing India in the bottom ten countries in the world on women's workforce participation, alongside countries such as Egypt, Somalia, Iraq, and Syria.

Like other Latin American countries, India has had a history of vibrant NGOs, social movements, and feminist groups who have been active at the transnational and local levels on advancing gender equality (Alvarez 1998; Narayanaswamy 2017). Also like other regions, the application of the SRHR framework 'on the ground' has not been fully realised. The policy approaches to SRHR in India regarding sex-selective abortion, as well as the decriminalisation of the termination of pregnancies, have had a unique history. SRHR became a part of the Indian postcolonial state's agenda of rights at its conception, with an initial emphasis on population control (Simon-Kumar 2007). The Indian state's approach to reproductive health has historically focused on population control rather than on the enhancement of individual autonomy. At the policy level the discourse on SRHR shifted from this earlier focus on population control to the rights-based framework approach, following from the successes of Cairo's 1994 International Conference on Population and Development (Sebastian et al. 2014). Thus, the continuous implementation of targets in family planning programmes led to egregious forms of violation of reproductive rights, particularly for women from marginalised communities. This Malthusian approach to governance has had a lasting impact on the provision of SRHR on the part of subsequent governments (Simon-Kumar 2007).

Combined with inadequate attention directed to human resources in public health institutions, poor funding has created severe shortages in the provision of public health, particularly for rural communities (Sharma 2015). India, however, is a signatory to international conventions and also has extensive legislation affecting access to maternity benefits, considered among the most liberal in the world, from domestic violence to harassment in the workplace, according to a 2018 report from the Partners for Law in Development and the SAMA Research Group for Women and Health.[5] Some of these have been enacted as a result of decades of feminist mobilisation around reproductive health; however, several challenges have persisted and millions of Indian women face difficulties translating these legal provisions into reality 'on the ground'. Unsafe abortion remains the third leading cause of maternal death (Singh et al. 2018).

As certain scholars note (Hirve 2004), despite decades of liberal legislation, most women in the country have difficulty gaining access to safe abortion care. Women in rural areas have a 26 per cent higher mortality rate due to the termination of pregnancies and their complications than do women who live in urban settings (Yokoe et al. 2019). Abortion is legal up to the twentieth week of pregnancy, the practice having been legalised in 1971 through the enactment of the Medical Termination of Pregnancy Act.[6] The past decades have also witnessed the increased privatisation and corporatisation of health care in the country due to the application of neoliberal economic policies, with India seeing the dismantling of welfare policies and the privatisation of state services. The emphasis has been on women fulfilling their own needs by resorting to the market (Sharma 2008). Because of this, the public health system has been under a lot of pressure, suffering from low public investment and poor infrastructure, including access to medications as well as inadequately skilled workers, and this has caused a deterioration in the accessibility, affordability, and quality of health care, including that for reproductive health.

Various NGOs in India alongside public-sector workers have directed resources towards improving SRHR outcomes, with women's rights organisations having been central in pushing for a rights-based framework that could better attend to communities (Datta and Misra 2000). The two co-founders of the NGO Ideosync Media Combine in India said that the 1990s and 2000s saw a lot of advancements in the field,[7] including working with the government to adopt sex curricula education. Many of these gains, however, were later reversed:

> In the 1990s there was a lot of hope and energy for change. The ICPD was a landmark moment for pushing rights-based discourse. The point was to hold governments accountable in the work that they have done within SRHR. From the 1990s till the 2000s was when a lot of progressive conversations were happening. We even worked with state governments to include sex education curricula, and we did a lot of work on this, but they were unable to adopt it eventually. All that work was lost. The rights-based discourse has been adopted by governments, but the approach is still the same. A lot of gains made during that moment have been reversed ... The conversation globally has regressed. There is a lot of self-censorship ... I heard of an organisation doing sex education without mentioning the word 'sex' because that is what the government wants. Twenty years ago, civil society organisations would have pushed back, they wouldn't decide to self-censor on primary aspects of their advocacy because that's what the government wanted. Now that is not the case.

Nonetheless, the director of programmes and the senior manager of Knowledge Management Partnerships from the Population Foundation of India highlighted some important achievements made in the field throughout the region.[8] She emphasised the placement of SRHR within the *feminist empowerment framework* and the role of the development sector in taking this forward:

> I think Southeast Asian countries have done very well, like Bangladesh, Indonesia, all these countries who have realised the importance of allowing women to choose from a basket of contraceptives ... India is also moving towards that system, the introduction of three new contraceptives in India's public

health system in 2017 is a right step in that direction. We have definitely made progress in maternal mortality and so have the other countries, in terms of reductions in infant and maternal mortality ... There is growing recognition of the fact that the two go hand in hand, the fact that giving women control over their reproductive rights and giving them that kind of agency is really the means to empower them. There is increasing evidence in that direction ... Of late we have been talking about family planning impacting all seven of the SDGS. This study is gaining a lot of momentum ... I would think that among the SRHR players there is growing recognition that women's empowerment is important when it comes to any of the choices in reproductive health ... PFI has been working within the women's empowerment framework. Anything that we do within family planning or reproductive health services must be within this ... including our social and behavioural change communications, recognising that social norms will impact the status of women ... Within the SRHR community there is a lot of recognition. If you're looking at feminist activity as a separate domain, there isn't that much recognition of the need for SRHR ... In that sense it's the development sector that has recognised the value.

Various NGOs in India working on SRHR, particularly those within the development sector or the more activist grassroots organisations, are continuing to play a vital role in the struggle for the enhancement of public policies on reproductive health, albeit under difficult circumstances and facing various funding shortfalls. Although to some extent new modalities – such as sector-wide approaches, basket funding, and budget support – have increased official development assistance to developing countries, women's organisations have often lost access to assistance funding (Aasen 2006) in a context within which certain areas, such as economics, education, and health more broadly, are privileged with regard to receiving development assistance and aid. This is the case even though family planning programmes started to figure more prominently from the late 1990s onwards.

There is also the issue of the limits of some of this work, from the more 'existential' crisis faced by the development sector itself with regard to the lack of funding as well as the allocation of resources to some areas to the detriment of others. Development funding through the public sector and NGOs has traditionally supported various programmes in reproductive health, from family planning to access to contraceptives and awareness-building campaigns (Sen and Mukherjee 2014). The concentration of funding for programmes around gender economic justice has also led to a shortfall in resources for areas that are not seen as a priority, such as SRHR, with programmes in the field being directed towards narrowly conceived conceptions of reproductive health, mostly limited to maternal and child health (Simon-Kumar 2007).

There has also been a wide range of development programmes that have been initiated by Indian governments in areas such as family planning, maternal and child health, contraception, and (more recently) adolescent health. However, in their design and implementation, these programmes exclude vulnerable populations and lack a focus on quality of care and SRHR (Datta and Misra 2000). This has been the case with organisations like the US Agency for International Development (USAID), which is geared towards family planning and maternal health programmes and sustains discourses around supporting an individual's right to make informed decisions regarding her body and reproductive health.[9] An analysis of these programmes consistently reflects the lack of a rights-based framework, with the resulting persistence of the exclusion of groups who still encounter sustained barriers to gaining access to quality health care.

Federal and state governments continue to maintain a target-based approach to sterilisation, coercing health workers to increase it by any means to meet predetermined targets, largely affecting low-income communities (Wilson 2015). This has been widely criticised by feminist activists as a form of systemic devaluation of the lives of marginalised women and even as a reflection of caste eugenics (Wilson 2015). Moreover, despite concerted efforts by feminist organisations, marital rape continues to remain outside the scope of criminalised rape (Makkar 2019). The World Bank has concentrated its efforts in rural areas, seeking to deliver programming through local community health networks and facility-based services. By leveraging these community efforts, the organisation claims that the goal of many development programs is to provide access to services as well as to shift social priorities.[10] However, the lens on reproductive health information and service availability here is seen as being too narrow, with an overt focus on enhancing technological solutions. This is the case with regard to the widely contested Digital ID programme, which is used to increase access to health care in India. Due to the Global Gag Rule, women who use or rely on services provided by organisations funded by USAID are prohibited from receiving any abortion-related care or information.

The senior adviser of the Centre for Catalysing Change stated that a lot of the NGOs working in the field have taken on an important role in the context of the 'loss of relevance' of development-sector organisations.[11] In line with what other scholars point out regarding the limits imposed by donors and funding on women's health organisations (Gideon and Porter 2016), she admits that their work is limited by donor compliance:

> We do get money from USAID. And we've had to – we cannot directly speak about abortion. And in other work we do provide information ... we are not an activist organisation. We mainly work as a technical partner with government ... In the states of Chattisgarh and Orissa we do a facility-level training of health workers, the doctors, and providers on their understanding of gender and social inclusion. These are those who support women to access services. So those are projects funded by the USAID, and that has certainly limited us ... We work on maternal health and preventable maternal mortality ... and we do orientations for our alliance partners as part of the White Ribbon Coalition on sexual health. If we are providing information and capacity building, or, in the school health programme, when we are talking to teachers, we do speak of rights and do talk about abortion. But we must – since its donor compliance, not to have direct programmes on safe abortion ... Over time the NGO universe has changed, and there are different kinds of NGOs. There are techno-managerial organisations and more development-focused organisations who are linked more closely with movements ... Development-sector organisations, like in the past, have lost their relevance, they have not been able to reinvent themselves to be leading players in the system. So, you see the rise of a lot of Indian NGOs ... certainly, a lot of organisations have become donor-driven. The Gates Foundation is one of [the] biggest donors ... and organisations that they must work with have to match that mandate. But it's a choice that organisations are making. Even earlier, there were social movements, and organisations that were leading those movements or working with the community. Many of them today are now languishing for funds, who have programmes that are focused on movement building.

Other health and feminist NGOs located in South Asia also underlined how their work has been affected by the Global Gag Rule. This was the case with the NGO Hidden Pockets, even though that policy was reversed at the start of the Biden administration in 2021. The director of Hidden Pockets underlined the problems that still exist in the conversations around SRHR,[12] which occur within a context of increasing neoliberalism and a lack of appropriate funding:

> At Hidden Pockets we work with a transnational organisation called RSRJ [Realisation of Sexual and Reproductive Health and Rights Justice]. It's a global alliance where fourteen Global South countries come together and use our studies, the ... data that we collect, to effect UN-based spaces. In the limited engagement that we have had ... we see the language being picked up ... But there is a lot of backlash, we see sex workers being left out of the conversation, disability rights is being left out ... A lot of articulation of SRH rights has happened. These are all international spaces where you were making states accountable ... So, we are a health referral platform for women who want abortion. But it was very clear that you can provide anything else, but not services on abortion. But that's what we do, so funding just got stopped ... we had to apply to new funders ... But as we reached the SDGs, there is mention of all these words, but they don't have enough impact. Targets don't have enough allocation of funding ... Funding allocation has happened for private-public partnerships, for technological innovation to improve SRHR. A lot of feminists have been criticizing this – the advocacy that happened during the ICPD has been diluted, and it is going more towards ... a future which is more of a technotopia.

Other organisations, however, have not been affected by this policy. This was the case with CREA India, whereas others, like Centre for Catalysing Change, stressed some of the difficulties they faced due to the lack of funding from USAID. According to their senior director for programmes and operations,[13] the NGO has been incredibly fortunate:

> CREA's work has not been impacted, because our work is not dependent on USAID or any other funding impacted by the Global Gag Rule. We know of organisations in East Africa

and South Asia, in places such as Bangladesh, where it [i.e., abortion] is already illegal, their work has been impacted ... When the ICPD happened and thereafter there was a lot of positive moves towards inclusion of language on rights ... We have moved to conservative governments. So that has impacted how much of sexual and reproductive rights gains we've had up until ICPD 10 ... One would think after so many years we would have moved forward. But we must constantly hold onto what we have ... So, people in the feminist movement that look at sexuality related issues have always had to push certain boundaries, whether it has to do with surrogacy ... how do you look at sex selective abortion ... how do you look at reproductive health technology from a feminist lens ... Technology has changed so much around us; how do you engage with that sudden change ... How do you do that in way that ... keeps possibilities of advancements open ... Also, pushing the boundaries of who you consider feminist and who you consider women, like trans women get left out or other groups like sex workers ... An NGO is not necessarily bad, but it depends on how you locate yourself and what are the questions you ask ... I think the problem is that you go out and work in these countries, South Asia, East Africa, wherever, and you're not located there. You come and do the work and move out – service delivery. It doesn't enable groups and movements ... to become stronger ... In the end when you're looking at rights, it's always strongest when the people that are affected can demand their rights. If as an NGO you don't have space for this, that is an issue.

However, the extent to which feminist and health NGOs in India have contributed to the advancement of women's rights, as well as to the field of reproductive health, and the precise nature of these contributions, have also been placed under scrutiny in the last years. There has been a debate concerning the credibility of NGOs in India in terms of their capacity to represent the grassroots and 'the poor', when many are still controlled by the higher strata of society, mainly middle-class Indian feminists. Narayanaswamy (2017) compares the situation of India with that of other countries of the Global South, underlining studies within the African context (e.g., Amadiume 2000; Creevey 2004; Gugerty and Kremer 2008) as well as within the Latin

American (e.g., Gonzalez de la Rocha 2007, 59; Alvarez 1998; Monasterios 2007) context. These studies make use of different epistemological inquiries but come to similar conclusions. They underscore how class-based inequalities often function to exclude the participation of lower-class women (e.g., Creevey 2004), further pointing out how this is often manifested in the power hierarchies at play between feminists within the third sector.

Influenced by the work of Alvarez (2009) on the process of NGO-ization, Narayanaswamy (2017, 96–7) outlines the experiences of a 'disconnection identified between feminists working in professionalized non-profit organisations from the poorer and less privileged women whom they seek to represent'. Here she points to the work of various postcolonial and feminist scholars (Mohanty 2000; Spivak 1988; Yuval-Davis 2010) who have questioned the conceptualisation of feminists as a homogenous group and the existence of a supposedly unified 'sisterhood' between women. Narayanaswamy (2017, 97) further cites Gore's (1993) work on how women build solidarity with other women based on shared gender/sex identity or other group identities (i.e., class or race), while oppressing those who do not fit into these categories.

Wilson (2015) is critical of the avenue to women's empowerment within development in the Indian context, problematizing, for instance, the case of the 'entrepreneurial Southern women' who are often still racialised and still seen as being the passive recipients of development assistance (i.e., 'the victims of patriarchy in need of saving'). Like Alvarez (2009) argument, and what has been discussed earlier, Wilson notes how women's collectives, including self-help groups, have been co-opted into a narrative that privileges discourses around financial growth, with membership largely facilitating financial services rather than demanding state action on policies relating to women's rights, or even challenging the dominant neoliberal model.

As signalled by many of the interviewees, dependence on donor support can make NGOs very vulnerable, with the best recipe for survival still being the support that these organisations can secure from governments or from large private grants. However, this can be project-based, short-term, and often top-down, and not necessarily community- or participatory-led. The dependence on funding from governments can thus be a double-edged sword, culminating in various NGOs shying away from confrontation or from taking more critical stances in relation to issues that are seen as controversial by whatever administration is currently in power. The reality is that funding for NGOs working in the Global South, as well as other parts of the world, is tight, with many resorting to original and creative communication strategies when encountering difficulties in advancing their communications portfolio because of the lack of resources. I now turn to examining how the NGOs that took part in this research used communications for advocacy and activism around sexuality and reproductive health. I also examine their communication strategies and practices and conduct a content and critical discourse analysis of their institutional websites and social media engagement on platforms such as Twitter and Facebook.

6

Development Communications and Advocacy for Women's Health and Rights

Why It Matters

Development communications has expanded considerably in the last decades and has become an important field within the discipline of media and communications, while the development industry and practitioners have recognised the importance of media and the ways in which the use of communications can be beneficial in advancing the aims of development programmes. Despite the different epistemological underpinnings of many of the theories and approaches in the field – from the social marketing perspective more associated with the modernisation framework to the emphasis placed on community media in the participatory tradition – at the core of the field is a concern with the ways in which media and communications technologies, systems, and tools, as well as content and discourses, can have a role in enabling social change across a range of development issues. This includes everything from poverty reduction to health outcomes and gender equality (Rogers 1976; Wilkins and Mody 2001; Huesca 2008; Serveas 2008, 2017; Dutta 2011; Hemer and Tufte 2016; Obregon and Waisbord 2012; Wilkins 2016).

Discussions on the use of communications for social change in development have tended to be cast within a dichotomy that, on one side, identifies with strategies that favour traditional top-down approaches and that are grounded in modernisation theory, or, on the other, bottom-up approaches that are largely supported by participatory frameworks that favour empowerment and community engagement (Servaes 2017; Dutta 2011; Manyozo 2012a; Tufte 2012).

As Dutta (2011) points out in his examination of social change, there have been a wide range of approaches, but these have operated within a dialectical tension between being an individual-level behavioural change approach, which emphasises changes in beliefs (e.g., social marketing campaigns), and being a more collective structural process, which focuses on structural redistribution and that is identified with the participatory framework (Manyozo 2012a).

Communications for social change has traditionally been used in international development programmes and interventions that favoured top-down approaches and strategies whose aim was to 'modernise' developing countries, making them 'catch up' to the more developed North. These assigned a role for communications as a key vehicle in the modernisation process for 'traditional' or 'backward' communities of the Global South who needed to 'catch up' with the 'modern' civilization of the Global North. Media and communications are seen as contributing to the development process by spreading the 'messages of modernity' to members of the population, inspiring them to want to develop. Communications is seen as crucial in changing the attitudes and beliefs of individuals from the Global South, cultivating in them a 'climate for development' (Melkote and Steeves 2001; Huesca 2008).

These criticisms led to the revisionist debate within the dominant paradigm and the acknowledgement that communications involved a *dialogical process* and was not solely about information sharing between sender and receiver (Waisbord 2001; Huesca 2008; Manyozo 2012b). Thus later authors, like Lerner and Schramm (1967), critiqued the limited view of communications as a 'one-way flow' that was more associated with the early development period, going so far as to proclaim the 'passing of the dominant paradigm' (Rogers and Kincaid 1976; Sparks 2007). The dominant paradigm began to be critiqued by Latin American dependency theorists and other critical European, postcolonial, and Marxist scholars for its top-down approach to development, including its emphasis on economic growth and its failure to fully take into consideration local cultures and histories (Huesca 2008; Manyozo 2012a).

There were also criticisms of the top-down development interventions of the early modernisation period, which was accused of having been designed on philanthropical principles by development programmes born in the North and of benefitting the richer countries. This perpetuated the dependency of the former colonies in what was seen as a continuous cycle of 'underdevelopment', albeit examined from different epistemological perspectives (Frank 1969; Cardoso 1972). Moreover, along with the rise of the human rights framework in development, the emphasis on participation and on more participatory forms of communications had a profound impact on mainstream development thinking and practice. This to the extent that, pretty much from the 1990s onwards, a form of 'participation' would be embedded in all development programmes. This included multilateral and bilateral agencies as well as NGOs and other grass-roots organisations.

All these development players, in some form or other, would incorporate participatory elements into their interventions and communication approaches. 'Participation' in development was thus 'co-opted' and became mainstream, being used across social marketing and entertainment-education development campaigns designed within the modernisation framework as well as in development interventions within the participatory framework. The aim was to use communication to combat long-term structural inequalities, without focusing on short-term behavioural change (Waisbord 2015; Dutta 2011; Huesca 2008; Serveas 2008; Snyder 2003).

The participatory framework thus emerged in opposition to the form of 'participation' found within social marketing development campaigns (Waisbord 2001; Melkote 2003; Wilkins, Tufte, and Obregon 2014; Serveas 2020). Participation was seen as an important component of the whole communication process and as central to development programmes that aimed to engage with local communities (Tufte 2012; Manyozo 2012b, 2017; Dutta 2011). However, a key debate concerns how participation has been used in development programmes and by multilateral agencies (Sumner and Tribe 2008). This has included looking at its different epistemological underpinnings, how it has been conceptualised in relation to social change, and how it is best implemented (Dutta 2011). From the Marxist perspective, social change requires the transformation of both the social and economic structures that perpetuate oppression and the marginalisation of less privileged groups (Dutta 2011). As Dutta points out, it is the agenda of international donor agencies (e.g., governments) and international organisations (e.g., the UN), and the commitments that these establish with recipient societies that ends up defining *how* social change will be interpreted and, consequently, how it will be implemented.

Following from his discussion of the agenda of international organisations, Dutta (2011, 39) underscores how participation functions as a 'strategic tool for ... achieving the development agendas of the founding agencies'. Dutta further divides the use of communications for social change into two frameworks: one is a *message-based approach* while the other is a *process-based approach* (32). The former focuses on the creation of effective messages aimed at reaching targeted audiences and having an impact on the population, whereas the latter stresses 'shared spaces of interpretation', in which individuals and collectives can exercise their agency in relation to social structures. Participation is used to 'improve the effectiveness of the campaign' and to communicate the messages of development, often combining these with entertainment-education (EE) programmes.

Various authors emphasise the centrality of understanding communications in terms of *justice* and as a *right* (Servaes 2017; Noske-Turner 2017; Enghel and Noske-Turner 2018). Following from the development of three generations of human rights principles, rooted in Western thinking and in individualism (Servaes 2017), the *right to communicate* has become almost as important as other collective rights, from civil and political rights to the right to education. Servaes (2017, 136–7) sees human rights as being 'vital for social change'; however, it is important to understand that these have grown out of the earlier rights of the 'sender to inform without restrictions' to the 'active right of the receiver to be informed and to inform'. He further argues in favour of a *communications rights approach*, which 'needs to be built into development plans and social change projects' (141).

Here I conceptualise and understand communications for development as being part of the process that aims to promote genuine transformative and structural change. Here I stand with what Enghel and Noske-Turner (2018) articulate in their book *Communication in International Development: Doing Good and Looking Good*. Quoting various theorists (including Gumucio-Dagron and Tufte 2006; Servaes 2007; Wilkins 2008), Enghel and Noske-Turner (2018, 2) state that the aim of communication should be to 'play a *positive role in the production of progress*' (emphasis in original). They go on to add to this the notion of *justice*, defining communication as a 'right to which citizens are entitled', while recognising that this is a 'capability that is socially distributed in unequal ways'. They further lament that the 2030 Agenda for Sustainable Development, adopted by the

193 member states of the UN in 2015, did not include communication as 'a right and a capability affected by global/local conditions' (2).

The understanding of communication as a *right*, and as being fundamental to development processes, has been incorporated by multilateral agencies into crucial documents. In line with its commitment to poverty reduction, the United Nations Development Programme (UNDP) (2009, 7) defines communication for development (C4D) as largely anchored in a human rights-based approach, one that incorporates equity and empowerment perspectives. It further alludes to Article 19 of the United Nations Declaration of Human Rights, which highlights the concepts of 'communication' and 'information', recognising that people are 'generators, users, and conduits' of information. Citizens are right holders and can place demands on governments and other sectors for accurate information on policies that shape their lives. They also have the right of participation and access to information and communication (UNDP 2009). C4D is addressed through four pillars that are part of its Access to Information (A2I) work, including the strengthening of communication tools available to vulnerable groups and the raising of awareness on rights of information access.

These communication frameworks and definitions provided by multilateral and UN bodies attest to the fact that there is scope for wider discussion of the role of communication in development. Some of the results of my research attest to this. Writing more than a decade ago in the journal *Communication Theory* on the role of communication in development, Wilkins and Mody (2001, 391) were already arguing that the use of new technologies within development was often for the purposes of information transmission rather than for promoting a more participatory dialogue. I believe that, despite advances since then, with NGOs and multilateral agencies more concerned with participations, as well as health advocacy campaigns more aware of the need to engage in dialogue with communities, the fact remains that communication is still used in its traditional form and continues to be under-utilised in development.

Wilkins and Mody (2001, 392) stress the importance of questioning the content of communication interventions, including the efficiency of messages, in terms of the 'relationship which exists between the mediated representations and the larger social circumstances'. This is crucial, for instance, in campaigns directed towards women in development, which can have a short-term impact for population programmes but which, in the long run, can function to 'curtail more progressive goals' aimed at changing ingrained gender norms and roles (Wilkins 2016; Gideon and Porter 2016). Moreover, in their assessment of the field of health communications, authors such as Obregon and Tufte (2017) note that it is important for development communications to pursue more interdisciplinary and qualitative research so that it can contribute to theory-building as well as to raising the epistemological status of the field. It is important to raise the bar of the field while at the same time assessing how communications used by social movements, NGOs, and institutional organisations working with development can be most effectively utilized.

The use of empiricist studies underpinned by quantitative methodology, including the use of surveys, to assess individual changes in the behaviour of citizens after they have been exposed to certain health campaigns, has been a common tradition in the field. However, I believe that, this is less about doing more quantitative measuring of development communication campaigns in order to assess their effectiveness (Synder 2003), as quantitative methods and the monitoring of development campaigns in terms of outcomes, impact, and inputs/outputs are already part of the results-based management tradition of the development field (Sumner and Tribe 2008). We should instead consider the relevance of more indirect long-term forms of 'effectiveness', many of which are more difficult to 'measure' from a short-term perspective.

In his discussion of development campaigns in the early 2000s, Synder (2003, 167–9) talks about how these began to be popular in the 1960s and how they initially drew from the *diffusions and innovations theory* (Rogers 1962), which had been used in the North through programmes that used the media to spread agriculture technologies to farmers in the US. These became central in campaigns directed towards health problems. Synder (2003, 167–88) identifies progress made regarding the planning, organisation, and coordination of the campaigns, although he points out that only a limited number of studies 'measured' the effectiveness of campaigns comparatively. He provides the example of the assessment of ten USAID child survival campaigns conducted in different nations, which found some positive effects, with entertainment-education showing itself to be effective (Tufte 2012; Dutta 2011).

I thus favour a more holistic understanding and approach to communication for development and social change (C4DSC), one that is not only grounded in 'measuring' the ability of messages to change individual behaviour but one that is also more concerned with communications (with all its contradictions). This includes understanding communication as a right and as something that can be part of a long-term process of learning, discussion, dialogue, and development for both the organisations and the communities involved as they attempt to tackle complex social problems – problems that can take years to address within local contexts. This understanding also places a central role on educational processes in assisting in the production of more effective change through the application of well thought out communication processes (Matos 2012).

I endorse Tacchi and Lennie's (2014) participatory framework for the evaluation of communication for development. They provide four concepts for evaluation, including stressing how it should be best considered and most usefully practised as an *ongoing learning and improvement process,* highlighting the need to shift from *proving impact* to *improving development practices.* They also underline seven components of the participatory framework, emphasising the critical and complex nature of these interventions and the ways in which one needs to be realistic regarding their long-term outcomes. Media content in development communication campaigns should not be solely concerned with short-term impact, one that can be 'measured' and produce immediate results. Instead, it should seek to tackle structural inequalities and to address all the factors involved in the development problem.

I believe that Tacchi and Lennie's (2014) intellectual perspective is part of a tradition that sees a connection between communication and a wider philosophical sense of self-improvement and learning, something that can be of benefit to the public good as well as to the individual. The influence clearly comes from the work of Paulo Freire (1970) and his use of participation in education as a form of 'conscious building'. In his discussion of the legacy of Freire's work, Waisbord (2020) seems to borrow from this idea when he defines communication as being rooted in a process in which we all *learn how to be human,* a view that I share. Thus, when it comes to 'rights', communication is closely interwoven with ideas of social justice. At the core of this is the idea that the type of communication matters, that it can contribute to learning and development and self-improvement on a continuous basis, having the capacity to be creative, innovative, and engaging, as well as being empowering and genuinely transformative.

All these different theoretical and epistemological frameworks on development communications are united in examining *how* communication can be best appropriated for development, for those who are already using it as well as for those who are yet to fully master it. Just as we need to problematise what constitutes an 'effective' development communication campaign and how we should measure it (Synder 2003; Tacchie and Lennie 2014), so we should examine *how* to go about developing more interdisciplinary research that would strengthen the epistemological underpinnings of the field. This includes carrying out more empirical work on media content and messages coming from development communication campaigns, programmes, and advocacy communication efforts. The objective is to seek to better understand *how* we can go about enacting wider and more structural social change in the field of gender equality, sexuality, and reproductive health.

In the next chapter I assess the field of health communications, particularly the growth in concerns with regard to applying human rights frameworks and participatory approaches to health advocacy communication campaigns. I then discuss the communication strategies, practices, and content of the NGOs that took part in this research.

7

Making Development Work for Women

Assessing Health Communications, Development Campaigns, and Entertainment-Education Approaches

The dominant understanding of communication within global health has been that it should transmit information, media content, and messages to targeted publics, with the strategic aim of changing individual attitudes towards a particular health issue. Health is thus seen as embedded in power dynamics (Lewis and Lewis 2015), with communication about and for health being a *political* process (Dutta 2011; Lewis and Lewis 2015). There has been quite a lot of debate within health communications regarding the 'effectiveness' of campaigns in the field, and none of this has led to a clear consensus (Sood, Shefner-Rogers, and Skinner 2014). This is similar to the examination of the use of entertainment-education methods in health promotion public campaigns (Obregon and Waisbord 2012a). As Lewis and Lewis (2015, 12) state, not only governments, NGOs, and interested groups but also individual members of the public are 'producing, sharing, and exchanging information ... about health in a variety of ways. Communities are taking action to ... influence their opportunities for healthy lives by using new modes of communication to form coalitions ... in strategies to influence decision-makers'. Thus the previous top-down model of health communications delivery, supported by the medical practice of providing services for people who need them (Rogers [1973] in Rimon [2001] in Sood, Shefner-Rogers, and Skinner 2014, 69), began to be challenged by wider community engagement and capacity building in the field as well as by other bottom-up participatory initiatives (Lewis and Lewis 2015, 12–13; Sood, Shefner-Rogers, and Skinner 2014, 69).

In their review of articles and books on health communication campaigns in developing countries, Sood, Shefner-Rogers, and Skinner (2014) discuss how many of the campaigns employed multiple strategies and forms of communication. They state that the consensus was that these health communication campaigns had modest rather than strong impacts and that this was due less to the communication process and more to the complex programming of the campaign. Quoting Rimon's (2001) *Four Eras in Global Health Communication*, they note the shift in the last decades from the 'social marketing era' to the 'strategic behaviour change communication era' (before this there was the 'clinic era' and the 'field era'), thus moving away from adopting commercial marketing strategies in health campaigns to using behavioural change models to influence social norms, facilitating both individual change *and* social change (Figueroa et al. 2002 in Rimon 2001).

The link between health and other social problems also has been recognised in mainstream development. Sood, Shefner-Rogers, and Skinner (2014, 69) quote the World Health Organisation (WHO), which states that 'health and the MDGs are linked: all the MDGs (*Millennium Development Goals*) influence health (these however have been superseded by the *Sustainable Development Goals* (SDGs) [emphasis mine]. For example, better health enables children to learn … Reducing poverty, hunger and environmental degradation positively influences … better health'. Thus, despite the shift to community-based communications and participation, when it comes to strategic communications for health, the language used by the WHO continues to be embedded in behavioural change concerns.[1] Sood, Shefner-Rogers, and Skinner (2014) also quote Wakefield et al. (2010) and the findings of their review to show that community-based approaches to health communication campaigns were the norm in developing countries. However, this did not necessarily mean that the campaigns were genuinely community- or participatory-driven.

In their *Strategic Communications Framework* (WHO 2017, 10), WHO defines communication as being a 'necessary component of any effort to achieve positive health outcomes'. It further explores the need for strategies to create effective messages focused on behavioural change, from raising awareness around a health issue to moving towards a behaviour change that could result in specific health outcomes. Thus, for a campaign to be 'effective', it needs to 'adapt to the context of the community that it serves' (14). The WHO text also reflects the concern with adapting health messages to the needs of communities, signalling indirectly to the importance of the participation of those affected by the campaign while stating the need to focus on behavioural change.

Health communication campaigns also began to improve, with campaigns using a multiple range of media, from community mobilisation to interpersonal forms of communication (Sood, Shefner-Rogers, and Skinner 2014). These became increasingly more sophisticated in their design and creation (Synder 2003), particularly from the 1990s onwards. According to Melkote (2003, 136–7), since the 1990s, the Regulation Communication Services, aided by USAID, began to adopt a strategic communications framework to overcome past weaknesses in family planning communication. Quoting Piotrow (2005) and her colleagues at the Johns Hopkins Center for Communication Programs, Colle (2008, 132) underlines how the researchers foresaw that the next decades would bring 'continuing rapid demographic, political and technological change' that would 'require family planning and reproductive health communication programmes to adapt' to various situations. These included changes in everything from the channels of communications to organisational structures as well as political environments and resources. Strategic communications were used to describe an operational framework that incorporated social marketing and behavioural change models into the design, execution, and evaluation of the communication strategy intended to influence any given change.

As should be clear by now, the roots of the discipline of health communications, with its focus on behavioural forms of communications, lie within the dicta of modernisation theory and the role it assigned to communications in development (Obregon and Waisbord 2012). The use of communications within the social psychology or behaviourist 'media-effects' tradition has marked the field of global health communications from breast-feeding to HIV/AIDS prevention campaigns during the 1950s and 1960s (Waisbord 2001; Huesca 2008). Social marketing and entertainment-education models are popular communication approaches used in health communication campaigns (Waisbord 2001; Tufte 2005; Huesca 2008; Dutta 2011). Despite criticisms, many argue that these approaches have proven to be largely effective in these campaigns (Lewis and Lewis 2015).

Thus health communication programmes, particularly those population interventions dealing with sexual and reproductive health and rights, have nonetheless largely remained restricted to specific social and gender policy interventions on the part of NGOs or multilateral agencies. These have not always been inserted within broader development interventions that understand gender development from a holistic perspective. As I argue, social, economic, and political developments are intertwined: we cannot talk about SRHR in a vacuum. Sexual rights and reproductive health are always inserted within particular political and economic paradigms, and this produces very particular types of health systems as well as health indicators and outcomes, including inequalities when it comes to women's access and their right to be informed of accurate health information.

As Lewis and Lewis (2015, 10) correctly point out, health is an unequal resource. In their edited collection *The Handbook of Global Health Communications*, Obregon and Waisbord (2012a) note how in the last few decades various organisations, from the Melinda and Gates Foundation to the government of India, have made wider investments in international health and development to eradicate diseases such as polio. This includes the US's focus on the plight of HIV in poorer regions of the world. Obregon and Waisbord (2012a) further argue that communication has played a crucial role in advocating for healthy policies, mobilizing communities as well as promoting the adoption of new health behaviours, with the creation of campaigns aimed at preventing HIV/AIDS and other diseases (such as malaria) and reducing maternal and child mortality (1–2). The field is divided between theoretical debates on information/media effects and critical theories in development communications (i.e., the participatory framework) (Obregon and Waisbord 2012a, 10; Manyozo 2012a). Some scholars are concerned with the efficacy of messages that promote behavioural change, while others are concerned with examining the integration of communication strategies.

Many of these theories have been developed in the US, although their application has largely taken place in non-Western contexts, something that has raised accusations of intellectual imperialism as well as arguments that models that reflect local conditions are more useful to study health communications as these consider social inequalities in health disparities (Waisbord and Obregon 2012a, 647). Waisbord and Obregon (2012a) state that the examination of power structures within health communications has been largely neglected in favour of individualistic approaches and that we have little knowledge about how communications can affect policies capable of promoting health changes (643–7). They also underscore the need to understand communication as a tool to address the power relations that are implicated in health opportunities. They emphasise that communication is often not seen as a priority within development and health communications, something that I also identify in this research, with many organisations admitting to only recently taking up communications and including it as part of their strategic organisational plans and advocacy efforts.

Critical perspectives on health communications would eventually offer some important contributions, questioning the predominance of the behaviourist tradition and the neglect of power (Dutta 2011; Zoller and Kline 2008 in Obregon and Waisbord 2012a, 21; Tufte 2012; Manyozo 2012a; Airhinhenbuwa and Dutta 2012). These studies call out for more qualitative and in-depth methods as well as interpretive and discourse analysis approaches that are able to examine how societies understand health, how inequalities are formed, and how public debate plays a role in informing health decisions. These critical perspectives draw attention to the unequal structures under which health practices operate, further underpinning the importance of the role of governments in providing health programmes and assistance to citizens, including paying attention to the worldwide impact of the privatisation of health services, cuts to public health systems, and problems concerning quality and access of delivery, particularly to less privileged groups (Airhinhenbuwa and Dutta 2012; Manyozo 2012a).

Evaluating the field of global health communications, Tufte (2012) points to the continued weakness of this research tradition, identifying the gaps that could still be filled when it comes to theoretical inquiries and research. Tufte (in Obregon and Waisbord 2012, 609–10) argues for more interdisciplinary approaches to global health communications, making the case for the discipline to make more inroads into the social sciences, from anthropology to media and political science. There is a need to adopt a wider range of methodological and epistemological approaches, including more culture-centred studies, defended by scholars like Dutta (2011), as well as more interdisciplinary work that can re-evaluate the role of communications to better assist in the health concerns of citizens (Tufte 2012). Regarding the understanding of communications within the health communications field, Tufte (2012, 614–15) identifies it as a 'poorly explored societal force'. He further cites an example of good practice, the case of the participatory NGO Femina Hip, which made creative use of communications for advocacy around SRHR (616). This NGO adopted popular culture formats (including magazines, TV talk shows, and radio dramas) to provide Tanzanians with the information needed to make adequate choices regarding sexuality and reproductive health through what seems to be a clear application of entertainment-education strategies to their communication use.

It is through the notion of communication as the *mobilisation of community resources*, with the aim of transforming health conditions for citizens and embedded in a participatory framework, that various scholars (Manyozo 2012a, 643) understand the use of communications in health campaigns. Health activists have criticised the tendency to approach health from the individual perspective, emphasising the need for a more 'structurally based approach', one that can examine the structural factors that bar people's access to health and, in so doing, seek ways to change this (Airhinhenbuwa and Dutta 2012, 48). Similarly, with regard to the use of social marketing strategies in health communication campaigns, entertainment-education approaches are widely used in development communication campaigns in developing countries and are becoming popular in development projects concerned with social change (Waisbord 2001; Melkote in Mody and Gudykunst 2003; Tufte 2012; Dutta 2011; Singhal 2013). How entertainment-education can be effective in health communications has however been widely discussed (Obregon and Waisbord 2012a; Lewis and Lewis 2015; Sood, Shefner-Rogers, and Skinner 2014), with some criticising this approach due to its roots in the modernisation framework whilst others underscored its merits (Tufte 2012; Singhal and Rogers 1999; Singhal 2013). Entertainment-education, or 'EE', is thus defined as being the insertion of entertainment content into media messages with the intention of influencing behaviour towards a socially desirable objective.

Entertainment-education draws from a range of theories, including Bandura's (1977) *social learning theory*, which claims that individuals learn behaviour by observing role models in the media. EE became popular because of its applicability to family planning programmes, HIV/AIDS, and other health development interventions (Waisbord and Obregon 2012a; 2012b). Many scholars have praised EE's impact on collective agency and social change as well as the participatory nature of the design of many of its programs. EE principles are seen as having had positive consequences, including prompting conversations about health, reinforcing messages and social norms. If EE is embedded within a communication framework that is participatory and designed in a creative manner, so that it could appeal to people's lives, then it would be better equipped to effect wider long-term social change. Tufte (2012) argues that, if EE is designed with participatory approaches in mind, then it can be useful in health promotion campaigns. Lewis and Lewis (2015) note how popular culture and entertainment can provide avenues to send out messages that promote social change that is meaningful to the communities affected.

Scholars like Jacobson and Storey also discuss the potential of EE programs to bridge theoretical divides and promote participatory ideals, but again only if they redesigned on participatory premises (Waisbord and Obregon 2012b). One position argues that EE programs can offer opportunities for marginalised populations to think critically (e.g., Soul City in South Africa and the NGO Puntos de Encuentro in Nicaragua) (Tufte 2001). Dutta (2006) expresses reservations, stating that EE is grounded in 'individualistic and universalistic premises, as well as the overall limitations of health programs supported by international donors' (in Waisbord and Obregon 2012b, 24). Dutta (2011) equates the effectiveness of a health communication campaign with its capacity to facilitate 'participation' in social change (in Lewis and Lewis 2015, 9).

Evidence of impact on behaviour change is ambiguous (Melkote in Mody and Gudykunst 2003; Waisbord and Obregon 2012b). Waisbord and Obregon (2012b) underline the fact that health/social messages can be included without necessarily being part of collective actions. Various scholars (e.g., Lewis and Lewis 2015; Singhal and Rogers 1999) are more enthusiastic and argue that entertainment-education research is on the rise and that it is an effective way of reaching out to less educated or more marginalised groups who might disengage from the more conventional fact-based communication approaches traditionally used for health messages.

The importance of the use of storytelling techniques in development communication campaigns has been explored by various scholars. Hemer and Tufte (2016) point out how the communication of feelings through stories can permit the sharing of emotions, making them public. Singhal (2013) emphasises the 'power of storytelling'. Quoting the British novelist Gilbert Chesterton, who disputes the 'truth' of fairytales because they 'tell us that dragons can be beaten', Singhal (2013, 3) stresses the importance of stories and how they can create opportunities for *transformative dialogue*. He points out that, in the last decades, storytelling has become increasingly popular, being incorporated into various social projects, including those coming from the Johns Hopkins Center for Communications Programs, the Population Media Center, the BBC World Service Trust, and the Soul City Institute of Health and Development Communication. Writing within the context of the role that activism plays in social movements and advocacy networks in international politics, Keck and Sikkink (1998) note how the use of 'testimonials' can be influential forms of messages.

In her discussion of how storytelling has become a powerful marketing technique used by charities and other third-sector organisations from the Global North for fundraising campaigns, with a particular focus on the case of the NGO Kiva, Ascough (2018, 534) tells how stories can help us to think about the lives of 'others', building in people 'a sharpened sense of empathy and compassion'. This can contribute to altering views on a range of issues, from sexuality to race (Gottschall 2014 in Ascough 2018, 534). This is because stories can reflect the hardships that people face, with individual narratives that are explored in digital storytelling having the capacity to foster understanding across different groups, making private stories public.

Ascough (2018, 534–40) argues, as do I, that many stories and narratives within international development often provide problematic representations of people from developing countries, despite the criticisms articulated by various postcolonial scholars (e.g., Mohanty 2000). Storytelling is not always used to *enlighten*. It can also be that many of these narratives exist within neoliberal discourses of individual success stories, many of which end up *depoliticising* complex political problems (Ascough 2018), thus undermining the discussion of the impact of structural inequalities on issues such as gender inequality and reproductive health. This is the case of Wilkins's (2016) critique regarding some traditional population development programmes and their application in Egypt, where they target women and girls and frequently assign to them individual responsibility for their change in behaviour pertaining to reproductive health practices.

Thus the EE approach has moved away from the social marketing model towards the community-level involvement of targeted groups at all stages of the communication strategies (Tufte 2005). Some EE campaigns on SRHR considered successful by the NGOs interviewed for this research include examples provided by Amnesty International Argentina and La Mesa por la Vida y la Salud de las Mujeres. The director of press and communications for Amnesty International

Argentina talked about a campaign on YouTube[2] – one that generated quite an impact.[3] The campaign made use of popular culture formats, such as rap music, which resonates with young audiences. It included a young woman who demanded integral sexual education ('mi corpo es mi propriedad' [my body is my property]), with the lyrics of the song being used as a way of transmitting information. Another campaign that inserted itself within popular culture was Amnesty International UK's 'Repeal the 8th in Ireland'. According to the media and PR manager of the organisation,[4] who responded to the survey questionnaire, the campaign was seen as having succeeded in making a 'good online buzz', with 'lots of influences, clear messaging, well used hashtags, iconic images that were shared, and visible branding (Maser mural/image, 'REPEAL jumpers and T-shirts, #HometoVote etc.)'.

In videos, the organisations explored examples of the use of personal accounts of people who have suffered over difficult decisions. The former coordinator of the Colombian NGO La Mesa por la Vida de Las Mujeres (and current secretary of Las Mujeres de Medellin) talked about how the organisation sought to explore the use of artistic expression in its advocacy communications content. This included human interest stories that featured men and women who had lived through experiences of abortion. On its institutional website, translated from the Spanish, the organisation emphasised:

> *Unstoppable Women*, 20 years leading the way. This is an initiative of *La Mesa por la Vida y la Salud de las Mujeres* which, through different artistic expressions such as literature, illustration, and urban art, seeks to make visible the experience of women and men who have lived or accompanied related experiences with the *Voluntary Termination of Pregnancy* (IVE) in Colombia[5].

The executive director of the Peruvian NGO Centro de Promocion y Defensa de los Derechos Reprodutivos (Promsex) also affirmed that feminism has now become more complex,[6] interlinking many different factors beyond SRHR in its quest for the advancement of women's rights. She also gave an example of what she considered to be a successful health communication campaign for SRHR, which engaged with popular culture formats and made use of influencers with the aim of dismantling 'myths' propagated by conservative groups:

I believe that the commitment that feminists have maintained are with the themes and what has occurred is a widening of the complexity of the agenda ... not only with the expectations of women regarding having more choice over their own reproductive decisions, but also in relation to new emergent themes related to ... population changes. There is wider demand for assisted reproduction, sexual diversity, the changes in reproduction patterns ... from violence to human traffic ... The #EducaciónConIgualdad campaign, for instance, was part of the response to the onslaught of conservative groups to eliminate the gender approach from [the] basic education school curriculum. This campaign had three moments, in which different influencers joined to make a call to public opinion to be informed and to join #EducationWithEquality. You can check some of their videos. [7]

Thus health disparities and gender inequalities can be seen as being embedded in social structures and the structural dimensions of political and economic systems. Resources here play a crucial part in defining development interventions that move forward (and that can be successful) to those that encounter barriers and that – however well developed their health communication campaigns, entertainment-education formats, or multiple use of media and communication strategies for advocacy – are limited by external constraints or the inadequacy of the design of the development programme itself and its short-term focus. Other restrictions include social and cultural norms, economic limitations, and political will. The centrality of the role played by various actors is crucial, particularly the advocacy communication efforts and the mobilisation of feminists and health NGOs and activists to promote their causes and advance policy debate around SRHR, using various communication tools as well as taking advantage of some of the avenues opened by the media, despite the limitations of resources and the political challenges that they face. It is to the communication strategies and practices utilised by health and feminist NGOs working in the field, where advocacy communication efforts often blur with wider forms of feminist digital activism, that I now turn.

8

NGOs, Advocacy Communications, and Feminist Digital Activism on Sexual and Reproductive Health and Rights

In the last decades feminist research across the social sciences, from sociology, political science, to media studies as well as development, has attempted to examine how new communication technologies are being used by social movements and groups, including by individuals, for political mobilisation and digital activism. Different studies provide sophisticated analyses of and insights into the complexities of online engagement in the digital era (Grint and Gill 1995; Fotopoulou 2016b; Daniels 2009; Sassen 2002; Newsom and Lengel 2012; Khamis 2015; Youngs 2015; Mendes, Ringrose, and Keller 2019). Feminist theory within the field of science and technology has also made significant contributions (Wajcman 2000; Plant 1995; Haraway 2000; Michaeilidou 2018). The assumption that science and technology are 'neutral' and 'objective' spaces has been dismantled by various feminist authors (Haraway 2000; Harding 1993). The internet started to be seen as a site that is not exclusively 'masculine' and not merely exploitative of cheap women's labour (Wajcman 2000) but, rather, a realm within which women can make good use of its various webs and networks for their own empowerment, self-expression, and transnational feminist activism (Plant 1995; Harcourt 2011).

Feminist scholars from different fields, from development studies to political theory, from Harcourt (1999, 2017) to Youngs (2002, 2015), are enthusiastic about the possibilities that the internet offers transnational feminist movements and international advocacy networks, from opportunities for mobilisation around women's rights to the raising of awareness of the cause to reach a wider 'global' audience. Mendes, Ringrose, and Keller (2019) argue that 'new forms of feminisms' have been reinvigorated by the opportunities afforded by digital media technologies, with feminism becoming increasingly popular with its activism and online hashtags that challenge sexism, misogyny, and rape culture (e.g., Fotopoulou 2016a; Banet-Weiser and Miltner 2016; Keller 2012 and 2015 in Mendes, Ringrose, and Keller 2019, 2). This includes the ways in which online communications can enhance the networking capabilities of feminists across borders, making it possible to 'do politics' without the constraints of national borders and with the intention of increasing empathy as well as sharing the experiences of different groups of women from various localities (Harcourt 1999 in Youngs 2002, 25).

Arguably, many feminist campaigns have in fact been enacted locally, within what some scholars call a *politics of location* (Kaplan 1997, 139), with the intention of having influence at the global level. These have ranged from the Arab Spring protests (Khamis 2015; Newsom and Lengel 2012) to other demonstrations throughout the Global South, from the global SlutWalk (Mendes, Ringrose, and Keller 2019) to the #MeToo movement campaigns, to the FEMEN and Russian Pussy Riot rallies, as well as other women's campaigns that have called attention to violence and bodily control in offline spaces (e.g., the Latin American #NiUnaMenos hashtag campaign[1]) (Chenou and Cepeda-Masmela 2019).

In the case of sexual and reproductive health, many gender experts interviewed for this research drew parallels between different feminist campaigns on women's rights from across the world, in both developed and developing countries. For example, parallels were drawn between Ireland and Argentina with regard to grassroots feminist campaigns advocating for the decriminalisation of abortion, with links being made between both and the acknowledgement by some NGO advocates of how each campaign fed from the other. The programme manager of Women's Human Rights at Amnesty International UK, comparing different feminist campaigns, stressed how the solidarity among women from across the world has been building in the last years:[2]

> I think that the fact that the rise of the right is shaping, is kind of happening in very similar ways in different countries, and thus offering the opportunities to connect ... So basically the Italian movement #NonUNaDiMena, which is a movement which had called support from other European feminists, there were I think around 150,000 people from other European countries, and from Argentina. And if you see that #NonUNaDiMena has

adopted the green handkerchief that the Argentinians were wearing, how do you call it? The green handkerchief that the Argentinians were wearing? I think they call it panuelo? They did the same with ... pink ...? There is this spreading of iconography, for example the way that the costumes have been used in protests in Italy, in the US, also in Latin America, it kind of gives a sense of global solidarity from a visual and communications perspective?

At the core of the debate on feminism and online activism is the extent to which digital space can complement the offline world in terms of reach and influence (Earl and Kimport 2013; Fotopoulou 2016b; Mendes, Ringrose, and Keller 2019), especially how it can create possibilities for transformative change for women in the offline world, further contributing to deepening democratisation as well as providing more opportunities for less privileged groups to be heard (Haraway 2000; Youngs 2015; Fotopoulou 2016a). Studies have started to examine the paradoxes of the online environment, where women can be caught between *vulnerability* and *empowerment* (Fotopoulou 2016a), seeking forms of emancipation, political mobilisation, and transnational connections. As Fotopoulou (2016a) notes, most work on uses of online networks for activism has been done by social movement scholars and those working on alternative media, leaving space for further exploration of the experiences of women and girls and how they engage online. Digital activism has frequently been framed within a *cyberfeminist* utopia or dominant narratives of productivity and a progressive 'good life'. Fotopoulou (2016a) prefers to provide a more realistic assessment, defining 'digital engagement' as 'the adoption of a set of digital media practices (social media, email, websites) by both civil society organisations and individuals from marginalised groups' (991), which leaves the ground open for multiple possibilities, from contradictions and regressions to more genuine attempts at progressive change.

Online activism on social media platforms and elsewhere should not be naively celebrated, as if these tools permit the proliferation of a rational, critical Habermasian space of enlightened debate (Habermas 1992; Iosifidis 2011). Quoting the work of Jonathan Dean, Fotopoulou (2016a) further underlines how he has been among the scholars who have been more sceptical about the capacity of the web to deliver digital democracy, given the fact that online spaces are highly fragmented and do not necessarily contribute to the unification of causes. Online activism has limited capacity for changing the impact of the inequalities of the offline world (Kingston and Stam 2013). What is central are discussions on what it means to be an 'activist', including the preconceived assumption that an 'activist' is necessarily a 'male' as well as the potential of online activism to enact social change. Kingston and Stam (2013) identify two key schools of thought within the literature on online activism: the 'supersize model', whereby the internet increases reach and speed without affecting the process, and the theory 2 approach, which suggests that the web can advance change. They further add that scholars like Earl and Kimport (2013, 78) maintain that both outcomes can be possible, depending on 'activists' choices and ... abilities to leverage "affordances"', including the benefits provided by technologies as well as the ways in which activists can make use of these.

The reality is that digital access has remained highly unequal and democratic participation continues to be limited. Access to the internet, however – or 'digital inclusion', as is the preferred term for discussions on the 'digital divide' within development – is rapidly expanding in regions like Latin America, providing opportunities for both democratisation *and* regression. In Brazil, the use of the WhatsApp technology during Bolsonaro's 2018 presidential campaign was vital for his attack campaigning against his opponents, influencing various voters and assisting in his election. Despite the persistence of digital inequalities in countries like India, women there have started to emerge as avid users of the internet. Communication technologies have thus been seen as *both* enabling and constraining, while also being a vital tool not just for mobilizing feminists but for engaging in advocacy around a series of causes (Harcourt 2013; Kapoor 2003; Youngs 2015; Fotopoulou 2016b).

Within international development there has been an increase in studies on the use of cyberfeminism for gender and development in the Global South as well as on the role of information, communication, and new technologies (ICTs) on the part of NGOs, feminists, and other activists from Latin America to Southeast Asia (Gajjala and Mamidipudi 1999; Gajjala 2003; Friedman 2003; Wilkins 2016; Harcourt 2011).[3] Scholars highlight how ICTs have been celebrated within the development industry (Kleine and Unwin 2009; Vokes 2018; Mansell and When 1998; Mansell 2014). Arguments have been largely constructed within a *technological deterministic/modernisation* framework regarding their capacity to bring development to emerging democracies through the expansion of a particular nation's infrastructure and online inclusion. Development is seen as having largely favoured more 'exogenous' approaches to technology use as opposed to more 'endogenous' approaches, which could favour a more holistic adoption of ICTs – one grounded in *how* these technologies are being used and in determining the role of communications in terms of facilitating and expanding wider participation and dialogue (Mansell 2014; Wilkins 2016).

Wilkins (2016, 114) further points to the fact that much of the discussion of the literature on new communication technologies within development looks at how ICTs can enable the creation of small micro-enterprises by individual women in developing countries rather than at the role that digital media can have for political mobilisation and protests or how it can provide more avenues for participation and dialogue. Moreover, scholars from the Global South situate the discussion on ICTs within a larger narrative of development as capitalist, neoliberal, and patriarchal. Gajjala and Mamidipudi (1999, 9, 15) are critical here, stating how new communication technologies have tended to reinforce or merely reflect 'perceptions of Northern society that Southern women are brown, backward and ignorant' rather than promoting activism in favour of social change and with the aim of empowering less privileged groups of women.

Distinctions should also be made between what is understood as 'advocacy' and what is understood as 'activism'. As I mention in the methods section, some of the NGOs that participated in this research are not necessarily seen as 'feminist organisations', and many could be defined as service delivery health organisations that work on women's rights and on SRHR. However, developing on Alvarez's (2014) understanding of feminism as being 'discursive spaces of action', it is possible to situate most of these organisations as part of the broader 'global feminist movement' that operates within the development and NGO sector in the fields of sexuality and reproductive health. Within this context the term 'advocacy' may be seen as being more associated with public health advocacy efforts taken up by organisations that work from a more conventional or even *institutional* standpoint, whereas the term 'activism' may be associated with more militant initiatives and with the 'on-the-ground' activism of groups who are prepared to push boundaries, work outside official norms, or from more grassroots or marginalised positions (Lewis and Lewis 2015), thus seeking to transgress norms.

Both these forms of engagement with SRHR are present here, and both make use of media and communications. Despite the differences between what is understood by 'advocacy' activities on the part of health and feminist organisations and more 'activist' forms of advocacy communications, it is often the case that these communication practices can be distinct in some cases but quite blurred in others, particularly for NGOs working on human rights-based gender equality issues or with other political issues within local and global contexts. This is regardless of the differences between more evidence- and medical-oriented service-delivery NGOs from the more single-issue feminist networks that advocate in favour of decriminalizing abortion through to more 'transgressive' activism.[4] Thus, although a media message from an organisation regarding SRHR, conducted through its conventional communication platforms, could be classified as being part of 'official health advocacy' in favour of reproductive health, it can also be used, or seen by others, as a form of activism around that particular issue. This is because it is being used in the pursuit of raising awareness or seeking to influence policy-making, thus having the intention of pushing for wider social change.

In the case of development programmes designed for the area of reproductive health, Colle (2008, 131) argues that advocacy has become a core term 'in developing reproductive health communications strategies'. He quotes Servaes (2000, 104), who underlines how 'advocacy' aims to foster 'public policies that support the solution of an issue'. Servaes and Malikhao (2010) further note how communication strategies have shifted away from the previous *behavioural change communication* approach, moving towards understanding policy-making as a fundamental process in social change, one that is expressed through a commitment to *participatory forms* of advocacy communications. Writing about the use of advocacy in development campaigns, Synder (2003) states that 'advocacy communications' should be understood as including the strengthening of community awareness through various media events, from capacity development programmes to community-led health research. Quoting the work of Keck and Sikkink (1998), McPherson (2015) also emphasises how advocacy can be seen as being a *communicative act*. However, it is important to stress that the communications with which NGOs engage differ from the communications used by news organisations. These organisations vary significantly in their aims, as well as in their diverse communications activities, which frequently results in the blurring of the distinctions between 'advocacy' and 'activism'. This is the case, for instance, for activities such as fundraising and the use of media to appeal to emotions.

Thus advocacy communication practices – including the use of information and facts to inform citizens or to mobilise around certain issues as well as other practices, such as mimicking professional journalistic cultures associated with media organisation – have become central to the activities of many third-sector organisations working in the field of civic and human rights (Powers 2014, 2017; McPherson 2015) and in the development sector. Here I draw from the work of Keck and Sikkink (1998) as well as Stroup and Murdie (2012) in their understanding of the term 'advocacy'. These authors point to the differences in advocacy tactics among organisations, showing how some can use information strategically through either partnering with powerful actors, holding governments accountable, or targeting different publics – from officials to the general public (Stroup and Murdie 2012, 427).

Advocacy communications for NGOs working with SRHR should be seen differently from other civic organisations, many of which produce news for consumption across media platforms (McPherson 2015, 125; Powers 2017; Kingston and Stam 2013). Thus, when thinking about the use of advocacy communications by health and feminist NGOs working in the field of SRHR, it is important not to assume that this is simply another expression of digital feminist activism at work; rather, many of these organisations are adding online communications to previous offline advocacy and media efforts, seeking to find ways to potentialize the capacity of digital communications. At the same time, they recognise the limits. These understandings around what SRHR means can be confusing (not just for the public but also for those working within the field), for here lie deeper philosophical and personal debates on definitions of motherhood and women's sexuality. The 'advocacy' in favour of sexual and reproductive health and rights can thus be widely misunderstood by sectors of the public. These could consequently end up endorsing largely simplistic narratives that do not provide an adequate understanding of the connection between sexual rights and poverty and reproductive health, showing how this is a human rights issue and is crucial to the advancement of gender equality.

Many of the gender experts from the NGOs interviewed for this research admitted that they would like to make better use of communications in their advocacy work on SRHR, including investing more money and resources into communications as well as hiring more staff, building advocacy communication plans, and elaborating communication strategies for their health campaigns and media messages. The director of communications of the US NGO Family Planning 2020, for instance, admitted that, after having worked for various decades with gender equality and SRHR in the US, it was only in the last five years that she began to take communications more seriously.[5] She also talked about the close links between the 'advocacy' and 'communications' teams around the construction of messages and media content on SRHR:[6]

> For a long time, there was no alignment on messaging. People said whatever their organisation wanted them to say. Consequently, the public perceptions of family planning were quite skewed because there was no common language ... In the last five years I would say people have gotten smarter ... and are being better about lining messages ... It is impossible to do communications without an eye towards advocacy. We have a wonderful person in the office ... so the two of us got to work together. The tools that we create are designed to drive advocacy, so it goes hand in hand ... So the advocacy goals around this, the results, have to do with ensuring that women's ability to choose what method that they may use is not narrowed by the results of this study, and in order to succeed in that, we needed to create good strong messages so that the communications community of practice is doing work at the moment to develop good top-line messaging, which we will then turn over to the advocacy team to disseminate and explain to all the advocacy people that they work with globally so that when the results of this clinical trial are announced, women are not hurt ... There is a misperception in the world that everyone can do communications ... But they do not understand that it is an art, in the same way that advocacy [is an art] ... It requires a certain level of knowledge and skill ... You know there is still a long way to go. I have seen a lot of organisations, particularly globally, if they have a small staff, communications is not representative.

The former CEO of CHANGE,[7] who is currently chief global advocacy officer at IPPRF WHR, also underlined how 'communications is the key to all advocacy'. She also explained how the area of 'advocacy' is being covered by communications:

I think that convening a piece of advocacy is so important, and this is covered by communications. It is creating safe spaces to try out new ideas, to have conversations, to bring together groups that typically do not come together, if it is convening just to share ideas. People are much more willing to come to the table together, and talk, so I think that has been an important strategy, that we talked about and used to advance SRHR, to really show. And these convening[s] are important, SRHR as well, whether it is to put together health advocates, or women peace and security advocates to really show how this framework is and to get more sectors to adopt this frame of work.

The coordinator and the executive director from the NGO Mujer y Salud both emphasised the central role that communications has had for advocacy on SRHR. Both provided very detailed information on how they use communications in their advocacy work and how this can be utilised for social change and for the advancement of progressive policies. According to them, it is important to examine *how* each message is going to be shown:

Being transversal, communication is one more dimension of all the activities that are carried out, even regarding advocacy. Communication must be carried out strategically so that we can give visibility to our political positions, but at the same time make them a translation of our field to reach all audiences. This implies an effort to work together with all areas of the organisation to maintain the essence and achieve a discourse with an accessible and clear rights approach. It is essential to emphasise that communication crosses all areas and works together because if the communicational products are not produced as a result of a process, we cannot have the necessary power and it becomes a service ... When we do advocacy, communication is essential, so we do the exercise of working on how we are going to show each message for the process and each action regarding political incidence ... Speeches and actions are defined according to the population to which you want to communicate, whether they are public officials ... and in turn to the objective that we have defined for each of them. The promotion of rights is fundamental. For this reason, communication works together with advocacy so that the political advances registered in the matter of rights in Uruguay that have been the result of ... the historical demand of social organisations can be defended.

Thus a key aspect of using communications for advocacy on such a complex topic as SRHR is *how* media content and messages need to be constructed and thought through carefully to ensure credibility and clarity within a global environment that is increasingly hostile towards gender and reproductive rights. A lot of communication content in SRHR seeks to persuade specific publics, including through the appeal to emotions and use of digital storytelling alongside reports and facts related to the public health argument. In the following chapters I examine these findings by discussing the content, and providing a critical discourse analysis, of the institutional websites, social media engagement, and the communication practices of the NGOs that participated in this research. This even when the messages put forward are supported by facts and endorsed by public health arguments and by medical evidence. Like other human rights NGOs, those working in the field use communication with different understandings of what this entails, adopting different practices, including restoring journalistic devices like 'fact checking' (McPherson 2015; Powers 2014) or simply sharing information and messages with the intention of generating impact.

Civic and human rights organisations compete for funds as much as they compete for media publicity and public attention (Powers 2014, 2017; Thrall, Stecula, and Sweet, 2014; McPherson 2015). They do this with communication strategies as well as through the use of online networks for advocacy, which is crucial for these organisations in their efforts to have their voices heard, influence policy, and reach targeted publics. Although digital technologies might have reduced the costs of distribution of information, working to assist in fundraising activities and mobilisation, they have not lowered the costs of producing information and the need to hire skilled people to produce media messages and content, particularly in areas that deal with complex global challenges that require sophisticated development programming and strategic thinking as well as communication campaigns.

In a further study that draws from Keck and Sikkink (1998), Thrall, Stecula, and Sweet (2014) examine the difficulties that NGOs have in engaging in publicity work within a highly competitive environment – one that seeks to gain 'media attention' as much as 'public engagement' for specific causes. McPherson (2017) alludes to Thrall, Stecula, and Sweet's (2014) study, which emphasises the existence of online inequalities and the ways in which organisations depend on resources for investment in media and communications. The budget of the NGOs that participated in this research, for instance, show that very few are in a position of surplus, with many reporting deficits or just barely managing. This attests to the fact that many of these organisations are not in principle profit-driven and do not use a lot of their communications to advocate for fundraising activities, as this research have shown.

Kingston and Stam (2013) state that, although NGOs engage with social media technologies, research has shown that many use the web to enhance already existing activities, thus being less likely to adopt creative new ones. Quoting Weberling (2012) on the use of email messages by large NGOs known for their advocacy work on women's health, Auger (2013) points to three types of messages that are most frequently used: *advocacy*, *fundraising*, and *news type*. She stresses how different rhetoric is employed for each of these: for example, advocacy is used to inspire logical decision making while fundraising is deployed to appeal to people's emotions. As I argue with regard to the differences between and the blurring of the boundaries between 'advocacy' and 'activism', including the ways in which facts can be used for advocacy and to persuade publics regarding particular issues (thus appealing to some emotional engagement with the cause), Weberling notes that advocacy messages often include 'facts': 'Advocacy messages included facts and figures and in depth information, while fundraising messages focused on hope' (Weberling 2012, 114 in Auger 2013, 371).

Lovejoy and Saxron (2012 in Auger 2013, 372) also found that NGOs' use of Twitter can be divided into three core functions: *information*, *action*, and *community*, while other research indicates that organisations are not using social media platforms like Facebook to their full potential (Waters et al. 2009 in Auger 2013, 372). This study contributes to some of these results, expanding on how advocacy communications can be used in accordance with different media channels as well as be inserted within a variety of contexts. This alludes to the fact that both traditional media and online communications can be combined to generate more impact. Arguably, the NGOs that work in this field operate within very difficult circumstances in which opposition from anti-choice, conservative, and populist groups has added pressure to their activities in an already highly competitive third-sector environment in which people's attention, commitment, and interest is scarce and uncertain (Thrall, Stecula, and Sweet 2014). Challenges range from the scarcity of resources to not always having public support for their causes.

NGO efforts with regard to advocacy communications in SRHR are thus inserted into larger struggles over meanings and discourses because these are ultimately connected to socially gendered norms and cultural practices, to specific political climates and economic contexts. Moreover, understanding around sexuality and reproductive health and rights is deeply intertwined with wider philosophical, religious, and moral questions pertaining to the role of motherhood, women's bodies and sexuality, infertility and reproduction. Advocacy for SRHR thus walks a thin line between adherence to the 'hard science' on the public health argument, on one side, and adherence to stronger feminist militancy around women's bodily autonomy, on the other. Thus, where 'advocacy' stops and (feminist) 'activism' begins can be difficult to identify with precision. It is to the empirical findings of the content analysis and the communication strategies and activities of these health and feminist NGOs that I turn next.

9

Content Analysis of Institutional Websites and NGO Communication Strategies

From Family Planning 2020 to Anis Brasil

Carolina Matos with Tatiane Leal

The responses from the interviews as well as from the communication questionnaires, combined with the results from the content analysis of the institutional websites of the NGOs and the critical discourse analysis of the social media engagement of these organisations on Twitter and Facebook, reveal great diversity in the use of communication strategies and practices as well as in the online communication tools for advocacy on sexual and reproductive health and rights. All the responses from the survey and the in-depth interviews confirm the difficulties of SRHR advocacy within a challenging climate of political and religious opposition as well as scarcity of funds for projects and investments in communications. Here I examine the results of the content analysis of the institutional websites; in the chapters to follow, I present the findings of the social media engagement of these organisations on Twitter and Facebook, including the results of the analyses of the blog samples.

The survey-style questionnaire applied to the communication experts of the organisations followed some aspects of the logics behind the factors shaping NGOs' advocacy communications work on SRHR. Participants were asked to outline their key principles and to indicate their offline communication activities, including what they had in their institutional websites (which was complemented by the content analysis of the institutional websites of the organisations), how long they had been using online communications, and which ones they preferred

(Facebook, Twitter, Instagram, etc). WhatsApp was not included as an option, although some organisations named this in the questionnaire's 'other' option. This was the case of the Latin American NGO Fundacion Desafio. The participants for the NGOs were also asked to respond to what type of challenges they encountered in advocating for SRHR, including what measures they set in place to deal with these difficulties. They were asked to name successful campaigns and the strategies used to compensate for lack of funds, whether they intended to invest in online communications and media activities. The representatives of the organisations were further asked to comment on their offline communication practices and whether they thought online communications was more effective than, or if it was a complement to, their engagement with the mainstream media.

The NGOs and networks whose members filled out the questionnaire were: Amnesty International UK and Argentina; Promsex; Coletivo de Salud Feminista; Family Planning 2020; Fundacion Desafio; Global Fund for Women; Ibis Reproductive Health; Ideosync; Inspire Euro NGO; International Planned Parenthood Federation; La Mesa por La Vida; Movimento Nacional das Cidadas Positivas; Muyer y Salud; Population Foundation of India; Reprolatina; Sexual and Reproductive Health; Swasti and Youth Coalition for Sexual and Reproductive Rights. A total of eighteen organisations answered the survey questionnaire only; another three did the interviews (CARE International UK, CHANGE, and YouAct); and Family Planning 2020 did both (i.e., filled out the questionnaire and participated in the in-depth interviews).

I here build on Powers' (2014) discussion of the components that shape civic NGOs' publicity and communication strategies, some of which resemble the news production processes in journalism (Waisbord 2015; McPherson 2014) (such as the focus on resources to desired impacts), to examine how the theoretical frameworks and epistemological positions are defended by the organisations and translated into their everyday communication practices (see table 9.1). The factors that shaped the organisational dynamics of the NGOs include: (1) *the feminist theorizations and approaches to sexual and reproductive health and rights*; (2) *the targeted publics*; (3) *the resources*, and (4) *the communication strategies adopted* (e.g., were these offline or online, or both?). Next to the 'factors', I add three rows, including 'information and communications', the 'intended outcomes', and the 'challenges' (e.g., of advocating for SRHR within the current geopolitical context of misinformation on women's health issues).

So the question that I ask is how the organisation's SRHR framework translates into its communication strategies and practices. This leads to the question of *how* this is presented (e.g., whether messages are used to 'deconstruct myths' as an intended outcome) as well as of how this is inserted within a series of challenges (e.g., attacks against a 'gender ideology' or the proliferation of 'fake news' on women's rights). In the case of the 'targeted publics', who are these (e.g., who is the organisation seeking to influence, media or policy-makers?), and, under 'information and communications', how can these have a wider impact (e.g., what are the intended outcomes)? Moreover, what are the challenges in reaching out to wider publics (e.g., engagement)? In terms of 'funding and resources', this has been divided into different types (e.g., fundraising or funds for advocacy work), and, in the case of 'communications', this includes the need for more investments. Regarding the use of communication strategies, this includes (1) determining whether this is offline (i.e., engagement with traditional media), (2) online, or (3) both. This is followed by the need to further embed communications in all of the organisations' policy and advocacy processes (the 'intended outcomes'), including the broader challenges that make communications in SRHR difficult and that require wider attention to language and discourses. This refers to the 'framing' and construction of the media messages in order to make them more accessible (e.g., through avenues such as entertainment-education formats). All these factors shape the information and communications used in SRHR as well as the organisations' intended outcomes and the various challenges that they face (see table 9.1).

The content analysis of the websites shows how organisations share extensive and detailed resources online, from papers and reports to videos. There was little use of online communication tools like Instagram and podcasts, some use of videos, and not a lot of sharing Plugin or LinkedIn. Video use was at 57.1 per cent, Instagram at 34.7 per cent, blogs at 36.7 per cent, and RSS/newsletters at 42.9 per cent, indicating that there is space, for instance, for the wider use of Instagram, which has become quite a popular social media platform with the younger audience and with social media influencers, as well as blogs. Unsurprisingly, the use of emails is quite high (87.8 per cent), while LinkedIn clocks in at 30.6 per cent, which could be seen as a high number for such a platform and an indication of its being increasingly adopted with the intention of 'branding' and taking care of the organisation's image, further building networks and partnerships.

Table 9.1
Factors shaping NGOs' SRHR communications strategies and advocacy

Factors	Information and communications	Intended outcomes	Challenges
1) SRHR framework	Single issue/ gender/health	Construct/ deconstruct SRHR	Understanding/ 'gender ideology'/ misinformation
2) Targeted publics	Media/policy/ 'general public'	Widen reach and impact	Engagement (emotion/reason)
3) Funding and resources	Fundraising/ lobby/ advocacy	More investments/ funding	Global Gag Rule/ under-funding of project/COVID-19
4) Communication activities	Online/offline	Embed comms. in policy	Language and discourse/accessible

Table 9.2 also shows the forty-nine NGOs examined and their web features, with the exception of the Brazilian organisations Acoes Afirmativas em Direto e Saude and Cidadas Positivas, as well as the European Inspire Euro, as these did not have their websites functioning at the time of analysis. The results show a strong presence on social media, with the organisations making use of social media platforms such as Facebook and Twitter for advocacy communications, with 100 per cent and 98 per cent for each, respectively. Some of these organisations are also among the most active on Twitter and Facebook, as I explore in the next chapter.

The total income, expenditure, and deficit/surplus figures of the top ten NGOs with the largest revenues appears in *Table 3* on the budget information of the organisations (see table 9.3). The revenue data are reported annually. Most organisations included information from 2018–19, except for International Planned Parenthood (2016) and Population Foundation of India (2017–18). There was also a disproportionate difference in budgets, and it was not possible to provide a fuller picture of all the organisations as those with fewer resources basically disappeared from the histogram. The table in appendix C further includes a total of twenty-two organisations, from the total of fifty-two, as these NGOs made their budget information available on their websites during the period of analysis (in alphabetical order and GBP).

As the table in appendix C indicates, those who appear in 'red' under the deficit/surplus section reported losses, while those in 'blue' had a surplus. The organisations that are listed in red include

Table 9.2
Forty-nine NGOS' web features

Website features*	Facebook	YouTube	Twitter	Emails	Instagram	Videos	Podcasts	RSS/ Updates/ Newsletter	Blogs	E-learning link	Discussion Forums/ Comments/ User's area	LinkedIn	Sharing plugins	Other
Akahatá	1	1	1	1	0	1	0	0	0	0	0	1	1	0
Amnesty International UK	1	1	1	1	1	1	0	0	1	0	0	0	0	0
Anis	1	1	1	1	1	1	0	0	0	0	1	0	0	0
Asap	1	1	1	1	1	1	0	1	1	1	0	0	0	0
Asia Pacific Alliance	1	0	1	1	0	0	0	1	1	0	0	0	0	0
Care International UK	1	0	1	1	1	0	0	0	1	0	0	1	0	0
Católicas pelo Direito de Decidir	1	1	1	1	0	1	0	0	0	0	0	0	0	1 (Flickr)
Center for Catalyzing Change India	1	1	1	0	0	0	0	0	1	0	0	0	0	0
Center for Health and Gender Equality (CHANGE)	1	0	1	1	0	1	0	1	1	0	0	0	0	0

Table 9.2
Forty-nine NGOS' web features (Continued)

Website features*	Facebook	YouTube	Twitter	Emails	Instagram	Videos	Podcasts	RSS/ Updates/ Newsletter	Blogs	E-learning link	Discussion Forums/ Comments/ User's area	LinkedIn	Sharing plugins	Other
Center for Reproductive Rights	1	1	1	1	0	0	0	1	0	0	0	0	1	0
Centro de Estudios de Estado y Sociedad de Argentina	1	1	1	1	0	0	0	1	0	0	0	0	0	0
Cepia	1	1	1	1	1	1	0	0	0	0	0	1	1	0
Cfemea	1	1	1	1	0	1	0	0	0	1 (Universidade livre feminista)	0	0	1	0
Colectivo de Salud Feminista	1	0	0	0	0	1	0	0	0	0	0	0	0	0
Consorcio latino-americano contra el aborto inseguro (CLACAI)	1	1	1	1	0	1	0	0	0	0	0	0	1	0
Crea India	1	1	1	0	0	1	0	1	1	0	0	0	0	0

Family Planning 2020	1	1	1	0	1	1	0	0	0	0	0
Feminismo Plural	1	0	1	1	1	0	1	0	0	0	0
Fundacion Desafio	1	1	1	1	0	0	0	0	0	1	0
Global Fund for Women	1	1	1	1	0	1	0	0	1	0	0
Guttmacher Institute	1	1	1	0	0	1	0	0	1	0	1 (Tumblr)
IAW (International Alliance of Women)	1	0	1	0	1	0	0	0	0	0	0
Ibis Reproductive Health	1	0	1	0	0	1	0	1	1	0	0
International Planned Parenthood Federation	1	0	1	1	1	1	1	0	1	1	1
La Mesa por la vida de las mujeres	1	1	1	1	0	0	0	0	0	1	0
CLADEM	1	1	1	0	0	1	0	0	0	0	0
Mujer y Salud Uruguay	1	1	1	1	0	0	1	1	0	0	1 (app)

Table 9.2
Forty-nine NGOS' web features (Continued)

Website features*	Facebook	YouTube	Twitter	Emails	Instagram	Videos	Podcasts	RSS/ Updates/ Newsletter	Blogs	E-learning link	Discussion Forums/ Comments/ User's area	LinkedIn	Sharing plugins	Other
Population Foundation of India	1	1	1	0	1	1	0	0	0	1	0	0	0	1 (Google Plus, now defunct)
Promsex - Centro de Promocion y Defensa de los Derechos Sexuales y reprodutivos	1	1	1	1	0	1	0	1	0	0	0	1	0	0
Realizing Sexual and Reproductive Justice (RESURJ)	1	1	1	1	1	0	0	0	0	0	0	0	0	1 (Vimeo)
Rede Feminista de Saúde, Direitos Sexuais e Reprodutivos	1	0	1	1	0	0	0	0	1	0	0	0	0	0

Reproductive health supplies coalition	1	1	1	0	1	1	0	1	0	1	0	1	0	0
Reprolatina	1	1	1	0	1	0	0	0	0	1	0	1	0	0
Safe Abortion Women's Rights	1	0	1	1	0	0	1	0	0	0	0	0	0	0
Sexual and Reproductive Health Matters (RHM)	1	0	1	0	0	1	1	1	0	1	0	1	0	0
Sexual Policy Watch	1	1	1	0	1	1	0	1	0	0	0	0	1	0
Sexual Rights Initiative (SRI)	1	0	1	0	0	1	0	0	0	0	0	0	0	0
SheDecides	1	0	1	1	0	0	0	0	0	1	0	0	0	0
Sos Corpo	1	1	1	0	1	1	0	0	0	0	0	0	0	0
Swasti	1	1	0	1	1	1	0	1	0	1	0	1	0	0
United Nations Population Fund	1	1	1	0	1	0	1	1	0	1	0	1	0	0
Universal Access Project	1	1	1	1	0	0	0	0	0	0	0	1	0	0

Table 9.2
Forty-nine NGOs' web features (Continued)

Website features*	Facebook	YouTube	Twitter	Emails	Instagram	Videos	Podcasts	Newsletter	RSS/ Updates/ Blogs	E-learning link	Discussion Forums/ Comments/ User's area	LinkedIn	Sharing plugins	Other
White Ribbon Alliance India	1	1	1	1	1	0	0	0	0	0	0	0	0	0
Women Deliver	1	1	1	1	0	1	0	0	1	0	0	1	1	0
Women's Global Network for Reproductive Rights	1	0	1	1	0	0	0	1	0	0	1	0	0	0
Women's Learning Partnership	1	0	1	1	0	0	0	1	1	1	0	1	0	0
Women's Link Worldwide	1	1	1	1	1	1	0	1	0	0	1	0	1	0
You Act	1	0	1	1	0	0	0	0	1	0	0	0	0	0
Youth Coalition for Sexual and Reproductive Rights	1	0	1	1	0	0	0	1	0	0	0	0	1	0
Total	49	33	48	43	17	28	3	21	18	5	4	15	13	5

*Inspire Euro, Movimento Nacional das Cidadãs Positivas e Ações Afirmativas em Direito e Saúde websites not found.

Akahata, CARE International UK, Guttmacher Institute, Ibis Reproductive Health, Swasti, and YouAct. Some of those with the largest budget, such as CARE, with 65.079.000.00, also reported a deficit of -1.803.000.00, while Guttmacher Institute appeared with 7.614.748.60 and with a deficit of -13.863.494.94. Some of those with a large income, such as Amnesty International UK (20.122.000.00), reported a surplus of 118.000.00, as well as the Centre for Reproductive Health, which reported 510.603.99, and the US's Global Fund Women, which reported 32.199.35. The organisation that appeared in the strongest position was International Planned Parenthood Federation (IPPF), with 197.812.547.87 and a surplus of 4.908.968.51, while Women Deliver (with 10.235.368.88) had a surplus of 3.652.630.39. IPPF is a global NGO with regional offices in Africa, the Americas and the Caribbean, Asia, the Arab World, and Europe. The data here also reveal what would be previously expected, mainly that most of these organisations have a relatively small surplus, operating with some level of annual deficit. The findings also show a low level of use of communications for fundraising activities and for lobbying in contrast to a wider use of media activities for advocacy communications on reproductive health, particularly for activities such as engagement and mobilisation.

The organisations had links to their vision and mission statements, in which they clearly stated their approach to SRHR. The exceptions here are CEPIA, La Mesa, and Centro de Estudos de Estado y Sociedade de Argentina. Most organisations expressed a commitment to a human rights framework on SRHR, situated within wider concerns with advancing women's rights and seeking gender equality and social justice on sexual and reproductive rights and on 'women's empowerment'. Most focused on all areas of sexual and reproductive health, with a few being more issue-focused, particularly on safe abortion and family planning (e.g., Movimento Nacional Cidadaes Positivas – HIV, Population Foundation of India, Family Planning, ASAP, and Safe Abortion Women's Rights).

As explained in the methods section, the communication practices of the NGOs were examined through a focus on the type of communications activities. This led to adding five categories to the codebook as a means of sorting out the data – *information, advocacy, community engagement, fundraising and resources,* and *mobilisation.* Under each of these five categories, five to seven subcategories were developed to make sense of the diversity of the communication material collected

Table 9.3
Budget information of ten largest organisations

NGO budget (GBP)	Period	Total income	Total expenditure	Yearly surplus/deficit
International Planned Parenthood Federation	1 January–31 December 2016	97,812,547.87	-92,903,579.00	4,908,968.51
Care International UK	1 July 2018–30 June 2019	65,079,000.00	-66,882,000.00	-1,803,000.00
Center for Reproductive Rights	1 July 2018–30 June 2019	26,337,046.04	-25,866,442.05	510,603.99
Amnesty International UK	1 January–31 December 2018	20,122,000.00	-20,004,000.00	118,000.00
Global Fund for Women	1 July 2018–30 June 2019	14,197,774.39	-14,165,575.04	32,199.35
Women Deliver	1 January–31 December 2018	10,235,368.88	-6,582,738.49	3,652,630.39
Guttmacher Institute	1 January–31 December 2018	7,614,748.60	-21,478,243.54	-13,863,494.94
White Ribbon Alliance India	1 January–31 December 2018	5,692,049.51	-3,003,539.33	2,688,510.18
Population Foundation of India	1 April 2017–31 March 2018	3,236,807.95	-2,656,567.36	580,240.59
Ibis Reproductive Health	1 July 2018–30 June 2019	3,102,580.62	-5,009,772.65	-1,907,192.03

for communications advocacy on SRHR. This included the information and communications material put out by each NGO during the period of analysis, both on the online platform and offline. This was further complemented by the responses given in the questionnaire and in the interviews. To identify the presence of each category, a specific sheet in the codebook included the organisations on one side and the categories/subcategories on the other, with a '1' given when the presence of the category was detected and a '0' when it was absent. This was done by combining the data from the results of the content analysis of the institutional websites with the responses given by the communication professionals.

Most of the organisations showed themselves to be active in all five categories. Amnesty International showed presence in all categories (ticking all the boxes and receiving a '1'), whereas other NGOs were stronger on 'information', like CHANGE and the Centre for Reproductive Rights. Organisations like the Global Fund for Women scored more strongly in the categories of 'fundraising' and 'mobilisation', and less in 'information'. These results are in alignment with the NGOs' aims. Some of the smaller organisations focused more on the 'advocacy' category (with a series of activities such as information and campaigns, conduct of events and workshops) as well as on 'community engagement'. This was the case of Akahata, for instance.

Not surprisingly, however, the findings show that the most active organisations on social media, specifically on Twitter and Facebook, are the same ones that use communications across all categories. These include the Centre for Reproductive Health, Family Planning 2020, Global Fund for Women, Guttmacher Institute, International Planned Parenthood Federation, Fundacion Desafio, La Mesa, and Muyer y Salud. This was also the case of Amnesty International, which made use of press releases and information (under the 'information' category) and ticked all the boxes in all of the subcategories for 'advocacy' and 'community engagement', from the realization of events and campaigns to discussion forums and workshops. The Brazilian NGO Anis also scored quite strongly on 'information', some 'advocacy' activity (information and discussion forums were the most popular subcategories), as well as on 'community engagement' (through workshops and events).

Table 9.4 gives the thirteen most active organisations on Twitter and Facebook (Inspire Euro had to be excluded as it did not have an active website) while table 9.5 gives the six most active. In order to develop the two graphs below, data were selected concerning the organisation's media engagement on Twitter and Facebook. Comparing these tables, it was possible to identify the fourteen most active organisations on these platforms (Amnesty International UK, Anis, Asia Pacific Alliance, Centre for Reproductive Rights, CEPIA, CREA India, Family Planning 2020, Global Fund for Women, Guttmacher Institute, Inspire Euro NGOs, Promsex, Sexual and Reproductive Health Matters, Sexual Policy Watch, and Women Deliver). The six most active organisations are CREA India, Center for Reproductive Rights, Global Funding for Women, Promsex, and Women Deliver. As table 9.4 (thirteen NGOs) and table 9.5 (six NGOs) show, there is a growing use of videos (61.5 per cent and 66.6 per cent, respectively), whereas when it comes to blogs, the percentage is slightly lower, at 46.2 per cent and 33.3 per cent, respectively. However, this indicates a pattern of increasing use of blogs for advocacy around SRHR.

The use of communications can be seen as operating very much in a *one-way flow* process, judging by the low percentage registered in the discussion forums and comments (7.7 per cent and 16.6 per cent, respectively). This attests to the need for organisations to engage in more communicative dialogue and discussion with their targeted publics, as well as with the wider public, when it comes to SRHR. YouTube, however, proved to be a popular platform for engagement with the younger audience, registering 84.6 per cent use among the top thirteen organisations and 100 per cent among the six most active NGOs. Instagram emerged as another platform that showed potential growth, registering a use of 38.5 per cent among the top thirteen NGOs and 50 per cent among the top six (see tables 9.4 and 9.5, respectively).

From the graphs it is clear that digital communications is mostly associated with the social media platforms Facebook and Twitter, followed by YouTube, emails, and videos.[1] According to the results of the communications questionnaire, in the category 'fundraising and resources', many included 'donations' and 'funding', with the use of communications to 'lobby politicians' or 'policy-makers' being less frequently identified. This was not the case of Akhata, Amnesty International, Anis, CARE International UK, Católicas pelo Direito de Decidir, Global Fund for Women, Guttmacher Institute, IAW, and Mujer y Salud. Not all of these listed campaigns that they organise; however, many indicated that they do have them. Again, this was the case for some of the larger and more well-known NGOs as well as

Table 9.4
Thirteen NGOs' web features and social media engagement

Website features	Facebook	YouTube	Twitter	Emails	Instagram	Videos	Podcasts	RSS/ Updates/ Newsletter	Blogs	E-learning link	Discussion Forums/ Comments/ User's area	LinkedIn	Sharing plugins	Other
Amnesty International UK	1	1	1	1	1	1	0	0	1	0	0	0	0	0
Anis	1	1	1	1	1	1	0	0	0	0	1	0	0	0
Asia Pacific Alliance	1	0	1	1	0	0	0	1	1	0	0	0	0	0
Center for Reproductive Rights	1	1	1	1	0	0	0	1	0	0	0	0	1	0
Cepia	1	1	1	1	1	1	0	0	0	0	0	1	1	0
Crea India	1	1	1	0	0	1	0	0	1	0	0	0	0	0
Family Planning 2020	1	1	1	1	0	1	0	1	1	0	0	0	0	0
Global Fund for Women	1	1	1	1	1	1	0	1	0	0	0	1	0	0
Guttmacher Institute	1	1	1	1	0	0	0	1	0	0	0	1	0	1 (Tumblr)

Table 9.4
Thirteen NGOs' web features and social media engagement (Continued)

Website features	Facebook	YouTube	Twitter	Emails	Instagram	Videos	Podcasts	Newsletter	RSS/ Updates/ Blogs	E-learning link	Discussion Forums/ Comments/ User's area	LinkedIn	Sharing plugins	Other
Promsex - Centro de Promocion y Defensa de los Derechos Sexuales y reprodutivos	1	1	1	1	0	1	0	1	0	0	0	1	0	0
Sexual and Reproductive Health Matters (RHM)	1	0	1	1	0	0	0	1	1	0	0	1	0	0
Sexual Policy Watch	1	1	1	1	0	1	0	1	0	0	0	0	1	1
Women Deliver	1	1	1	1	1	0	1	0	1	0	0	1	1	0

Table 9.5
Six NGOs' web features and social media engagement

Website features	Facebook	YouTube	Twitter	Emails	Instagram	Videos	Podcasts	Newsletter	RSS/ Updates/ Blogs	E-learning link	Discussion Forums/ Comments/ User's area	LinkedIn	Sharing plugins	Other
Anis	1	1	1	1	1	1	0	0	0	0	1	0	0	0
Center for Reproductive Rights	1	1	1	1	0	0	0	1	0	0	0	0	1	0
Crea India	1	1	1	0	0	1	0	0	1	0	0	0	0	0
Global Fund for Women	1	1	1	1	1	1	0	1	0	0	0	1	0	0
Promsex - Centro de Promocion y Defensa de los Derechos Sexuales y reprodutivos	1	1	1	0	1	1	0	1	0	0	0	1	0	0
Women Deliver	1	1	1	1	0	1	1	0	1	0	0	1	1	0

the more active-led ones (Ações, Amnesty International, ASAP, Asia, CARE, Católicas pelo Direito de Decidir, Centre for Catalysing Change, CHANGE, Centre for Reproductive Health, CEPIA, CREA India, Global Fund Women, and Fundacion). Most made use of the same type of communications, such as policy reports, publications, press releases, and media articles.

The strategic use of communications to present a particular view on SRHR, one that aligns with both the organisation's image and its mission, with the intention of emphasising its credibility to stakeholders and to the public, was something that a few NGOs clearly stated that they engaged in. It could be argued that some of the advocacy communications work of the NGOs on SRHR could overlap with the 'branding' of the organisation and how it seeks to portray itself. This was the case with CARE International UK and with the US organisations CHANGE and Family Planning 2020. Both the former CEO of CARE International UK and its head of communications commented on some of the CARE's priorities in the field of sexual and reproductive health, within the wider framework of combating poverty and gender inequalities.

The former CEO of CARE International UK emphasised the adaptation of language and communications around SRHR according to the particularities of local contexts,[2] underlining the private-public partnerships and the relationship with governments and health providers in some of the countries of the Global South in which CARE operates. Like other larger NGOs working with SRHR within the humanitarian or international development field, the main work that CARE does is in family planning, making contraception available. Some would question the focus on this area for, as we have seen, there is some controversy within international development concerning SRHR's emphasis on fertility, which is seen as rooted within the Malthusian framework of equating sexual and reproductive health with 'birth control' and the need to engage with this as a way of combatting poverty and inequality.

However, this is far from the full picture, as contraception and family planning remain part of the wider discussions concerning SRHR throughout the world and are closely connected to issues of gender inequality, women's autonomy, and better access to reproductive health. Despite differences in political perspectives, funding, resources, and focus, NGOs share many similarities, whether they are larger organisations or grassroots and activist-led – for example, common concerns, terminology, and emphasis on the 'empowerment' of women and their agency in developing countries.

The former CEO of CARE International UK further underlined the attention given to language pertaining to SRHR in accordance with specific local contexts:

> No, it is [i.e., SRHR] a very big part of our programming. And that it is because we see it as so fundamental for women's empowerment in general and to gender equality. If women who do not have access to contraception and the right and practical ability to have kids, you know, a lot of another empowerment is impossible ... And we in the past had many programmes in India, but also quite a lot in West Africa, which is a long way behind in terms of access to contraception ... [What] we have done in India ... where a group might be a long away from expert doctors, is have a kind of mobile system whereby the community health workers have a mobile phone ... There are lots of numbers when they are visiting a patient, they can download a number and listen to expert advice ... Our approach is that we might tweak our language in different places. It is partly about not being misunderstood, knowing that words carry ... different meanings ... And it is partly about not being heard at all ... And the fact that we are a confederation ... and part of our structure is that there is room for variety in the way that it is described ... So I think you know you will see us turning at the family planning summit hearing in London, possibly using much more global kind of language ... the emphasis is still to bring SRHR services to people who have least access ... So in parts of Bangladesh, where the government system does not really reach at all, the way we work with government is training private health providers to the same standard that the government would have ... making sure there is referral into the government system for more serious cases ... But essentially it is doing things like the government would do ... but in places where the government is not reaching ... Is it about attitudes of women in the home? Is it about attitudes of community leaders? Is it about resources in the health sector? ... And you can design programmes that try to address that ... So we see advocacy in that sense ... and I guess we use whatever communications tools will work for a particular advocacy strategy in a particular place.

Regarding the use of communications for SRHR advocacy, the head of communications stated that there is a team of six people who cover social media, websites, press and PR, communications, and events.[3] This does not include digital advertising, which is done by a separate team responsible for social media posts. She admitted that the field of SRHR has not been a priority in their press work and has been even less of a focus for their advocacy activities. She also pointed to the ways in which communications is seen as key to the construction of the CARE 'brand':

> There isn't like a gender equality group, if you see what I mean ... They may be regionally specific or globally specific ... so my understanding is that a lot of the SRHR, some of the best work done has been really focusing on some of the advocacy work done in the US ... As I say, SRHR specifically has not been a top priority for our press and PR work. It is been one that we have covered a lot, in fundraising, in human interest stories, but it has been less of a specific focus for our advocacy, except perhaps in emergencies ... So there is some support for SRHR, but I think there needs to be a job to be done to make people realise that this is a key issue in emergency response in development programmes. As I said, you almost take it for granted, the ability to manage your birth control ... Within digital, we want to have a network of people on social media who are engaged ... They are talking to us, and to each other in conversation ... On our many websites we want to tell people what CARE is. We want ... to inspire them to raise funds or give money. And then we have a third area of digital, which is a policy and programme's website, and that is very much talking to the second audiences, and especially the third sector and the government. We are not looking for huge figures on that website ... Facebook ... is changing a lot these things ... At the moment we are using it less for advocacy pieces and more essentially for fundraising, who we are, and human interest stories ... Instagram, very much human messages so very powerful images, and for that we draw across the board ... Image-led, human-led, sometimes like slogans, so trying to set out who we are as an organisation, and perhaps being set apart from the advocacy campaign ... So while communications can change opinion, as you say, it is critical in raising awareness,

critical in *brands*, people might know us and they might give money, critical in raising brands across the sector, so other agencies want to work with you, so the donors want to fund your projects.

Another organisation that stressed its advocacy communications work in SRHR, and its connection to the 'brand' itself, was the US organisation CHANGE. Its head of communications explained how it engages with the topic and how it is looking for ways to make this more accessible to the public:[4]

Yeah, that is a challenge that we are facing, and we have talked a lot through our re-brand, to make sexual and reproductive health and rights more accessible ... because it is a complex issue ... The public is not familiar with the terminology, what I have been trying to do since my time is to try to break down how we communicate with our topics in our way which is plain language ... When I joined they were in the process of developing a strategy for communications ... I worked with them to finalize that ... And in communications this falls into our impact model, so we have four areas ... advocacy, conveying, research and policy analysis, and strategic communications ... With the conversations with the organisation at the time, we got four goals to achieve through our strategy: our first goal in our strategic communications plan is to strike in our activism to advance SRHR rights globally ... One of the big projects is a big focus for our communications team [and] is actually re-branding the organisation ... and how our community and our target audiences understand who we are and what we do ... We also prioritize our target audiences, and as I look through them they are listed in order of priority, our primary audience is US policy-makers, opinion leaders, US-based organisations, global organisations, our current donors ... As you were saying with advocacy, certainly the most immediate way we are able to do that is via social media in real time, we do that individually as an organisation ... We identify those opportunities and amplify across all of our channels, whether it be participating in a Twitter storm, or doing a joint statement ... Obviously communications ... is the key to all advocacy ... Since my time here we have been trying to build on our existing presence, on some social media platforms we do not have really a solid following, that continues to grow on Twitter and we have a hectic following on Facebook ... LinkedIn and Instagram are growing ... Most of our interaction with the public has been of pushing messages, rather than pushing and pulling messaging, so it has not been like a two-way conversation.

The feminist and health organisations and networks interviewed here acknowledged the importance of online communications for advocacy, despite having underlined the limits of online media. Many stated that offline lobbying, or face-to-face advocacy with stakeholders or decision-making people, was more 'effective' than online tools, but they nonetheless signalled to the possibility of combining the two and making use of online communications to reinforce their reach and generating more impact. Many claimed that their online communications were 'very effective' or 'somewhat effective'. The categories that received ticks were 'mobilisation' and 'information'. Amnesty International Argentina considered online communications to be 'somewhat effective' for advocacy, community engagement, mobilisation, and information. The South Asian organisation Centre for Catalysing Change in India chose the option 'very effective' for advocacy and information, whereas Swasti underlined the same option for advocacy but indicated that it was 'not effective' for fundraising and community engagement. Both CHANGE and Family Planning 2020 chose 'very effective' for advocacy, engagement, mobilisation, and information, whereas Ibis Reproductive Health chose it for all of them. The latter organisation also selected the option 'more effective than offline lobbying', whereas La Mesa indicated that 'both are combined', stating that online communication was 'more effective' than offline lobbying.

In terms of targeted publics that the organisations seek to influence through their online/offline communications, the options given on the questionnaire included networking and building connections, the goal of influencing policy-makers, politicians, the media, or public opinion. There was also the option of choosing 'all of the above'. Most, however, included the options 'influence policy-makers' and 'public opinion'. Some included 'networking and connections', 'influence politicians', 'influence the media', or 'all of the above'. This was the case of organisations like Ibis, Inspire, International Planned Parenthood Federation, La Mesa, Mujer y Salud and Reprolatina. The South Asians Asia Pacific, ASAP, and Centre for Catalysing Change opted for 'influencing policy-makers' and 'public opinion', whereas CHANGE included 'politicians' and 'the media', opting for 'all of the above'. Other organisations that also selected 'all the above' for the targeted publics included Ibis, Inspire, La Mesa, Muyer y Salud, White Ribbon Alliance, YouAct, and Youth Coalition.

Most if not all the NGOs opted for 'b' and 'd' on the question on the use of offline communication media ('press releases and contact with media and journalists' and 'face-to-face conversations with affected participants and stakeholders', respectively). The option on the 'need for more investment' in communications was also quite popular. It was underlined by practically all the organisations, from the larger ones to the more grassroots and/or issue-based, with many indicating their intention of expanding the use of online networks. Some of the measures proposed and considered essential ranged from the hiring of more staff to the adoption of a wider set of communication tools.

Various NGOs also included the embedding of communications in their future strategic plans, underlining a wider need to connect policy to advocacy processes. Amnesty International Argentina stated it seeks to make use of all forms of online communication tools, underlining the difficulties it has with communications within the growing political polarisation around SRHR. On the question on their key principles, the head of press and communications wrote that this entails planning the year 'in coordination with all the areas ... Communications is a 'Cross' area, so our plan is fed by the contents of the different ... areas.'[5] She also highlighted that online communications is not necessarily more effective, depending very much on the issue tackled. It was the only organisation to have answered 'no' on the need for more resources, indicating, however, the desire to attend more to online communications. Among the key communication and interactive features included were 'urgent and cyber actions, support AIAR, access to media channels' and 'youth participation.'[6] The NGO also made use of all online communication tools and social media platforms; however, it viewed the latter as 'somewhat effective'. It makes use of these digital tools to 'create awareness around the topic for the public' as well as to influence 'the media and public opinion.'

The head of the communications campaigns for Amnesty International UK explained in her response to the questionnaire the centrality of communications in achieving the organisation's aims.[7] She underlined how there is a 'need for a strong and clear unified message about human rights, a constant message about the things that define us as human beings':

> Communications is a vital mechanism for achieving our aims (not just a way of *saying what we've done,* but vital to achieving our goals) – we don't communicate to talk about the change we make in the world. We communicate to make change happen.

Amnesty International UK makes use of all online communication tools, with a preference for Facebook, Twitter, Instagram, and emails. The head also indicated how the use of social media for SRHR advocacy can result in attempts at intimidation and censorship on the part of oppositional groups, stating that the organisation receives 'negative backlash, trolling in comments'. 'We've seen this especially in relation to communications around sex worker rights, abortion rights, and trans rights', she wrote. It also wants to 'avoid confrontation', aiming to 'positively promote our message', with the top priority in communications being to protect 'the rights holders who we are speaking with and advocating for' and using them in a manner that 'keeps them [i.e., rights holders] safe and does not put them in difficult situations'.

The programme manager of women's rights at Amnesty International UK emphasised what she saw as an important role that traditional media should have in seeking to better understand the historical struggles for women's rights across the world, including in reproductive health:

> I think the media needs to be better educated on women's struggles and basically understand that rights cannot be taken for granted. The connections between SRHR and bodily autonomy, and women's status in society, and why some women are more scrutinised than others in their bodies and in their choices, and how that connects to pressure systems like racism. There needs to be much more recognition that women's achievements have come through struggle. For example, last year [2018] it was one hundred years since the first women in the UK won the right to vote, and there were celebrations of the suffragettes everywhere. The government put money for the celebrations across the country ... And now we have women imprisoned in Saudi Arabia who want to drive ... Women have had to fight, we see that in the US with the change in the

administration ... And I think there is still this white supremacy idea here, of superiority, that says 'we are better, we treat women better here'. We have gender equality etc. That fuels the argument, what about the men? The only benchmark is the white middle-class straight professional women rather than looking at what is going on in our own country. The movements are using that to find themselves in the global struggle.

As mentioned in previous chapters, organisations are beginning to make more use of WhatsApp's technology, particularly in Latin America. The organisation based in Ecuador, Fundacion Desafio, strongly emphasised how it makes use of WhatsApp as a digital communications tool for advocacy on reproductive health. The director of the NGO answered the communications questionnaire and stated that the aim is to position Foundacion 'before the community, the media, social networks and financing and human rights organisations as a reference institution, with its own institutional identity and image'.[8] This is done through the dissemination of vital information to the targeted groups, from 'women, youth, decision-makers' to 'politicians, social, feminist, and human rights organisations'. She also mentioned that Fundacion Desafio has someone who specifically 'produces daily messages, slides, videos according to the situation and according to the projects that are being executed'. Like other NGOs, it has been making use of online communications in the last five to ten years, growing its presence on social media. It further aims to provide information related to 'research, training, and political advocacy actions'.[9]

Like Brazil's Reprolatina and some other South Asian organisations, Fundacion Deasfio was one of the few to specifically stress the limits of digital communications due to its lack of reach in poorer rural communities. The director sees this as a barrier to the wider dissemination of accurate knowledge about SRHR. Despite this, the organisation makes use of *all* forms of online communications, considering these to be more effective than traditional lobbying. It would like to invest more in communications, underlining that the combination of several 'different instruments' is the 'key to their success'. This includes using Instagram to reach out to young people and Twitter to reach out to the adult population, including decision-makers and politicians. The use of YouTube is also seen as useful for broadcasting longer videos or life stories. As she further wrote:

> It seems to me that if there is enough information, perhaps access to a smart device, a smartphone, could be an obstacle. In Ecuador 30 percent of the population is young, therefore they must have access to information. The excluded and poor population groups can have obstacles, having a cell phone, for example, is not a guarantee of access. In this field I believe that women of mature or 'older' ages may have less access to information ... The issue of abortion is undoubtedly a space that needs to be worked in greater depth ... The issue of sexuality, the right to pleasure and the possibilities of self-care to avoid infections is important ... Access to information in this field is very important ... The Foundation executes its projects in the provinces that are far from the political centrality of Quito ... We communicate through WhatsApp, which is a good form of communication ... and transmission of a lot of information as well as coordination of actions.

The programme director of Global Fund Women talked about the fear of visibility and the threats posed to activists working in the field. Like the director of Fundacion Desfio, she also identified the potential of the use of WhatsApp technology for advocacy communications on reproductive health:

> I think that yes, activists are fearful. We are talking about individual lives, when we see murders and executions and forced disappearances ... it becomes very real. If you are a face of the movement, you will be under threat. There is definitely fear of visibility ... I think that also women's movements are using technologies to the extent that they can, I believe that funding is an issue, but they use it to create a network, and to create those spaces where they can continue to strategize across their movements ... and utilize whatever social media and communication technologies that they can ... For example, WhatsApp is a way I communicate with so many people, people use it all the time, people use it to provide information, at the same time, it is not secure, when we are looking at Facebook ... So women are moving to other forms of technology. I think what is interesting, not only from a communications perspective, we need to think ... not just about women and girls utilizing it, but also, we need to think of *how* women and girls can get more control

of it ... Of course these communication tools have been dominated and operated by men. Right there and then we are going to see a gender gap, and it is the Global North, black and brown people in the South who do not have the control of these ... We are starting an initiative just in Kenya to talk about these issues, to support women's organisations.

The communications regional adviser for Latin America and the Caribbean from LAC UNFPA also noted how digital communications has facilitated the inclusion of the rights framework into the everyday conversations about SRHR:

The declaration of the consensus of Cairo, the consensus of the international population and development, said population is not about numbers, it is about people. So we need to look at the holistic approach ... the rights of the human being, everything that surrounded the human being in terms of what it is to live ... At that moment, when we introduced the terminology of 'reproductive health and rights', and that is very well understood by technical people, but for the overall public, that is something that does not sit ... There is a lack of understanding of a very substantive and technical language ... Since 1994, we have been doing a series of *advocacy* work ... gaining a sense among the public what this term is. However, in the last ten years, since 2010, 2009, because of the advent of the internet ... in different societies, communication means that the word we brought was adapted to sexual rights, the work of rights has been more adapted to the ... daily conversation in everything that we do. Rights to education, rights to migration ... The public has a very good and strong understanding of the terminology on rights.

Some organisations included the investment in communications as part of their strategic plan. This was the case, for example, with Ibis Reproductive Health. The communications lead of the organisation pointed out that a key aim was to ensure the wide dissemination of its research.[10] The NGO develops specific websites for projects; however, it also admitted that online communication platforms like YouTube are still little used, while Instagram is slowly expanding. Similar to organisations like CHANGE, Ibis sees an increase in the level of public discourse and debate around SRHR. This can be seen as a good opportunity for health and other feminist NGOs in the field to push for change. At the same time, this raises challenges, such as the need to ensure that 'evidence-based, information is disseminated by the media' to other policy-makers globally.

Ibis also stated that online communications is 'very effective' and can involve more than traditional lobbying with politicians. The organisation's core offline communication activities include contact with media and journalists, and face-to-face discussions and meetings with the participants that are affected. In the questionnaire, Ibis's communications lead stated:

> In our five-year strategic plan, we have identified as a goal the expansion of our communications in order to increase our impact and reach. To achieve this ... we will need to identify additional resources, including by building dissemination/communication into research grant proposals and pursing communication-specific funding opportunities ... Funders invest in NGOs communications and we need to ensure that NGOs have the capacity/training/staffing to effectively use online communications in the SRHR sphere.

Like CARE International UK, one of the larger organisations, Ibis also has six people on its communications staff. According to the communications lead, they regularly post news and announcements, as well as research projects and supporting materials, on their website and update the 'principal partnerships'. They also use all communication tools and social media platforms, particularly Facebook, Twitter, and Instagram, and consider online communications to be 'very effective'. She stated that they aim to use online communications for all of the options provided, from the intent to create awareness to the exerting of influence. The communications lead argued that communications around SRHR could be more effective if people could find more 'evidence-based information online from trustworthy sources' and engage in 'lifting up the voices of impacted communities through research and campaigns.' Among the campaigns mentioned were 'Free the Pill',[11] operated with the aim of 'educating and engaging the public' in support of an over-the-counter birth control option in the US. For its part, Mmoho uses a 'positive, rights-based approach to advocate for comprehensive and accessible SRH services for young people in Southern Africa'.[12]

The communications lead for Ibis went on to underscore the challenges for advocacy communications within the current geopolitical context, emphasising the need to build 'stronger relationships with the media':

> The level of public discourse around SRHR continues to increase, especially as the current US administration continues to impose restrictions and create barriers to people exercising their human right to live ... a healthy sexual and reproductive life. This increase in conversation presents a greater challenge in ensuring evidence-based information is disseminated by the media, advocates, policy-makers ... Yes, unfortunately there is a lot of misinformation, lack of knowledge and understanding, and prejudice related to sexual and reproductive health ... This is evident in media reporting, which is why having a strong earned media strategy is so important ... It's also very clear based on conversations happening on social media ... We have also found a lack of knowledge about SRH among participants in our research studies ... We continue to enhance our earned media strategy to leverage the current social and political environment in the US and around the world, want to build and strengthen our relationships with the media, to insert evidence-based information into broader cultural conversations. We continue to enhance our use of digital media to more effectively reach and engage our key audiences around our bold, rigorous research and advocacy to advance policy and service-delivery solutions that transform people's reproductive lives.

Most of the organisations responded that they have been working with communications 'for the last five to ten years', with only a few indicating that they worked with volunteers. The communications specialist from the NGO Global Fund for Women stated that among their key aims was to 'extend the reach and influence of the organisation', as well as to 'strengthen the movements to adhere to women's human rights and accelerate fundraising'.[13] Key communication features that were stressed included the use of news articles, statements, and press releases, and the signing up to newsletter buttons and donation links. The organisation constantly updates its website and social media, making use of all communications tools, particularly Facebook, Twitter, and Instagram. It sees online media as being 'very effective', although, like other organisations, it recognises the limits of their reach.

Emphasising the Global Fund for Women's appeal to both 'intellect' and 'emotion' in its advocacy communications work, its communications specialist underlined the key difficulties in advocating around SRHR within a growing climate of 'censorship' and crackdowns on the internet on sex education material. She underscored the efforts of the NGO to transcend these challenges:

> Educating the audience; finding relevant calls to action; making connections for US audiences to international issues … All include helpful information about SRHR: our website articles, which are creative, story-driven campaigns, news-driven, explaining core work that we do. Social media posts with website article content. E-mails (movement news …) with fundraising appeals. We hope to appeal to both intellect and emotion to understand these issues. We seek to change attitudes so that we hold up women's voices so they can be heard … Sexuality-related content has been the subject of removal and crackdown on the internet (e.g., Instagram, FB … all blocking 'sexually explicit' material; shutdown of Backdoor; blocking of sex workers on social media while white supremacists have been allowed to organize and find audiences with little pushback) – all this … points to upcoming crackdowns on sex education.

The NGO Inspire, formerly known as EuroNGOs, the European Partnership for Sexual and Reproductive Health and Rights, admitted that all three members of its staff participate in the communication process, with funds being sought for other activities. Inspire emphasised in its response to the communication questionnaire that one of its key objectives is to 'create spaces where organisations can meet'. The lead of Inspire noted that its main aim is to use social media to communicate with the public,[14] attempting to be more 'inclusive' and to bring more men into the conversation. Inspire did not classify itself as an 'advocacy organisation' but, rather, as an NGO whose purpose is to organise conferences with the community, 'to provide a space for people, from funders to policy-makers, to strategize and get together'. She also outlined the strategies used to secure wider 'inclusivity':

So our key principles, I would say, are to (1) create content and communicate, (2) not being political (in terms of advocacy), and (3) being available and accessible for all ... We use social media accounts to communicate with the public ... But the thing we do the most is go to the place to get information, what are the trends, statistics ... And we make sure to be inclusive, for example, because we know it's not a women's issue, so we try not to exclude men ... We organize conferences, it's one of the main things ... All the topics that are hot in the community right now, people go there to be inspired about new ideas ... As we are not an advocacy organisation, we try to focus on creating the space where the exchange can happen ... Even inside the bubble people tend to default back to 'it's a women's issue' ... Men also need to have information about gender-based violence ... We try to make sure we are inclusive in videos and posts we make ... We try to feature the less featured groups to make sure we are inclusive in our communications ... Maybe it's about breaking the bubble, but I am not sure what's the strategy for that, maybe collaboration with organisations that reach greater audiences, but I am not sure I have a solution ... I think communications are more visual than they used to be ... It's not necessarily a challenge but it's formatting the news in a way that is picked up. But also, to make sure we don't lose ourselves in Facebook and Twitter because the face-to-face interactions that we create for our members are the most valuable thing.

Working with three communications professionals and one intern, Inspire was one of the few NGOs that admitted to 'monitoring the traffic on its website' through analytical tools in order to see how people spend time with information. It sees online communications as being 'somewhat effective' and makes full use of digital communications, particularly Facebook and Twitter. It stated, however, that 'face-to-face' communications was more effective. Its lead also admitted that a key challenge on social media is still to go 'beyond the bubble' and to engage with people beyond the 'already converted'.

The communications manager for Sexual and Reproductive Health Matters (SRHM),[15] previously known as Reproductive Health Matters, talked about how the organisation aims, above all, to be a source of trustworthy knowledge. Its objective is to combine research with advocacy, building partnerships as well as making use of communication opportunities to inspire and generate knowledge about SRHR. The organisation does this by using peer-reviewed and rights-based evidence as an advocacy tool, which it sees as a way of engaging a global policy discussion on the topic. She also stated in the questionnaire that the communications staff is composed of two consultants and one intern, with the main forms of offline communications being the press releases and face-to-face contact. Blogs are extensively used.

When it comes to online communications, all forms are used, with Inspire defining this as being 'somewhat effective'. It is used mainly to influence key actors, including the media. Popular social media platforms are not only Twitter and Facebook but also YouTube videos, emails, and blogs. She also underscored the importance of working with the mainstream media to raise the visibility of reproductive health. Although the question about misinformation and prejudice towards SRHR was not answered, she admitted difficulties in advocacy work, including in the effective creation of communication content. Among the challenges encountered, the need to 'educate the audience' and to 'change attitudes' was highlighted, as was the centrality of making connections to permit US audiences to understand issues, including fundraising. She discussed the need for more resources, underlining the strategies used to compensate for lack of funds, such as the dependency on the work of interns:

> Understanding where to reach different advocates for different issues within SRHR and creating material which can be used in advocacy effectively ... I think that working with mainstream media is an important method for ... gaining visibility for the evidence in question ... While knowledge generation and transfer are essential in advancing SRHR, knowledge must be translated into action through policy and practice. This is one area that SRHM intends to focus on in the coming years and under its strategic direction in 2019–22.

Some organisations talked about how they seek to embed communications in all their activities, while others pointed to the desire to have more 'conversations' about the topic of sexual and reproductive health as a means of improving the quality of communications in that area. Organisations like YouAct (European Youth Network on Sexual and Reproductive Rights) and the Latin American Ela (Equipo Latinoamericano de Justica e Genero) made similar points. The lead for communications at the NGO Ela argued that discourses around reproductive health need to be better formulated. As she correctly noted, a lot of these conversations have been 'framed' around the ideas articulated by more conservative groups that work to impede progress:

> I think we have the legal, the scientific, and the medical arguments that prove that abortion should be legal. I believe that we have to find a better way *to communicate* those arguments. Mainly because of what the conservative and anti-rights groups managed to do very well for the past few years – decades – is to associate abortion with murder. They were good at doing that. And we need to change that speech because we know that when a woman goes to the hospital and asks for an abortion, if she gets that abortion denied, she's going to find some other away to get it done. And sometimes that pushes hard to unsafe situations that have consequences for health … There is a communication thing that we need to improve to have a debate at the Congress, to really show that we need legal abortion not because women are spoiled or because they want to have sex without taking care of themselves. And it affects their bodies and affects their health both physically and emotionally … And we need to be able to do that … I think that is important for the different organisations … to have an improvement of communication basically because of that. Because we know that everybody who is against abortion has been working for decades with gory stories, gory pictures and basically established the idea of death. It was common, during the debate, to hear people scream to women with the green scarf: 'you're a murderer!'

The coordinator at YouAct further highlighted the centrality of evidence-based arguments, emphasising the importance of adapting communications according to an organisation's needs:

> I mean obviously this makes advocacy around this work more challenging, but with challenges also comes creativity. We do have to be more creative when it comes to wording, but at the same time, we have to be careful … I feel that we need to stand for whatever the organisation believes in or is advocating for. We cannot tip toe on the wording on abortion: it is what it is. And we also must remain evidence-based, medically accurate …

And this we cannot change in the advocacy ... So, I kind of understand the needs of some ... but I also see other organisations that are rooting their feet in the sand and saying, 'No this is what we are talking about, and these are the words that we use'. Whether they receive more backlash or not, I do not know ... I just think that from YouAct's point of view, we must be clear on the way that we say things ... that we do use the right terminology, and that we do not dance around and use incorrect words ... I think that we in YouAct have very much tried to integrate communications in our day-to-day work. From a strategic point of view, especially working with young people, if you do not have Facebook, and you do not have a specific place where young people can seek information, your organisation is probably not doing that great. You must get your message out ... All types of media are legitimate if you want to focus on documentaries ... I think they are a great way of advocating on different topics. Or through Instagram you get an overview, it really depends ... For us, we work with young people. I also see many organisations just creating a website, like for one project ... And then what? That type of advocacy and form of communication is for a short period ... So, it is something that you consistently must feed ... It is a two-way dialogue.

A *two-way dialogue* is something that the organisations are trying to do more work on, as some of the interviewees indicated, aligning their messages to pursue ways of generating more impact. In the communications questionnaire, which the director of communications of Family Planning 2020 answered (as well as having participated in the in-depth interview), it was noted how the communications and advocacy teams work closely together to achieve the organisation's communications strategy plan. Some of its key principles included the aligning and supporting of messages of the FP global community as well as the gathering of communications staff around the world to work on pooling resources. This includes planning for major events. Family Planning 2020 also makes use of social media platforms, from Twitter and Facebook to YouTube videos.

The director also talked about how SRHR is understood differently across countries, underlining that family planning can work in some countries but not in others. She pointed out how, in some countries in Northern Africa, they would not talk about contraceptives, but they would talk about 'birth control'. As she stated, the change of a term could lead to a disconnect with the audience. Thus, in order to overcome the numerous challenges of advocating SRHR across sectors and different local contexts, she underscored the need to have more 'counselling and individual knowledge sharing' on the issue. This is important in order to 'integrate across sectors – from contraception to HIV for dual protection'. She further emphasised the problem around language barriers when it comes to SRHR:

> So when organisations get involved in personal decisioning, as we do [at] FP2020, you have to temper the communication strategy so that you keep your messages sane, and easy to understand, so that they resonate with the greatest amount of people, and so you are also protecting the privacy of people who benefit from your work ... It does not matter if the woman is in Ghana, Bogota, Bangkok, it is all the same, she deserves her privacy ... So most of the communications work that we do now ... is walking the fine line between coming up with those stories, so other people will be touched by them, but also respecting the fact that this is a very private decision. And our mission here [at] FP2020 is to safeguard the rights of women ... Predominantly we work in Africa and Southeast Asia, we do have a few countries in Latin America ... The successes are not ours, because the way we work is that the countries make commitments in terms to family planning ... They decide numerically whether the commitment is to increase the number of women using modern forms of contraception; they decide whether it is to provide more comprehensive sexuality education for young people under eighteen, so the commitments vary ... We are here to help ... We offer technical assistance and some small amounts of money ... In terms of communication, well, the countries do not always understand the power of communications. They use it, and they may call it 'advocacy', they may call it 'outreach', they call it different things, but they are using communications. Some of it is for social behavioural change, some of it is for campaigns, some of it is to promote new clinics or new methods of contraception. But communication play a role in every aspect of advocacy.

Another interesting case is the Youth Coalition for Sexual and Reproductive Rights (YCSRR),[16] which, despite limited funds, developed a quite professional and detailed advocacy communications plan whose purpose was to make the most use of communications in offline and online spaces. In its *Communication Guide*, YCSRR defines itself as being 'a youthful and inviting personality with a voice of knowledge', a place where content 'is friendly, knowledgeable, and definitive', and a tone that aims 'to be conversational, credible and direct'. At the core of its communications strategy is the desire to maintain 'a strong social media presence', creating original content to be shared on different media. The head of communications said that YCSRR had eight core goals, among them to 'engage more people in YCSRR's work', to strive to maintain a presence on Facebook and to be active on Twitter, as well as to 'create original quality content to be shared on different media'.

In its advocacy communications plan, the organisation included its core goals. These were divided into *ultimate goals* (e.g., 'to protect and promote young people's SRR at the international and national levels'), *intermediate goals* (e.g., 'to strengthen strategic communications within the movement, strengthen its capacity to advocate for young people as well as increase knowledge'), and *immediate goals* (e.g., 'to strengthen the delivery of YC content, the brand's identity, the partnerships for communications and the evidence-based knowledge for advocacy'). The organisation, which relies on three volunteers for the communications work, was among the few that admitted that it lobbies 'with policy-makers and politicians' on SRHR, stressing that lobbying with policy-makers and interaction with stakeholders was its core offline communication strategy. It also makes use of *all* forms of online communications, from creating awareness around the topic to influencing key political actors, although it stated that it sees online communications as being only 'somewhat effective'. The organisation further underscored how it considers it important to have an online presence to show 'funders that we are active'.

In the questionnaire some organisations referred to censorship practices and to the negative feedback that they receive on their media content. Some raised concerns over the opposition groups and their increasing harassment and intimation of some advocates working in the field. This was the case with Youth Coalition and Global Fund for Women, whose communications lead affirmed that it was necessary to talk about SRHR to naturalize the conversations around the topic, making them less 'controversial':

In SRHR, specifically topics like abortion and LGBTQIA+ are considered as ... 'taboo'... in some countries. Sharing or liking any social media content containing these topics often encounters serious political, socio-economic, cultural barriers associated with legislation gaps, dominating patriarchal culture values, cultivation of homophobia, and other factors ... For example, one of our members from Russia got persecuted because they shared a Facebook post about the LGBT community. This person was persecuted under the 'homosexual propaganda law' in 2017... We should mainstream SRHR issues more and not shy away from it. Not talking about it or posting about it would reinforce the idea that SRHR issues are taboo.

The vice-chair of the Youth Coalition for Sexual and Reproductive Rights talked about the threats that some health and gender NGO advocates face,[17] something that is sometimes not taken as seriously as it should be. She also pointed to the difficulties of advocating for SRHR within the Russian context:

And coming from Russia (but I don't live in Russia) ... we see a huge regression of human rights ... but especially women's rights ... It's very difficult to judge at the global level ... but at the same time what makes me happy is the cross of the woman's rights movements that you can visibly see in the discourses ... And also, not only in regard to women's rights but also to people of all gender identities ... It makes me respect more also Global South movements and see how powerful they are because, for example, the movements in Latin America are perhaps the most powerful examples of how women's activism could be done ... Because to be underfunded and under-resourced and having language barriers they still managed to do such amazing projects and things that are so inspirational ... People get really confused about what we are talking about. And so, this is why ... fake news [is] really strong because it seems like it's very hard to educate the population, and these strong conservative politicians are really against educating the population at school about sexual and gender rights ... We always try to explain from different dimensions ... what is the gender identity and how is it connected to ... But I don't know if everybody should have such deep knowledge ... Perhaps just awareness that people can be different regarding their sexuality ... Just the awareness and the tolerance [of] these topics can be highly appreciated ... Sexuality is a topic that is extremely taboo in most ... countries ... and even where it is not strongly taboo people still don't really talk about it ... At the same time, you have this problem for NGOs who don't really engage with the public ... In my country the work of NGOs is restricted. We had over half of NGOs being shut down just because of the government actions, and because they did not go together with the opinion of the governments on how we wish to have sex and reproductive health ... There are just a couple of NGOs in my home city ... Everybody is underfunded ... Not being able to exercise our freedom of speech, being careful what you talk, with whom, you face fatal consequences ... So I think personal safety ... is also something that people very often forget.

A key issue raised by many of the interviewees is the dependence that the organisations have on the funding and resources provided by donors. The scarcity of funds to invest further in communications obliges many organisations to think creatively about how to advocate for SRHR, partnering with other NGOs to share content and messages to amplify impact as well as resorting to other digital formats, such as personal interest stories through videos on YouTube. To compensate for lack of funds, many tweet and post news reports on sexual and reproductive rights on Twitter and Facebook, which have been published in the mainstream media. The vice-chair of the Youth Coalition further emphasised the importance of funding for the NGOs:

When I think about the feminist movement, for example, it's really about certain topics that bring people together. Becoming sustainable with the funding which can be difficult to achieve ... I really think that the funding model should change because with the current model the NGOs are so depending on funding from donors and funders, and unfortunately this can lead to less freedom on project management for some of them. So sustainable funding is so important for me where NGOs can manoeuvre how they get the money so they can do the projects they want to do.

As we have seen, the NGOs' dependence on funding, and the impact this can have on project management and on how the organisations engage with SRHR, including their capacity to advocate from a more holistic perspective, is something that has been identified by researchers working in the field of international development and women's health (Gideon and Porter 2016). It is to the results of the critical discourse analysis of the NGOs' social media engagement with SRHR on Twitter and Facebook that I turn next.

10

Deconstructing 'Gender Ideology' Myths and Digital Storytelling through Critical Discourse Analysis

A Case Study of NGOs' Social Media Engagement on Twitter and Facebook

Carolina Matos with Tatiane Leal

The results of this study show that there were lots of differences in the organisations' social media engagement as well as in their online presence on platforms such as Twitter and Facebook. This research examined the social media engagement of the organisations on these two main platforms during a two-week period of analysis, from 25 March to 7 April 2019. It reveals that, overall, the organisations are increasingly making use of online communications and strategies for all the categories concerning the type of communications (*information, advocacy, fundraising, community engagement*, and *mobilisation*) relating to sexual and reproductive health and rights. However, the findings also indicate that many organisations can still make better use of these platforms and online resources, including by investing in strategic thinking on communications as well as by making better use of these tools for advocacy on reproductive health.

The critical discourse analysis of Twitter and Facebook seeks to make sense of the media content posted on the platforms, including assessing where it fits into the categories of 'reason' or 'emotion'. The posts from both these platforms have been placed under the categories developed for the different types of communications (*information, advocacy, fundraising, community engagement,* and *mobilisation*), with the category of 'lobbying' having been added here as well to connect to the questionnaire applied to the communication professionals (see appendix D). The organisations also engaged with topics around sexual and reproductive health, underlining specific concerns. These included the rebuking of myths regarding SRHR, the defence of comprehensive sexual education in schools, and advocacy around the decriminalisation of abortion. As we shall see, they frequently inserted their local demands within wider global challenges, thereby seeking to engage publics both 'on the ground' and transnationally.

There were a lot of differences between the NGOs in terms of social media engagement, with little use of online communication tools like Instagram and podcasts. Twitter showed itself to be more popular for advocacy and mobilisation around SRHR than Facebook. The results also showed that the frequency of tweets and Facebook posts were quite uneven, and it was not necessarily the larger organisations that were more active on social media. The preference for one social media platform over the other had a certain alignment with the geographical location of the NGO. When it came to the frequency of posts, the highest average shared on Twitter during the period analysed was by the US NGOs, while Facebook was used more by many Latin American organisations.

The total number of Facebook posts was significantly less than those found on Twitter, coming to 741 posts during the period examined. The region of Latin America had 298, US ($n = 162$), Asia ($n = 104$), Europe ($n = 161$), and the 'international' organisations ($n = 16$). The combined Twitter and Facebook tweets and post feeds totalled 2,164 ($n = 100$ per cent). Similar to the pattern detected on Twitter, Facebook also saw a predominance of content that could be placed under the category of 'reason' ($n = 415$) over 'emotion' ($n = 252$). The total amount for 'advocacy' was 474 (100 per cent), community engagement ($n = 138$), information ($n = 37$), lobbying ($n = 13$), and fundraising ($n = 10$). The total number of Twitter tweets was 1,505 (100 per cent), of which 358 were from Asia, Europe ($n = 265$), Latin America ($n = 327$), US ($n = 521$), and 'international' ($n = 34$).

Of the total tweets collected from the organisations, many mingled 'emotional' contents with the more 'rational' contents (e.g., emphasis on *facts-based evidence*), with some emphasising one more than the other. Of all the organisations analysed, a total of 433 tweets (100 per cent) were placed under the category of 'emotion' and another 922 were placed under 'reason'. This showed the predominance of advocacy practices and use of communications to promote the cause of SRHR through the appeal to facts. The total number of tweets placed under 'advocacy' was quite high, at 977, whereas the total placed under 'fundraising' was only 15, of which 11 were from CARE International UK (see tables 10.1 and 10.2).

Table 10.2 shows the ten most active organisations on Facebook, and their total number of posts. These were: (1) Sexual Policy Watch (n = 90); (2) Global Fund for Women (n = 58); (3) Anis (n = 53); (4) CREA India (n = 48); (5) Promsex (n = 46); (6) Centre for Reproductive Rights (n = 38); (7) CEPIA (n = 36); (8) Inspire Euro NGOs (n = 36); (9) Sexual and Reproductive Health Matters (n = 28); and (10) Women Deliver (n = 29). For Twitter (see table 10.1), the ten most active were: (1) Promsex (n = 168); (2) CREA India (n = 165); (3) Global Fund for Women (n = 135); (4) Centre for Reproductive Rights (n = 109); (5) Family Planning 2020 (n = 81); (6) Asia Pacific Alliance (n = 58); (7) Anis (n = 51); (8) Amnesty International UK (n = 50); (9) Women Deliver (n = 5); and (10) the Guttmacher Institute (n = 149). Not surprisingly, most of the organisations that were very active on Facebook were also among some of the top ones on Twitter. This was the case of CREA India, Global Fund for Women, Anis, Promsex, Centre for Reproductive Rights, and Women Deliver. However, a few that were active on Twitter were not among the top ten on Facebook, as was the case with Family Planning 2020, Asia Pacific Alliance, Amnesty International UK, and the Guttmacher Institute. The organisations that appeared only among the ten for Facebook were Sexual Policy Watch, CEPIA, Inspire Euro NGO, and Sexual and Reproductive Health Matters.

For Twitter, the higher number of tweets came from some of the larger research-led organisations, such as the Centre for Reproductive Rights (n = 109), CREA India (n = 165), Global Fund for Women (n = 135), and Promsex (n = 168). Many equally prestigious NGOs recorded a lower number of tweets, such as 34 for CHANGE, Ibis (n = 20) and Akahata (n = 3). Some of the tweets were placed under 'advocacy', such as those from CREA India (n = 134), whereas others relied more on facts and were placed under 'reason', as was the case with those from the Centre for Reproductive Rights (n = 96). Other organisations showed a more even balance between the content that was placed under 'reason' and that placed under 'emotion', reflecting what some gender experts and other communication professionals had mentioned regarding trying to combine both in their advocacy

Table 10.1
The top ten most active organisations on Twitter

Type of Information of NGOs Twitter feeds	Total tweets	Emotion	Reason	Fundraising	Advocacy	Mobilization	Community engagement	Information and Media	Lobbying
1 Promsex	168	63	105	0	126	15	1	6	20
2 Crea India	165	18	57	0	134	0	67	10	0
3 Global Fund for Women	135	55	80	1	100	7	27	0	0
4 Center for Reproductive Rights	109	13	96	2	83	9	3	0	12
5 Family Planning 2020	81	30	51	0	53	2	25	1	0
6 Asia Pacific Alliance	58	9	29	0	32	1	5	16	0
7 Anis	51	10	41	0	43	0	3	5	0
8 Amnesty International UK	50	29	21	0	26	9	12	0	3
9 Women Deliver	50	8	38	0	40	0	10	28	0
10 Guttmacher Institute	49	12	37	0	40	1	2	0	6

Table 10.2
The top ten most active organisations on Facebook

Type of Information of NGOs Facebook posts	Total posts	Emotion	Reason	Fundraising	Advocacy	Mobilization	Community engagement	Information and Media	Lobbying
1 Sexual Policy Watch	90	33	57	0	79	3	7	1	0
2 Global Fund for Women	58	25	33	1	49	2	6	0	0
3 Anis	53	17	33	0	48	0	3	2	0
4 Crea India	48	6	3	0	5	0	38	2	0
5 Promsex	46	26	20	0	19	17	0	0	7
6 Center for Reproductive Rights	38	4	34	2	35	1	0	0	0
7 Cepia	36	9	27	0	26	0	10	0	0
8 Inspire Euro NGOs	36	16	20	0	30	1	3	2	0
9 Sexual and Reproductive Health Matters	28	1	27	0	24	0	2	2	0
10 Women Deliver	24								

communications strategies. Promsex had 105 tweets under 'reason' and 126 under 'emotion'. However, the results of the analysis showed that, for both Twitter and Facebook, the balance tipped slightly towards favouring the category 'reason' over that of 'emotion', reflecting an emphasis on content that is evidence-based. Moreover, table 10.1, the Twitter graph, shows that 69 per cent of the messages were classified under the category of 'reason', whereas 31 per cent were classified under 'emotion'. For Facebook, the results were 65 per cent for 'reason' and 35 per cent for 'emotion'.

The results reveal that a lot of the advocacy communications material put out on social media was intended to appeal to the intellect, including more reports and facts surrounding reproductive health. However, the fact that 'emotion' scored around 30 per cent could also be seen as significant, indicating the increasing use of human interest narratives, digital storytelling, and other communicative devices that stress emotion and subjectivity in media messages. Other organisations that reflected a balance between the categories classified under 'emotion' and 'reason' on Twitter included Family Planning 2020, which had 30 under 'emotion' and 51 under 'reason', whereas Global Fund Women had 80 under 'reason' and 55 under 'emotion', with Sexual Policy Watch on Facebook having 33 under 'emotion' and 57 under 'reason'. On Facebook, Global Fund Women showed an equilibrium between the appeal to the intellect and the appeal to emotional content, with 25 for 'emotion' and 33 for 'reason'. This was similar to Inspire Euro NGO (16 for 'emotion' and 20 for 'reason').

For some organisations, however, the balanced tipped in favour of one category rather than the other. On Twitter, this was the case for the Centre for Reproductive Rights (96 under 'reason', 13 under 'emotion') and of the Latin American NGO Promsex (105 under 'reason' and 63 under 'emotion'). However, the situation was different on Facebook. Promsex published more posts under the category 'emotion' than under 'reason' (26 and 20, respectively). These findings show that there is space for growth in human interest media content, digital storytelling, and other communication content that emphasises emotion and that can be built within participatory-led and entertainment-education formats of health communication advocacy messages on SRHR.

Most of the posts and tweets on Twitter and Facebook were used for advocacy purposes. On Twitter more posts were used for 'advocacy' purposes, closely followed by 'community engagement', 'mobilisation', and 'information'. One hundred and twenty-six posts for advocacy purposes were tweeted by Promsex, 134 by CREA India, 100 by Global Fund Women, and 83 by Centre for Reproductive Rights. Facebook was also mostly used for advocacy, with the second highest number of post feeds being used for 'community engagement', followed by 'mobilisation' and 'information'. Sexual Policy Watch had the highest number of posts for 'advocacy' ($n = 79$), followed by Global Fund Women ($n = 49$), Anis ($n = 48$), Centre for Reproductive Rights ($n = 35$), and Inspire Euro NGOs ($n = 30$). The NGOs in Latin America showed less activity on Twitter, with ten not posting anything during the period examined, and another four posting neither on Twitter nor on Facebook. The results reveal a focus on using social media for advocacy and for encouraging dialogue with the community rather than simply sharing information or attempting to mobilise people to take part in events. This indicates how the organisations are seeking to influence their targeted publics.

The category of 'mobilisation' had fewer tweets than expected, with only 104, and these came from a small group of organisations: Consorcio latino-americano contra el aborto inseguro ($n = 15$), Promsex ($n = 15$), Realizing Sexual and Reproductive Justice ($n = 15$), Amnesty International ($n = 9$), Centre for Reproductive Rights ($n = 9$), and Global Fund Women ($n = 7$). There were a higher number of tweets in the category 'community engagement' ($n = 314$), with CREA India ($n = 67$), Reproductive Health System Coalition ($n = 39$); Family Planning ($n = 25$), CHANGE ($n = 19$), Global Fund for Women ($n = 27$), and UNFPA ($n = 18$). The category 'information' included a total of 100, whereas 'lobbying' had a lower number of tweets ($n = 62$). The results confirm what most of the NGOs stated in their responses to the questionnaires and the interviews – mainly, that lobbying is not one of their key activities and is not seen as a priority.

The themes tweeted by the organisations included a multiplicity of issues under the umbrella of SRHR, ranging from safe abortion to rape and sexual assault to child pregnancy and gender equality. Popular hashtags and phrases included #safeabortionisaright and #Todas Lasfamiliassonfamilia ('All Families are families', Akahata, and Asap); 'Young people have started speaking' (Centre for Catalysing Change) and #Family planning to achieve (Family Planning 2020). Other hashtags used included #SRHR, #WorldHealthDay, and #Healthforall. The US organisations tended to focus more on the Global Gag Rule as well as on the global impact of the policy on SRHR and on health care.

The hashtag #NinasNoMadres (GirlsNotMothers) circulated in many of the posts analysed, including on the front cover of Twitter for the Latin American NGO Promsex. The #NinasNoMadres hashtag campaign has been endorsed by many NGOs, not just Promsex and Fundacion Desfio. Virginia Gomez, of the latter organisation, cited this campaign as having been important in providing visibility for the issue of teenage pregnancy.

The NGO Promsex was the most active on Twitter, with a total of 169 tweets. In the communications survey answered by the organisation, Promsex talked about a strong communication presence on the institutional website, stating that it considers online communications to be 'very effective' for SRHR advocacy. The CEO of Promsex affirmed that some of its online pages had been jeopardised by attacks from specific groups.[1] She said that prejudice towards SRHR, including misinformation and lack of knowledge, pose complex challenges for the advocacy communication efforts of NGOs who work in the field. She also defended the use of more spaces for the online articulation of SRHR:

> We do it at various levels, through the development of programmes that are a sustained process ... We also include communications strategically ... as the idea is to sensitize the public about these issues whose systematic non-compliance is transformed into violation of human rights. We also develop specific campaigns, such as "girls not mothers", "with trafficking there is no deal", "education with equality" ...
> The #EducaciónConIgualdad campaign ... is part of the response to the onslaught of conservative groups to eliminate the gender approach from the ... school curriculum. This campaign had three moments in which different influencers joined to make a call to public opinion ... to join it ... Interaction on our website occurs through the press releases that we disseminate through social networks as well as the publications that we periodically publish ... Our pages have been affected at some point due to attacks by opposition groups ... We also develop research to generate evidence on the issues we work on, which is then distributed and disseminated ... The public health issue could be understood as a limited approach since its references tend to refer to aspects such as dimension of the problem, cost and ability to reverse, and the agenda can go much further, such

as the concept of citizenship ... I do not believe that the debates are in opposing fields ... Perhaps one of the issues that has managed to build some common bridges is violence, particularly institutional violence, as well as the issue of people's autonomy.

Another key characteristic of the communication activities used by many organisations on their social media platforms, and that was spotted during the period analysed, was the sharing of information on SRHR from the mainstream media. The organisations made use of stories from the mainstream media, adding to them a personalised angle. Here the organisations resorted to different forms of hashtag activism to advocate their cause. This was the case, for instance, with the #Mexico president and #Obrador hashtags with regard to the tweets posted by Safe Abortion Women's Rights on the possibility of an abortion referendum. NGOs in Brazil tended to reproduce media material from the mainstream press slightly more often than did other Latin American, European, and US organisations, most likely due to insufficient resources. That said, organisations like Anis and Sexual Policy Watch shared a lot of mainstream media content. In doing so they provided their targeted publics with less information on how exactly they as organisations were working on SRHR, instead opting to address the debates that circulated in the mediated public sphere.

Some of the media content shared online consisted of stories from the mainstream media that were reproduced by the NGOs for advocacy purposes, community engagement, and raising awareness around the topic. This proves that online spaces can be used to amplify engagement so as to generate wider impact (Keck and Sikkink 1998). Arguably, the more in-depth journalistic pieces on SRHR are produced by the traditional media, which has more resources to report on these issues and produce original content than do many smaller organisations working in the field.

The regional communications adviser from UNFPA stated that he sees the mainstream media as providing more in-depth reporting on SRHR than the digital online world, particularly when it comes to topics such as teenage pregnancy. The online space is seen as serving other communication and advocacy aims, including mobilisation and raising awareness, being a space where the 'old media' and the 'new media' intersect (Chadwick 2006). Tweets are thus utilised to advocate simple and direct messages on the topic through emphasising more journalistic media language. Moreover, a hyperlink leads to the original text of the International Campaign for Women's Rights for Safe Abortion (originally published by Reuters, while the original source is attributed to Al Jazeera).

Here the emphasis on women's rights as being 'beyond opinion' is on par with the veracity that is attributed to factual journalism. It places this tweet in line with other examples of *deconstruction of discourses and myths* around SRHR, particularly on the topic of abortion. Similarly, Women's Link Worldwide posted on Facebook a news article from the UK newspaper the *Independent* on the many women crossing the border from Venezuela to seek antenatal care, with the hashtags #Colombia and #Venezuela. This strategy was used by NGOs in all the regions examined. Although the use of journalism reports and other media content has its advantages, it could be argued that dependence on the mainstream media's material on SRHR is not a good strategy of advocacy communications on a complex issue that needs further discussion. There is thus a need to move beyond dependence on the mainstream media, or the tendency to 'preach to the converted', as some of the gender experts and communication professionals interviewed here argued.

The use of advocacy communications on social media can seek to influence public opinion through an appeal to more accessible language as well as to emotions and to the interest that people generally have in individual stories of suffering, struggle, and the overcoming of hardships (Ascough 2018). The aim is not to advocate for NGOs to adopt behaviourist-style models of health communication campaigns (Tufte 2012) for SRHR but, rather, to stress the use of communication content that emphasises experiences of individual agency, which can create possibilities of connecting to others without depoliticising the debate. This encourages the discussion of complex structural problems that lie at the heart of sexual and reproductive health. This needs to be done in order to advance policy and change in the field for women's rights and reproductive health.

The results also show that, despite the differences in their levels of resources, credibility, and influence, many NGOs shared some common strategic communications strategies regardless of different geographical locations, cultures, languages, and priorities pertaining to SRHR. Many expressed similar concerns regarding the lack of resources, particularly for communication initiatives but also for campaigns and SRHR programmes; the lack of understanding regarding what constitutes sexual and reproductive health; as well as the need to engage with the younger population by working to develop new communication practices and strategies that better suit the current digital environment and the growing worldwide hostility towards women's rights and reproductive health.

As we have seen, across the board organisations are making wider use of Twitter and Facebook for advocacy communications, expressing a desire for wider investment in communications and embedding these within their policy processes. Like the US organisation CHANGE, the Argentinian NGO Coletivo de Salud showed that it wants to make better use of social media platforms. In the communications questionnaire, the organisation underlined the problem of lack of resources, which has made it rely on the exchange of emails and mainly on Facebook, although it has made use of YouTube for information videos. The head of communications for Coletivo de Salud Feminista stated in the questionnaire that online communications is perceived to be 'very effective'.[2] It is used mostly to 'inform the public on the ground' and to 'create communications between the organisations' that work in the same field as other NGOs. Its offline communication activities consist mainly of press releases and paid advertising; however, the organization also stated that it viewed online communications as 'more effective' than offline communications. He acknowledged that there is lack of information and prejudice when it comes to SRHR and, like the representatives of other organisations interviewed here, he denounced the attacks that the NGO encounters online. He also provided an interesting example of a campaign in which the language of 'rights' and the obligations of the state to deliver SRHR services were combined with notions of individual 'choice' and agency. He referred to an example of a video with a simple and direct message that went viral on social media:

> Last year [2018] we made a video about the rights of patients and the obligations of doctors and health institutions when it comes to accessing a safe abortion, and we posted it on Facebook. In three days, I already had 2 millions of views ... One of our main aims is to occupy a strategic place on YouTube, to make informative videos that rank well in YouTube search engines. The other point is through Facebook ... (Sorry, but I don't know what 'advocacy' is.) Our strategic plan does not involve a daily activity because we don't have the resources for it. When we want to communicate something, we do it through

Facebook and ... through our networks ... The main difficulty that we have had historically is the censorship that we suffer in social networks. Generally, when we make a publication that is very successful and gets a lot of diffusion, anti-right groups appear that denounce these publications (on YouTube and Facebook) and those companies usually eliminate the publication or even cancel our accounts.

Mujer y Salud from Uruguay is another NGO that showed commitment to using strategic communications for SRHR advocacy. It was also one of the few that adopted a more philosophical approach to communications, viewing it as playing a fundamental role in the construction of social thought. It underlined the need for multiple strategies for communications, stating that the combination of digital communications with offline media efforts in legal abortion was fundamental. The organisation ticked all the options in the questionnaire on offline communication activities, including from 'pressure groups for politicians and policy-makers' to 'paid advertising' and 'visual communication campaigns'. This was in contrast to most organisations, who opted mainly for 'b' in the questionnaire (press release and contact with journalists) and 'd' (face-to-face conversations with the affected parties).

As with the Brazilian Reprolatina, the representatives of Mujer y Salud en Uruguay (MYSU) stated that it had used communications beyond the five- to ten-year period that most NGOs indicated in the questionnaire (fourteen years and nineteen years, respectively, for its Brazilian counterpart). It noted that the entire team at MYSU work directly with, or were connected to, communication tasks and strategies. It further underlined that the main function of MYSU's institutional websites is to 'disseminate activities and research results'; 'carry out campaigns and position themselves online'; 'replicate institutional presence on digital and other media'; 'upload publications of the organisations', and to receive 'citizens' inquiries and complaints.' Moreover, both the executive director and the director of the NGO,[3] who participated in the in-depth interview and answered the communications questionnaire together, underlined how communications has helped the organisation become more influential. Both also believe that it is through communications that they can reach out to targeted publics, engaging people in dialogue around SRHR. They emphasised how digital media has complemented the organisation's offline activities:

Communication is one of the strategic lines of the organisation, through it the other lines are promoted (observatory, advocacy, and education /training), which have always had a communication component. It is used to position the issues that are being worked on in relation to sexual and reproductive rights ... The inclusion of communications, in the lines of action of women's and feminist organisations, serves to strengthen the political advocacy plan ... Communication strategies have positioned MYSU as one of the most consulted ... organisations by national, regional, and international press media ... MYSU's communication line includes campaigns, product development, positioning, information, dissemination, interactive platforms, and distant courses on ... sexual and reproductive rights. Communication is one of MYSU's lines of sustained work because it fundamentally understands its role in the construction of social thought ... Therefore it is a priority to include information and communication technologies in the various lines of work of our organisation ... Advocacy work on sexual and reproductive rights, and particularly on legal abortion, had an imprint of the use of digital media that effectively complemented offline strategies. In this sense, I highlight the use of the Hacelos Valer website to coordinate and disseminate advocacy actions and disseminate information about current regulations ... in this field. You can check it here on the link.[4]

The organisation thus affirmed that it wants to make better use of online communications, considering it to be 'very effective'. It also cited some platforms that it is also using, such as Hace Click[5] and Sexualidapp! App for Android and Apple.[6] Mujer y Salud also underscored that it wants to further invest in communications in the future, stating that the 'lack of diffusion of accurate information and campaigns directed at diverse publics, which tackle openly sexual and reproductive health and rights and gender justice, is a crucial problem'. Both representatives of the organisation made a strong argument in favour of the wider democratisation of access to accurate information as a means of exercising one's citizenship rights. They further highlighted the problem of insufficient official data on SRHR as the main difficulty for communications:

We know that there are important inequalities between socio-economic and educational sectors and that the awareness of the population for the exercise of rights requires democratisation of access to material and symbolic goods ... We make multiple efforts to promote the citizen's exercise of rights ... The weaknesses in the official data registration system, particularly in the field of gender inequalities and SRR, is also a main difficulty for communication ... Disseminating information about existing services or programmes is the way for the population to take ownership of them, and our action as a movement is to promote citizen participation ... Sexual and reproductive citizenship should not be limited exclusively to the individual exercise of the right but to the collective effort ... The misinformation about the services is considerable, MYSU has monitored the implementation of sexual and reproductive health services ... and has been able to verify the misinformation of the user population that has not received information on the characteristics and conditions of services.

MYSU also made use of online communications to inform the public, influence media and public opinion, and to diffuse its activities and those of other institutions in the field. Like the other NGOs interviewed here, Mujer y Salud seeks to adopt various strategies to deal with the difficulties in communicating about SRHR. These range from disseminating 'information generated and surveyed by the National Observatory on Gender and Sexual and Reproductive Health that MYSU has installed for the monitoring of SRHR policy in Uruguay' to 'advis[ing] by phone, email and direct messaging in networks and in person.' MYSU's representatives underlined their desire to work more creatively with other organisations to overcome the dissemination of 'fake news' and disinformation on reproductive health put out by oppositional groups:

[We] articulated and networked ... with other organisations ... that work in the field ... for the dissemination of pertinent information ... and communication products ... We work with both national and regional organisations ... given the technological advances and the culture of information on the internet ... to find more innovative ways of creating content for social networks ... including greater accessibility in the language and elaboration of messages coded differently for different ... groups. The use of mobile applications (apps) is essential ... but still has a lot of untapped scope for action ... In a context of post-truth and direct attack on organisations and movements that work ... on health and sexual and reproductive rights from groups 'against gender ideology', one of the barriers to overcome is the biased use of social networks, the dissemination of 'fake news' and 'alternative facts' by these media and the use that political-party actors are making, taking advantage of the opportunities opened up by a wide segmentation of the user population of social networks and other novel means of communication (such as WhatsApp) through increasingly sophisticated algorithms. Another barrier to overcome is that of cyberactivism that does not translate into activism 'off the screens' ... Establishing links between different forms of activism would contribute to a greater impact for the cause. Finally, the difference in access to material ... technological and human resources on the part of women's social organisations, the LGBTIQ ... that work in this field versus that of the private sector ... that work against this agenda is a challenge for which ... creative strategies are required.

The Brazilian organisation Reprolatina was quite detailed in its response to the communication strategies that it uses for its communications advocacy on SRHR. It also make wide use of all the communication platforms available to it, including WhatsApp. It has three institutional websites, an official one for Reprolatina, another for teenagers, and another only for contraceptives.[7] Reprolatina currently has seven people working on communications, with five professionals responsible for the creation of content, one for audiovisual production, and another to manage social media. The CEO of Reprolatina affirmed that the misinformation on the topic occurs not just among the general population but is also a problem among health professionals and others working in the field.[8] Although online communications were considered 'somewhat effective', the organisation chose the option 'more effective' than offline strategies.

Among the main points listed in Reprolatina's strategic plan for communications were 'giving visibility to the institution and its activities on SRHR'; 'the promotion on social media of the organisation's activities as well as technical information and empirical evidence-based information on SRHR', and the 'use of social media for each separate project'. It also underlined all the options provided for offline communication activity, including the use of banners, leaflets, and posters as well as 'material for information, education and advocacy'. Some of the difficulties mentioned included a lack of resources for communications and capacity-building in the area. Reprolatina also stated that it wants to further invest in communications and is also currently working on an advocacy communications plan in collaboration with me.[9] In the communications questionnaire, the CEO underlined as a key barrier the 'lack of information and knowledge on the topic by an important part of society' coupled with the fact that NGOs have struggled to survive in a period in which 'there are no budgets to support projects in the field'.

The CEO talked about how she makes use of different communication tools to reach out to different publics as well as about her own personal experiences battling 'fake news' and unscientific evidence against SRHR on social media:

> Yes, there is a lot of misinformation ... Currently, there is also a lot of opposition to the issue of sexual and reproductive rights ... due to the conservative government and groups, especially those linked to the churches. The strategies that we have used to tackle this have included the increase [in] in-person training and educational activities as well as using social media to send information related to the concepts of DH, DS, DR, comprehensive education in sexuality (EIS), sexism, feminism ... However, I think that technology in recent years ... And here I notice that there is an inequality, let's say, of what technology is used for among different populations. So, for example, if I'm going to work with parents, I could only use WhatsApp ... We've been creating these posts to share with the people who train with us ... I have a number of WhatsApp groups ... People will have information and will spread it ... Because a person who took a course with us, he has several other networks: there is the family's WhatsApp ... This is an area that I would very much like to evaluate better ... Because I spent a lot of time a day logging on to Facebook ... There is a network called Catraca Livre which has a lot of access by teenagers, and they sometimes

broadcast false news ... For example they spread ... that emergency contraception is abortive ... so I spent many hours in these networks, contesting with evidence ... They weren't even talking about fake news at that time ... Maybe it's really this work that we do ... where people can see the video, we can look them in the eyes ... so, we have been working more with these women who go to churches ... Social networks ... are here to stay ... We need to better know how to use these ... And then we had the chance, with the IT youth ... we had the chance to think a lot about the risks ... of IT ... We found very interesting things ... things that even for us are unknown, such as these deeper networks ... And maybe it's the networks, the dark movements, that are firmer with these ... discriminations against women ... I would very much like our institution to receive training in this area to optimize the use of communications ... I think a good advocacy strategy, using social media, would be essential, because with that you reach a lot of people ... For that you need professional people, let's say people who know how to make a good campaign. We must do the marketing, just like Coca-Cola is sold.

Many organisations have made wide use of the popular journalistic tool of 'fact checking' to advocate for SRHR on social media, to work on discourses that aim to deconstruct prejudices and stigma around SRHR. This was the case of NGOs like Ibis Reproductive Health and CHANGE, both of which resorted to emphasising rationality, facts, and statistics in their advocacy communications practices on Twitter. Ibis Reproductive Health underscored that the discussion of women's bodily autonomy should not be understood as being 'all about abortion' and that this is one among many other methods in a debate that involves the complexity of individual choice combined with the impact of collective structures and inequalities on the lives of individuals (Correa and Petchesky 1994). In a direct reference to the journalistic practice, the US NGO CHANGE made use of the hashtag #SRHRFactCheck. And, using the hashtag #GlobalGagRule, it underlined the US's responsibility for having expanded this rule, including its role in the increase of deaths throughout the world due to illegal abortion practices. The use of 'facts' here is a way of emphasising the veracity and credibility of an overwhelming range of 'opinionated' (or subjective, even 'emotional') ideas about SRHR.

These advocacy communication efforts on Twitter implicitly allude to the 'common-sense' assumptions, myths, and preconceived ideas around SRHR that circulate in the public sphere and among the 'general public', mostly propelled by the actions of conservative groups. They also connect to the discourses that claim to attack the 'gender agenda', which, according to the 'gender ideology' argument, is spread conspiratorially throughout the world by progressives, policy-makers, politicians, and gender advocates (or 'the left'). In such a context, another core challenge for conducting advocacy communications, one that was mentioned by many of the gender experts interviewed here, is the increasing backlash, negative feedback, and even censorship that they sometimes receive regarding their posts.

According to the communications survey questionnaire answered by the communications lead from the NGO Youth Coalition, the organisation aims to provide one to two original posts a day. It depends on the support of its activists to share information on SRHR, mainly around issues such as LGBT rights, HIV/AIDS, and women's rights. Youth Coalition developed a detailed strategy to make the best use of social media engagement, ensuring that at least one original tweet is posted a day. It provides a set of rules and 'best practice' initiatives for engagement on social media on both Facebook and Twitter, including a list of 'dos' and 'don'ts'. For Facebook, this includes ensuring that texts posted are accompanied by images. Youth Coalition is also allowed to share posts from partner organisations. Members should avoid 'responding to trolls' but should seek to engage with the audience, answering its questions. Regarding Twitter, it is expected that the organisation tweet at least once a day, 're-tweeting and including likes generously', further tagging partners, and making wide use of hashtags. Popular hashtags suggested included #SRHR, #youthsRHR, #reprojustice, #youthrights, #lgbtq, and #SDGs.

The European NGO YouAct, whose gender expert and communications lead were also supportive of this research,[10] attempts to share a lot of relevant articles online. It seeks to build a strategy around the publication of communications output on Facebook and Twitter, and it assesses how best to make use of increasingly popular online communications devices, such as digital storytelling. The communications lead said that she had been working on communications since 2018 and was working alongside an intern external communications officer on something 'challenging'. She underscored their core strategy:

We have recently developed a communications strategy ... which is also in line with our organisational strategy ... We usually put out our activities that we are implementing on a daily basis, we put out pictures of our campaigns. We are advertising our resources ... sharing relevant articles ... on what is happening around Europe, around the world ... so that it's a balance of advocacy but also awareness raising, and ... some sort of motivation for young people to get engaged ... and to get involved with our work ... We usually use Facebook, so we develop this plan where we write out the best time to post on Facebook based on our business instincts, and that means which days are better ... We update that information every month ... We also blog about our conferences, our different projects, how it went ... We also share that on our Twitter, on our Facebook, and on our webpage ... the Unite for CSE – Comprehensive Sexuality Education, we used another hashtag, Advance Sex Act, it was a very good project in the sense that we collaborated with five different countries – that was Georgia, Romania, Bulgaria, the Netherlands, and Cyprus, and one more country ... And then we took these messages from the young people to the members ... of the European Parliament ... On each Thursday, we had a post, and it was so consistent ... on YouAct and on our partner's Facebook channels ... a lot of comments from people form Nepal, from all over the world. It teaches us that consistency ... is so important to raise awareness ... We have a YouTube channel but we have only used it for the Unite CSE project ... Our main use of communications is Facebook and then Twitter, and of course we aim ... to increase our audience, but it needs to be said that, because we are a volunteer-based organisation, it is not always possible ... We had a toolkit on abortion storytelling, it was very powerful because people came out and talked about their ... experiences ... A lot of people think that abortion is an easy decision, that they wake up and say, "OK, I am going to have an abortion" ... The stigma that exists around it, the fact that these people found the courage to make their voices heard ... And we can always relate to another person [more] than we can relate to numbers.

Another interesting initiative that also makes use of sharing personal stories is the 'Family Planning Voices', or #FPVoices, from the US

NGO Family Planning 2020. Here the activists share their own experiences regarding their work on SRHR. The stories are included in one page of the social media platform Tumblr and were also shared on Facebook and Twitter.[11] There were also many posts that were explicitly about mobilizing members around campaigns. Twitter was the preferred space for this. It gave an opportunity for the organisation, muck like media industries, to provide coverage of its own events in real time. When it came to protests, Family Planning 2020 made use of social media to mobilise people to join its campaign.

The UK-based movement SheDecides, on the other hand, posted a series of tweets to mobilise members around the #8WeekChallenge, launched on 8 April 2019. The posts sought to mobilise people to endorse the causes of the organisation and to move beyond being a mere 'clickactivist'. The main aim was to sign the online manifesto. Discussions about young people and SRHR were widely explored, including through debates on topics from family planning, to contraception, sexual abuse, and rights.

Another prominent theme that stood out among the organisations analysed here was reproductive health and rights in situations of humanitarian crisis, generated either by wars or natural disasters. These themes were dominant among European, international, and North American NGOs, which emphasised events such as Cyclone Idai, which affected Mozambique. The concern was to demonstrate how these events culminated in severe problems for women's health, especially for mothers, as UNFPA's post UNFPA showed.[12] These themes did not appear that often in the posts of the Latin American NGOs, which tended to focus more on local issues.

The organisations engaged with various themes pertaining to SRHR, including issues from abortion to pregnancy, rape, sexual education, contraceptives and, to a lesser extent, questions concerning female genital mutilation, sexual pleasure, male contraceptives, and menstruation. They also provided snapshots of how SRHR appeared in more general themes, including, for instance, analyses of the governments of Bolsonaro in Brazil and Trump in the US, and in issues involving humanitarian crises, the health of women prisoners, equal pay, and the impact of these on the access to health services. They also focused on the impact of pension reforms on Brazilian women, situating this within the legacy of Brazil's 1970s military dictatorship.

The NGOs examined topics on human rights and gender equality, including domestic violence, feminicide, female empowerment, LGBT rights, transphobia, racism, and xenophobia. The use of *digital storytelling* and human interest pieces, exploring issues from maternity and abortion to sexual harassment and gender-based violence (GBV), emerged as popular communication strategies. The communications head of CHANGE emphasised the organisation's increasing use of digital storytelling as part of its advocacy communications on SRHR:

> So we are really trying to revamp our blog content ... We are trying to integrate ... more storytelling. We have made a lot of connections with young women, especially in the Global South ... They have the desire to share their stories ... but they want to share their stories online as well. So, we have identified four advocates ... who we were initially intending to use for another blog that we got connected with ... So we are taking advantage of having these women engage, so we could share their stories on our own platform ... We related to these first four group of young women ... through a platform called the Clap ... focused on menstruation. When we were first talking to them, knowing that this was our tool, to get the placement on this platform, we focused on their experience in their countries and communities around their menstruation, and a lot has to do with access ... A woman shared when she experienced her period, she is a working professional, but unfortunately in places where she lives there are no places to throw her sanitary napkins away. So there are times when she needs to walk around all day with sanitary napkins, and how that makes her feel ... We are working with her to share that story, most of it is around access ... We will get to know their stories a little bit more when we do our communications training with them ... Because they are such an important voice that needs to be heard ... And similarly ... we did a communications training for advocates of sexual and reproductive rights for sub-Saharan Africa, and we did a communications training with them for, basically, the tools of communication not only to communicate with the media but also with policy makers and with the public.

The Brazilian NGO Anis came up with an interesting campaign called #Euvoucontar (I will tell). This shared some similarities with other more high-profile internet campaigns like the #MeToo movement and the Brazilian version #MeuPrimeiroAssedio (MyFirstHarrassment) (Matos 2016, 2017). The picture is of anthropologist Debora Diniz, known for her work on abortion, who left Brazil due to death threats. Here the campaign consisted of videos in which activists read anonymous confessions of women who have had abortions, the idea being to grant marginalised women an opportunity to voice their experiences. These social media platforms also created the means for the organisation to promote its campaigns through specific hashtags, permitting it to share personal stories to sensitize people so that they would support the cause and become activists.

The use of human interest pieces and digital storytelling on the vast experiences of women and abortion offer examples of the *personal* becoming the *political*. Here questions of motherhood, a woman's role in society and within the family, as well as parental commitments regarding childcare as well as fertility come to the foreground. SRHR is understood as being something deeply personal, an emotional commitment that is dependent on an individual's choice as much as on external forces and wider collective structures, including different philosophies of life and ways of seeing the world.

Like other organisations, the International Planned Parenthood Federation underlined the sensitivity of the topic and the challenges that NGOs face in engaging in advocacy communications regarding SRHR. The director of advocacy of IPPF for the UK and Northern Ireland explained its advocacy strategies and the threats that it has faced.[13] She believes that this is a complex issue that cannot mobilise people only through access to medical knowledge; she also emphasised the importance of 'framing' language around SRHR:

> We have a strategy called the Advocacy Common Agenda –
> which has some of the specific priorities that we work, the focus
> of that centre is national change – national political change
> and accountability, we call it. Supported by international work
> that we do in the UN and Africa and EU ... We have offices
> in six regions ... to produce national and subnational change in
> five main thematic areas: What is universal access with SRHR,
> which includes access to modern contraception, universal health
> coverage, and leaving no one behind; the second prioritises safe
> abortion; the third is ... comprehensive sexuality education; the
> fourth is gender-based violence; and the fifth is having SRHR and
> gender equality in the political architecture ... We have created

three centres to work in two of those pathways which are ... supporting social movements and countering opposition. We have three centres that are led by different parts of the Federation ... The second centre is on countering opposition, which will work ... on ... creating a think tank on countering opposition, bringing together intelligence ... but also putting together some systems for ... the security of our member associations ... because many of our member associations have been attacked, physically attacked, death threats ... You know, something that's happening more ... digital advocacy ... has created an emotional relationship with some lived experience. That we NGOs are very bad at ... We are very technical, we show figures and, you know, curves ... We are constrained in a way by donors who want you to develop ... But the human story ... is the one which [is] always going to impact the most in people ... So we have one advocacy function and the other director of communications ... We work together ... yes, but as I always say, we don't do campaigns as such from the global level ... Because we do think that it needs to be more – and on that side, I think, the work with the media is ... you know, we have a relationship with major ... media ...we have a communication strategy, which is mainly a focus on amplifying the voices of what's happening on the ground.

IPPF is a well-known name in the field and has been around for sixty-seven years. The head of digital communications of IPPF admitted that the organisation was slow in taking up digital communications.[14] In the communications questionnaire that she answered, she underlined how social media is key, also indicating that the organisation engages in lobbying and tries to influence politicians and policy-makers, largely within Europe. However, she also admitted that it is only in the last two years that IPPF has increased its usage of online communications for advocacy activities. On the question on the uses of online communication technologies, she stated that she has been 'fighting' to make this 'a priority'. She further noted how it was crucial to engage the public in any process of social change, as 'we can only create real change ... if we can engage the same public who vote progressive or regressive governments'.

In her response to the questionnaire, the head did not include an example of a successful campaign, although she did state the need to 'invest more in digital communications' and said that, 'along with advocacy', the hope is to make everything 'digital first'. She underlined the organisation's use of Twitter and its growing use of LinkedIn, saying that online communications through them were considered 'very effective'. Moreover, she mentioned abortion as a challenging issue, further stressing the need to present content in an 'engaging manner', such as through storytelling or animation:

> We have a key messaging brief for journalists, donors as well as other external audiences. Abortion care is also at the forefront of the 'essential health care' argument, so we are heavily involved in media relations in ensuring that abortion is *framed* and considered essential health care. We are also sharing practical information on sex and COVID-19, pregnancy and COVID-19, and HIV and COVID-19, as our website search engine tells us people are actively seeking this information. You need to ensure you collate relating content onto a landing page so that it is easier to find for people visiting. You need to present content in an engaging way – through GIFs, quizzes, animations … People looking for practical information on sex will not want to read a PDF. We need to look at how other industries are communicating and take inspiration from them. Simplicity is key along with strong visuals … The opposition are well funded and better organised and prepared in the digital sphere as well as offline. I also think attitudes towards larger NGOs are changing – our audiences are changing, and we need to be better at audience mapping to attract like-minded millennials … We also need to be braver and stronger in our communications … From a comms perspective, we have heavily invested in reframing the language and narrative around SRHR, and specifically on abortion care. We use frames based on *care* – and we have done some research … in Ireland on how it has been used successful[ly] on traditional conservative politicians and it works.

Many of the organisations are making use of blogs to engage in discourses on reproductive health. The intention is to use these blogs to reach out to a more knowledgeable and more active public, a strategy that has not only positive results but also important limits in terms of generating more impact and creating more awareness around SRHR. It is thus to a critical discourse analysis of the NGOs' blogs that I now turn.

11

The NGOs' Blog Posts and Digital Storytelling on SRHR

A Critical Examination

Carolina Matos with Sarah Molisso

The results of this study show that, despite the growing popularity of blogs in the activist community, and despite their being seen in many ways as a key feature of citizen media within a wider participatory democracy, the reality is that this form of communication is not always widely used by NGOs and does not necessarily reach out to larger audiences. Of the fifty-two NGOs studied here, be they in the North or in the South, only twenty-one organisations had some form of blog posting on their websites. These included blogs with regular as well as infrequent postings, outdated blogs, 'stories', and 'chapters'. Blog posts that were published during this study's core data collection period (25 March–7 April 2019) were examined, but ten were not updated during the analysis. However, due to the limited sample,[1] an extra year was added to this time frame (25 March 2019–7 April 2020). Of the twenty-one NGOs that had some form of blog on their websites, five of them had blogs that were outside of the time frame, with organisations not posting after 2016, 2017, and 2018 (Anis, CREA India, Rede Feminista de Saúde, Women´s Global Network for Reproductive Rights, and Youth Coalition for Sexual and Reproductive Rights). Of the fifteen blogs analysed, six are from within the time frame (ASAP, CARE, FP2020, IPPF, SRHM, and WLP) and the other nine are not (Amnesty International, APA, C3, CHANGE, International Campaign for Women's Rights to Safe Abortion [ICWRSA, or Campaign], RESURJ, Swasti, Women Deliver, and YouAct).

All the blog posts could be placed under different styles of communications. They can be situated under the five categories developed for this research: *advocacy, information, fundraising, mobilisation,* and *community engagement*. The blog posts were placed under three core themes: (1) sexual and reproductive health and rights (SRHR), (2) gender-based-violence (GBV), and (3) comprehensive sexuality education (CSE). Most of the blog posts (eight out of fifteen) focused on an issue pertaining to SRHR, with six being included under the topic of GBV and one under CSE.[2] The blogs that fell outside of the original time frame were chosen based on whether they related to the core themes and were selected close to the original time frame. Several posts by the NGOs examined in the second stage of the collection process focused on issues faced during the COVID-19 pandemic,[3] although in the end these were not selected since other posts were better placed within the core themes developed here and were published closer to the research's time frame.[4]

Some of the organisations attempted to attach their blog posts with research expertise as a means of seeking credibility for their information, including naming the respective authors. Three blog posts, those of CARE, WLP, and YouAct, were co-authored publications,[5] while IPPF's blog post did not recognise any author. All the other blog posts credited an author. Seven of the blogs included tags or filters to categorise their posts, such as the one from FP2020 (which used the online publishing platform Medium), which had the tags 'Refugees', 'Family Planning', 'Women's Health', and 'Reproductive Rights.'

IPPF is listed under the subject 'abortion', whereas CHANGE is listed under 'contraception' and could also be tagged under 'human and sexual and reproductive rights'. WLP fell under the categories of *'Advancing Human Security'* and *'Empowering Refugee Women'*. The other blog posts had tags or filters that were not explicitly related to the themes of SRHR, GBV, or CSE. Campaign's blog post was posted in three separate places: 'Africa', 'Blog', and 'South Africa', while Women Deliver was tagged with 'Humanitarian Crises/Emergency Response' and 'Peace & Security'. The remaining eight blog posts did not have any tags, even though some appeared on blogs that did have tags, topics, or filters on them, including the organisation Sexual and Reproductive Health Matters (SRHM), whose blogs had topics such as 'book reviews', 'press releases', 'resources', 'SRHM in the news', and 'SRHM staff blog.'

The critical discourse analysis found that the communications strategies and the ways in which the NGOs used the blogs, as well as their approaches to sharing the posts, were quite varied. The NGOs CARE UK and WLP's sharing capabilities were numerous. At first glance, only two sharing links are shown on CARE UK's blog page (on Facebook and Twitter), whereas four are shown on WLP's page (Facebook, Twitter, Pinterest, and LinkedIn). However, upon clicking on the 'more' link, the reader is met with 179 possible ways to share the post. Some of these include Kakao Talk (South Korea), Line (popular in Japan), Nasza-Klasa (Poland), and *Kledy* (Germany), all of which highlight the ways in which the organisations sought to reach a global public in their attempts to generate impact.

The NGO YouAct had the option of sharing via VK, a Russian social networking site. Some blog posts did not have any options for the reader to share the post, reflecting the inequalities among the organisations and the ways in which the larger NGOs, and those with more resources, had the means of making their messages and content heard by a wider audience. These included the blog posts for SRHM, CHANGE, and Campaign. The most frequent options for sharing were also via Twitter (twelve), Facebook (eleven), LinkedIn (seven), and email (six). The diversity in the use of blog posts, as seen by their sharing capabilities (or lack thereof) also revealed that blogs are not a priority for advocacy communications pertaining to SRHR and that they are not necessarily used as a means of engaging with a wider public.

However, without access to the analytics of digital reach, it is obviously difficult to measure how often these blogs have been viewed. In this case, engagement and reception can most visibly be captured through the analysis of the number of 'likes', 'claps', or comments related to the blog posts. The examination of these blogs revealed that there was little engagement with the messages and content posted. None of these had any comments, with only Amnesty International UK and FP2020 enabling the posting of comments, while ASAP, C3, APA, CARE, CHANGE, Campaign, IPPF, RESURJ, SRHM, Swasti, Women Deliver, WLP, and YouAct did not. The only blog that had any visible engagement was that of FP2020. This may be because it is available on the online publishing platform Medium and therefore is subject to the same reception as other posts on the site in the form of responses and 'claps', which are akin to 'likes' (the post in question received three 'claps').

There were several ways that some of the blog posts could have been shared, yet there was seemingly little engagement with the actual posts. Some of the blog posts had either been posted before or afterwards on other platforms or shared via other social networking sites. APA's blog post (30 April 2019) was originally published via LinkedIn on 2 January 2019, although this post too received no comments. This post, unlike the one on APA's website, included a link to a YouTube video, 'CSO Joint Statement-Progress on ICPD in Asia Pacific', delivered by the communications representative of YCSRR, which has had 121 views,[6] two 'likes', but no comments. ASAP's blog post (26 March 2019) was later reposted on the personal blog, thatwhichiam,[7] having received one comment. This was also tweeted by ASAP on 10 April 2019 and was retweeted once.

Despite the problems with wider engagement, some of the blog posts – particularly those from the larger NGOs – were referenced by other organisations, showing how a lot of the discussion and communications on SRHR happens among the professionals themselves, creating 'echo chambers' or raising questions about why so much of the information here is about 'preaching to the already converted'. This was the case with CARE UK's blog post (28 March 2019), which was referenced in a policy briefing via the Africa Portal, as well as FP2020's content (1 April 2019), also reposted on 5 April 2019 on reliefweb[8] and on UNFPA Bangladesh.[9] This showed that from here it had been shared via Twitter twice. The NGO Women Deliver's post (10 July 209), like APA's, was originally posted on another webpage (the news site TheNewHumanitarian[10]). The post received a much more visible engagement, being shared among others via Twitter[11] and by Women Deliver on Facebook[12] on 10 July 2019, receiving twenty-four likes and two shares.

Although overall the blog posts received little engagement, this same material could be reposted on different websites, such as on ASAP's or on Campaign's blogs, or be taken from other sites and from other previous posts, such as those from APA and Women Deliver. It did not appear that these NGOs used blog posts as part of a *cohesive* communications strategy. The composition of the blogs did not show much uniformity, which suggests that blogs in general were not seen as the key component in the online communications strategies of the NGOs. This has been confirmed by the findings of this research as well as by many of the gender and communication experts. ASAP's blog was the only one to display its references at the end of the piece (albeit only three), while others' references were disseminated as hyperlinked words throughout the post. This was seen in posts from Amnesty International UK to FP2020 and RESURJ, which included a single link to a news article upon which the blog post was based on.

The results showed that various blogs are specifically targeted at a younger public. We have seen throughout that members of the younger public are major recipients of communicative material on SRHR and that most NGOs are seeking ways to engage them more in these debates. YouAct's single link was to an advocacy toolkit that the reader could download, and within this toolkit there was a series of supporting links. The toolkit explicitly stated that it was 'An Advocacy Toolkit Developed by and for Young People'. The toolkit was posted on YouAct's blog and promoted on Facebook. YouAct's blog post pointed to its advocacy toolkit, with a separate link allowing the reader to download it. The toolkit discussed the ways in which young people can advocate for CSE. It was developed as part of the 'The European Parliament, Our Ally' project, funded by Generation Now: Our Health, Our Rights, which was launched by the International AIDS Society (IAS) and Women Deliver to promote an 'interconnected agenda', including CSE programmes to prevent unintended pregnancies and HIV. The toolkit underlined the reasons advocacy should focus on CSE, linking parts of the text to different sources.[13] YouAct's toolkit also showed how smaller NGOs can be creative and maximise their outreach and impact by establishing partnerships with other organisations in the field (Yang and Saffer 2018).

This communication strategy aimed at reaching out to younger audiences, creating awareness and mobilisation around SRHR issues, was also detected in the discourses and narratives used in other NGO blogs. ASAP's blog post's title was repeated at the end (i.e., 'mantra for the new age: Keep Calm and Take the Medical Abortion Pill!'). This was clearly a play on the popular slogan 'Keep Calm and Carry On', taken from British Second World War motivational posters, and which has made a commercial comeback in the 2000s.

Some blogs had no references, such as those of the organisations APA, CARE UK, C3, and CHANGE. However, the latter did link the video it was talking about in the blog. Not all of the posts were written by or reviewed by the NGO. SRHM's blog included a disclosure stating that the posts did not necessarily reflect the views of SRHM as an organisation, yet calling for guest blog contributions. The CDA of the blogs revealed that updates were very sporadic. C3 only had four blog posts, dated 1 and 13 July 2016, and then on 2 and 13 March 2020. However, the media content available for the website included news and wider media coverage, various other publications, and the blogs, reflecting a dominant tendency among the NGOs to share mainstream media reports and stories. This might suggest that C3 did not see blogs as being an effective communications tool for advocacy on SRHR issues.

The use of an informal and conversational tone was a predominant feature of many of the communications outputs of various organisations, although some were more formal, making wider use of evidence-based research for advocacy and to raise awareness. The NGO FP2020 made wide use of statistics and quotes from experts. WLP also made frequent use of numbers, further showcasing an interview with two Nigerian Women, Peace and Security activists. Campaign's blog also resorted to the use of statistics in its advocacy communications, but this time as a means of appealing to the reader's emotions. This was the case with the post '105,358 illegal abortions were carried out in the Western Cape in 2016/7'. Unlike either FP2020 or the WLP, Campaign did not have any sharing capabilities on its blog, thus diminishing the extent to which its messages and content could reach a wider audience and generate impact. It was also possible to identify a thread of common themes on SRHR explored by the posts, and this is what is examined next.

THEMES EXPLORED IN THE BLOG POSTS

All of the blogs included topics concerning SRHR, but they also explored areas such as GBV and CSE. Four core themes appeared frequently within these broader topics. These were: (1) abortion (through ASAP, Campaign, IPPF and CHANGE's posts); (2) sexual and domestic violence (Swasti, CARE, WLP, and C3); (3) human rights (Amnesty International UK, Women Deliver, and FP2020); and (4) pregnancy (RESURJ and SHRM). Discussions of motherhood were explored in some posts, such as SRHM. The ASAP post weaved a narrative about how the oral medical abortion pill is linked to the wider oppression of women, showing how patriarchy is responsible for seeking to control women and their fertility. This was then connected to ideas of marriage and motherhood as supposed milestones in a woman's life. It also delved into issues of marital rape, child marriage, and the lack of CSE in schools.

The blog also advocated for the rights of sex workers or those seen as outside traditional relationships. The reader is directed towards three references at the end of the blog post: WHO's (2014) *Clinical Practice Handbook for Safe Abortion*, a news article on birth control in the US,[14] and a medical abortion factsheet published by ASAP (*ASAP's: Medical Abortion Factsheet*). This factsheet makes use of cartoon graphics and references WHO guidelines to answer questions regarding medical abortion, such as which drugs to use, who can use them, and their side effects. The factsheet directs the reader to ASAP's social media accounts, including Facebook and Twitter, as well as to its website. ASAP's blog post was unique in that it combined an anecdotal and conversational-style blog post, written by a gynaecologist who talked about the societal structures of patriarchy and their consequences, with other materials, like ASAP's factsheet.

This can be seen as being in line with the entertainment-education formats used in health communication campaigns (Tufte 2012; Lewis and Lewis 2015), in which factual, evidence-based medical knowledge is made attractive and engaging by using more direct language, conversations, and talk relating to the everyday reality of women's concerns with contraception, taking pills, and with abortion more broadly. ASAP's factsheet resorted to a comic-book style of communications to 'tell a certain story', showing texts and images of a young woman using her mobile phone and being very inquisitive.

ASAP's blog post also talked about the oral birth control pill, but this was situated specifically within the Asian context. While YouAct focused on the European Union, other blogs examined issues related to South America, Asia, and Africa. Four of the blog posts were focused on specific topics from Asia (APA [the Philippines], C3 and Swasti [India]; and FP2020 [Rohingya refugees]), while the remaining five blog posts focused on Africa (WLP [Nigeria], CARE [Malawi], Campaign [South Africa], RESURJ [Rwanda], and Women Deliver [connecting activists in Sudan to those in Syria]).

The US organisation CHANGE had a blog post whose aim was to promote knowledge on the global implications of the Global Gag Rule (GGR). CHANGE's post focused on the GGR and was centred on the making of it as well as on the rationale behind it. Out of eleven paragraphs, two were directly related to the GGR. These paragraphs, which were at the beginning of the post, included facts about the GGR, underlining how it had been a presidential memorandum that had been signed by every Republican president and rescinded by every

Democratic one since the Reagan government in 1984. However, when coupling the blog post with the documentary (the form taken by the project), there were a lot of references to facts whose purpose was to raise awareness of the US's Global Gag Rule policy and how it was undermining SRHR at home and abroad. The documentary featured expert voices, including that of the director of policy research at CHANGE, making further reference to the statistics obtained from the polls administered by CHANGE and PAI, with figures provided by IPPF, such as how the GGR will limit $100 million in funding.[15]

Campaign's blog posts also focused on abortion. However, rather than including a piece that linked the practicalities of medical abortion to theoretical concepts like ASAP's, Campaign's post concentrated on disseminating the politics surrounding the provision of medical facilities. It criticised the lack of centrality in the South African government's approach to reproductive justice. Like ASAP's post, Campaign's referenced outside sources, such as news articles on politics and reproductive justice.[16] Making use of a communication strategy similar to ASAP's, which makes a connection between theory and personal anecdotes, Campaign highlighted the need for more abortion facilities by providing personal stories related to the outcomes of illegal abortions. This included an article provided by the National Department of Health (which is not referenced) and that describes a disturbing situation whereby 'it was not uncommon for new-born foetuses to be found discarded' or in a bush or a communal toilet. The aim was to raise awareness of the severity of the problems caused by unsafe abortion practices, including health risks and social problems associated with the criminalisation of the termination of pregnancies. The situations outlined here may be seen as being integral to the reality experienced by less privileged women across the world.

However, the use of such narratives could function as a double-edged sword as they could evoke strong emotions from the public: rather than bring activists together around the common cause of reproductive justice (Pieck 2013) or even get people to favour the legalization of safe abortion. They could thus play into conservative counter-discourses against the advancement of women's rights in sexuality and reproductive health by equating (unsafe) abortion practice with criminal behaviour and actions committed by 'sinful' and 'promiscuous' women.

IPPF's blog post also aimed to reach audiences transnationally. The post discussed its *I Decide What Happens to My Body* movement, which advocated for universal access to safe abortion by including mobilisation anecdotes from countries such as Malaysia, Yemen, Morocco, Eswatini, Ireland, and Sri Lanka. It also included the use of radio and social media platforms, such as WhatsApp, Facebook, and Twitter. The blog posts further highlighted that these measures promoted '(normally unheard) voices', further enabling a wide variety of people to be *agents of change* in a democratic process – in this case, the activists in Eswatini who stimulated a 'country-wide debate on the provision of abortion that ha[d] got them invited to consult with the Ministry of Health'.

The I Decide movement capitalised on the idea of the individual as the agent of change, with its website being linked within the blog post, further enabling the reader to 'pledge your voice' by signing up online with her/his/their personal details. This practice was a good strategy for actively engaging the reader in conversations around abortion, women's agency, and individual choice. The reader is offered the possibility of signing up and agreeing with statements such as 'I believe that: all decisions regarding pregnancy must be voluntary. No woman should be forced to carry a pregnancy to term' as well as signing the pledge: 'I pledge to: Use my voice to challenge abortion stigma by having conversations about it with my family'.[17]

Similar to both ASAP's and CHANGE's blog posts, IPPF's blog posts included links to other resources in order to provide the reader with the opportunity to watch activist videos, all of which had been uploaded to Facebook. The link to the I Decide website also gave more information, with links in ASAP's and CHANGE's blog posts. These included animations explaining the difference between medical and surgical abortion as well as questions and answers that refer to specific facts on a range of issues from universal access to legal abortion. There were personal anecdotes in the form of stories as well as links to posts on social media and to the report *Her in Charge: Medical Abortion and Women's Lives – A Call for Action*, available to download in English, French, and Spanish.

The NGO Swasti included blog posts in the form of chapters, posting fifteen on a single day. These chapters covered topics ranging from investment in social development programmes to India's AIDS response, sexually transmitted infections, gender conformity, and hygiene. One topic examined was the gender differences in health care. This was framed in terms of sexual violence against female health workers, with some of the problems outlined including denunciations of how sexual favours can be used for career progression and how female community health workers can be sexually harassed on their way to work. This has implications for their capacity to attend to the obstetric needs of patients at night. Unlike the blog posts on abortion, however, this post did not include any external references to support its narrative, although it did refer to certain facts, including informing the reader of the existence of the gender pay gap for female health workers in India.

CARE UK's post, unlike that of Swasti, used a single narrative to raise awareness of the issues of gender-based violence in the aftermath of Cyclone Idai. In an effort to raise funds for the cause, it made reference to a human interest story and underlined the possibility of a woman refugee being the victim of sexual violence. The woman in question was referred to as 'Mary'. According to the stories: 'Many young men have been hounding her [Mary] for sexual favours in exchange of food. She says the advances have been increasing every day and now she fears that she may become a target of sexual abuse'. Furthermore, 'they [CARE's protection committees] are leading sessions in the camps, telling people to be aware of sexual abuse risks ... and how to report sexual exploitation and harassment'. It could be argued that here the image of the 'helpless woman victim in need of saving' is played out somewhat stereotypically. Because the post is dedicated to fundraising, the blog concludes by calling for donations to help CARE support people affected by the flooding, framing this within the narrative of gender-based violence. Like Swasti's post, CARE's did not include any links to external sites, but it did include some figures about the organisation's work (e.g., 'CARE has distributed plastic sheeting for roofing temporary shelters, water and sanitation items such as water buckets').

C3's (Centre for Catalyzing Change) blog post also touched upon domestic violence, discussing it through references to a film. The film's title, *Thappad*, is Hindi for 'slap', and the director contextualises domestic violence within the overarching notions of patriarchy and how these are deeply rooted in people's lives. This approach is similar to that of ASAP's blog post, which depicts the themes of abortion in the light of patriarchal structures that hinder women's lives. However, unlike ASAP's post, C3's does not include any external sources or facts on domestic abuse in India.[18] Amnesty International UK, Women Deliver, and FP2020 also explored the violation of human and women's rights. All three of these posts made various connections between gender-based violence and other political and societal issues.

Amnesty International UK published the only blog post on a specific problem related to the region of South America, in this case Ecuador. It linked gender-based violence to the environment and Ecuador's indigenous communities, documenting how indigenous women are defending their homes against threats from the oil industry and describing how some of these women have been psychically or verbally attacked. Just as CARE's post makes use of stories, so Amnesty International UK's post makes use of personal stories from two indigenous women from the provinces of Sápara and Pastaza. Its post, like WLP's, also includes one link to an external source, a research report on 'the brave women protecting human rights.'[19] The emphasis is on the image of women in development as agents of change, however oppressed by their social settings and political and economic circumstances.

RESURJ's blog post, like those of Amnesty International UK, Women Deliver, and FP2020, also attempted to discuss teenage pregnancy in the context of GBV. The author criticises the cuts to funding for vulnerable girls and then goes on to discuss the Rwanda's problematic framing of sexuality, showing that it is easier (and more common) to 'punish' girls for getting pregnant than it is to dismantle structural gender inequalities. This strategy is similar to that used by ASAP and C3 in their blog posts. And the argument is supported by the data, which indicate that, although many teenagers are already sexually active, the discussion of sexuality is usually targeted to married adults, resulting in a lack of information for young people, including on premarital sex and pregnancies. The linked news article provides further evidence, which frames teenage pregnancy as a gender-violence-based issue, underlining how, as of 2017, '17,444 teenagers had unwanted pregnancies across the country'.

The centrality of motherhood, and the social meanings associated with it, were also examined widely. SRHM's blog post, for instance, was essentially an advert for an art book that documents representations of fecundity. The author was a former UNFPA adviser for maternal health and rights who describes her professional life within international maternal and reproductive health,[20] having engaged in the prevention of 'complications of pregnancy and childbirth' and having facilitated the 'conception for women who wished to conceive', as well as having assisted in the avoidance of 'pregnancy for those who did not wish to have a child'. The blog underlined how 'the world over, women hope to conceive, then wait during pregnancy before finally giving birth'. It highlighted how 'Motherhood ... is beautiful'.

These statements were in contrast to some of the language used in other blogs, such as ASAP, which emphasised that 'sex happens, and pregnancy isn't always a wanted outcome'. This shows the complexities of the topic and how the organisations attempt to examine reproduction from various aspects, from fertility treatment (and infertility) to the reality experienced by women who do want to conceive but struggle to do so, or those who do not think the timing is right or that their socio-economic circumstances are adequate. It is also good to note that SRHM's blog post is an art book devoted to representations of fertility, coming from the perspective of someone who worked in the field of maternal health.

SRHM's blog post stressed the importance of motherhood, underpinning its universality and centrality to women's lives and bodies by focusing on objects, stories, and images of fertility, pregnancy, and childbirth. The image of women in their maternal bodies is something that is lived out in public and yet can take away from the individual self through 'the trap of essentialism', which can 'lurk at every turn' (Chase and Rogers 2001 in Miller 2005, 139). This post could be read in different ways, either as a reinforcement of patriarchal values and Western assumptions about motherhood or as a critical appreciation of reproduction in all its glory and miseries. This shows that SRHR is not synonymous with the 'defence of abortion' but, rather, that it serves as an umbrella for a range of complex themes. These are dealt with differently by the organisations not just in their practices, aims, and main strategies but also in relation to how they position themselves geographically, how they make use of communications, how they access funds and resources, and how they deal with various challenges, as discussed in previous chapters. And so it is to how these blog posts are used for advocacy communications purposes and for mobilisation that I turn next.

COMMUNICATIONS FOR ADVOCACY AND MOBILISATION

NGO agenda-building can take the form of NGOs blogging or using other communications strategies to boost the coverage of certain issues, with these then identified by the public as important (Yang and Saffer 2018). In the case of the communication strategies of the NGOs regarding their blog posts, it is possible to argue that their media content explores various types of communication styles and messages.

With some overlaps, all the blog posts fell within the following type of communications categories: *advocacy* (ASAP, Campaign, WLP, YouAct), *information* (FP2020), *fundraising* (CARE), *mobilisation* (Amnesty International UK, Asia Pacific Alliance [APA], C3, CHANGE, IPPF, RESURJ, Swasti, Women Deliver), and *community engagement* (C3, CHANGE, FP2020, SRHM).

Issues around medical abortion, and the impact of patriarchal structures on the oppression of women within the context of their sexuality and reproductive rights, were explored by some organisations in clear advocacy communication strategies. ASAP's post took a stance in favour of the oral medical abortion pill in such a way that it simultaneously vilified the patriarchal oppression of women. The author further appealed to human interest stories, a common journalistic strategy, by emphasising her personal experience (such as attending meetings with groups of women's rights activists).

WLP's blog post showed how its NGO had formed relationships with other civil actors and organisations, CEADER, and the two Women, Peace and Security advocates whom they interviewed for the blog post. These advocates were able to discuss what the issues were and how they were overcoming them through training workshops. Campaign's post tried to make use of advocacy around medical abortion as a means of setting this agenda in the public sphere, linking the post to a news article to call on the government to ensure that adequate provision and other reproductive health commodities are implemented in a timely fashion. Swasti's post is slightly different from that of the other advocacy strategies of the NGOs. While the others were published as single blogs posts, Swasti published fifteen 'chapters' on the same day as part of a series on strengthening health workforce-related practices across states and non-state actors.

The blog posts that were mobilisation pieces generally utilised emotional stories or language to engage the reader. Amnesty International UK's post highlighted the struggles of indigenous women leaders in Ecuador against the oil industry and its potential environmental impacts, linking it to a few personal stories that showed the abuse that women activists had suffered. This blog post issued a tangible call for mobilisation – asking readers to sign an online petition and to write to the Ecuadorian attorney general. Other posts, like IPPF's and RESURJ's, also fall under the category of mobilisation. These blog posts utilised stories that relied on moral and emotional language. IPPF also made use of phrases such as 'it has been truly phenomenal', 'it's been an incredible journey for us all', and 'we were even fortunate enough to', all of which encouraged the reader to address the stigmas surrounding abortion.

The NGO RESURJ focused on an online debate about the rescinding of scholarships to pregnant teenagers. Here the author clearly made an attempt to persuade the reader, using sentences such as 'It sparked a hot debate among many people (myself included) with different positions.' Like RESURJ, Swasti's blog post also concentrated on a localised issue, stressing the inequality faced by female health workers. With sentences such as 'they [i.e., women] compensate for the shortcomings of health systems through individual adjustments, at times to the detriment of their own health', and 'there are no special policies to address their parallel needs as mothers and wives, whether it is childcare', the post called for a change to the treatment of female health care workers by focusing on the discrimination that they faced.

APA's blog also called for mobilisation. It focused on the International Conference on Population and Development Program of Action (ICPD POA), highlighting some cultural factors that challenge its implementation in the Philippines. The post called for an adoption of policies that were 'human rights-based and gender responsive', addressing readers and asking them if they wanted to be involved. It also evoked emotion, though in a slightly different way than did RESURJ or Amnesty International's posts. APA's blog was more similar to IPPF's, which incited positive emotion in order to achieve mobilisation. This may be seen in sentences such as 'Why is it important for us to be involved in the process and make our governments accountable?'

Thus the problem of low engagement with the blogs, with the conversations around SRHR happening mainly among professionals already working in the field, may be seen as a testament to the difficulties that NGOs working with reproductive health continue to encounter in building wider public engagement, mobilisation, and a more indepth, knowledgeable interest in the topic. Without the space to comment on blog posts, and with little other engagement available for the reader (e.g., the 'likes'), the public's engagement can only be measured via analytical information on how many people actually accessed the blog posts. Knowing that 'the competition for attention is a zero-sum game' (Thrall, Stecula, and Sweet 2014) and that more attention is preferable to less, it does not appear that the NGO blogs are effectively using communications to gather more attention. Some posts were aimed at disseminating sensitive and often delicate issues (such as the oral contraception pill), and therefore sought to avoid bad publicity, be it from internet trolls or from readers who strongly disagreed with their ideas.

It appears that blogs also generally made use of emotions to disseminate their viewpoints and that this was seen as useful for both mobilisation and advocacy. The advocacy content in particular connected emotions with personal stories, inviting direct submissions, sharing different stories through campaigns (like IPPF's I Decide campaign), or 'trawling their social media feeds to identify story ideas' (Trevisan et al. 2020, 148). This was seen in the posts by RESURJ, Women Deliver, ASAP, Campaign, and FP2020, all of which had links to news articles. Some of these, including ASAP, CHANGE, CARE, and Women Deliver, also used personal stories to convey the writer's message. The use of personal stories further combined major debates with the writer's own experience, producing 'grassroots "expert" views' (Trevisan et al. 2020, 148), a strategy that was also used on social media.

Blogs are also a useful tool for both finding and disseminating topics of interest. Although blogs provide a space within which to explore different themes, NGOs employ different approaches, with some employing facts and figures and others striving to appeal more to emotions. Some link smaller topics to wider theoretical issues, while others focus on personal stories. When considering the discrepancies between NGOs' blog posts, such as their (in)frequency, their sharing capabilities, and their readers' comments, one may conclude that the NGOs working in the field of gender equality and reproductive health do not make full use of blogs as a major part of their communications strategy for SRHR advocacy. It is to the empirical results of the social media engagement of the South Asian NGOs that I now turn.

12

Social Media and Advocacy Communications from South Asian NGOs Working on Sexuality and Reproductive Health

Carolina Matos with Ambika Tandon

The critical discourse analysis of the social media engagement of the South Asian NGOs working in the field focused on nine organisations. Like those in the previous chapter, the results show that there is still room for more engagement and communications investment, particularly when it comes to the use of online communication tools for SRHR advocacy, from the raising of awareness around the cause to mobilising for action. A common finding for all the NGOs is that they highlighted two important aspects of their work on social media: (1) their advocacy work as a means of indicating problems and critiquing policy frameworks across different Asian countries and (2) their strategies for raising awareness of SRHR. They primarily targeted policy-makers, other civil society organisations, and the general public. Throughout the period of study, there was little media messaging addressed to donors and activists, and no fundraising communications was posted through the period of study. This confirms the finding that fundraising through social media is not necessarily a priority for these organisations.

All nine NGOs were more active on Twitter than on Facebook. Apart from ASAP, which was equally active across platforms, all eight South Asian organisations posted more frequently on Twitter than they did on other platforms, with Facebook having the second highest number of posts. This is in line with the social media engagement of many of the Northern NGOs. Many of Twitter's hashtags also made use of slang and popular language, with examples including #WhatWomenWant by White Ribbon Alliance on 30 March;[1] the #MainKuchBhiKarSaktiHoon (I can do anything) by PFI,[2] on 3 April 2019; and #SpeakUpIndia by Center for Catalyzing Change India, on 25 March.[3] YouTube videos and blogs were scarcely used, with only two videos posted in the two-week period by Women Deliver and ASAP, and only one blog posted by ASAP and APA.

Twitter's content consisted of a considerable number of retweets as compared to original posts, except for CREA, which had a higher proportion of original ones. APA posted fifty-six tweets, of which fourteen were original while forty-two were retweets aimed at amplifying the voices of other partners and allies. The latter can obviously contribute towards sustaining a network of actors working towards achieving shared goals. The NGO Centre for Catalyzing Change engaged on Twitter on 3 April 2019 to celebrate #WorldHealthWorkersWeek by posting about the 'frontline village level health workers', whose work can be credited for the success of several health programs across India, from the reduction of maternal death rates to the increase in vaccination programmes.[4]

There were also some posts that explicitly demonstrated that many organisations were building a network of collaboration between themselves. For instance, on 5 April 2019, Women Deliver tweeted about a rally in which thirty international communities would get together to collectively advocate for upholding the rights of women in emergency settings. Making use of hashtags such as #NotOptional and #Humanitarian4Her, the NGO engaged in appeals to its younger audience to raise awareness about this network collaboration.[5] Some of the communication practices of the South Asian organisations, as well as of their social media engagement, matched a few of the advocacy communication strategies identified in the work of other NGOs. This is a consequence of pressure due to underfunding and lack of resources.

Most of the South Asian organisations focused on sharing other NGOs' content rather than building their own social media presence. This provided their targeted public with little information on the organisations themselves, their type of work, and their priorities. It could be argued that this weakens the presence and advocacy communications engagement of these organisations on the internet and costs them an opportunity to effectively achieve their goals and raise awareness beyond local contexts. Most posts were shared across Twitter and Facebook with little to no change in the language or hashtags used. Moreover, most NGOs from the region, albeit not all, had a 'one-post-fits-all' strategy for each of its platforms rather than adapting media content to suit social media networks. Almost all of CREA's Facebook, Twitter, and Instagram posts analysed here were about Reconference, and they used hashtags such as #rethink, #reimagine, and #reboot.[6]

However, some NGOs showed creativity in the advocacy communication efforts despite a lack of resources. The founder of Hidden Pockets underlined the different strategies adopted for each platform:[7]

> There is a connection between service providers, information, and clients. NGOs and community-related start-ups can make this more efficient because the government, with its limited skill and capacity, can't seem to reach everywhere. That's the idea of being a good citizen digitally ... Especially local NGOs – problems need to be defined locally. For me, digital is not social media, it's the internet, where information is accessible to them ... Digital citizenship does not have rights and duties yet and has its own connotations. So, for instance, we work with SRHR, where if you come onto the digital it's because you didn't want citizenship ... Twitter is usually used to look at policy spaces, interact with ... policy-makers who are important ... Instagram is directly talking to the public and having a personal connection with the masses. Facebook, on the other hand, is more about throwing out bigger campaigns as it has the power to reach thousands of people.

One of the core objectives of the posts on social media platforms was the sharing of information to create awareness about various SRHR topics in a manner that could be accessible to a wider public. This goal was set by ASAP in a Facebook post on 27 March, which reiterated the importance of information sharing to deconstruct myths and misconceptions around SRHR and abortion. As emphasised in previous chapters, the stigmatisation around sexuality and reproductive health, and the spread of misinformation and 'fake news', is not restricted to Latin American, or even Eastern European or American, contexts. Many medical professionals have singled this out as a problem. For example, the president of the Federation of

Obstetric and Gynecological Societies of India Fogsi, talked about how 'misinformation, myths and stigma remain a formidable challenge for the medical fraternity.'[8]

Like North and Latin American organisations, South Asian NGOs attempted to build awareness among the public by sharing academic literature, making use of research-evidence reports to make authoritative claims. The NGO ASAP, for example, shared an informative post on its Facebook page on 2 April 2019 that discussed the disproportionate burden of reproductive health on women and girls. It did so by featuring an academic paper, published in a leading medical journal, that offered ethnographic insights into contraception, antenatal care, and cervical cancer, along with a link to the paper.[9]

Another commonly used strategy to share information and raise awareness was the use of clear language that would be easily comprehensible to a non-knowledgeable audience. Some organisations also used this strategy to challenge myths, misinformation, and stereotypes that are attached to marginalised groups within discussions on sexuality and reproductive health. Attempts to deconstruct the image of 'women as victims and in need of saving' were observed among some of the NGOs' posts. These organisations posted narratives of women and girls from the Global South as being in positions of strength as opposed to being dependent on international development organisations. ASAP in particular posted narratives of women as agents who fight to protect their rights. The use of storytelling devices and other visual material by the organisations is further examined in the next section.

STORYTELLING AND USE OF AUDIO-VISUAL MATERIAL

Like other US and Latin American organisations, many of the South Asian NGOs made use of direct language to make their communications more accessible to a larger audience. Overall, audio-visual material was used by all the NGOs except for Women Deliver and ASAP, both of which posted one video each on their YouTube channels. A majority of the posts by most organisations were text-based, with some accompanied by visual material (such as graphics). Many of the NGOs examined here made wide use of the increasingly popular communication strategy of *digital storytelling*, with Women Deliver using it to advocate for changing social norms. Women Deliver posted a poem that examined the difficulty of hiding one's gender, identity, or sexuality. This post was accompanied by pictures of a young girl standing in front of a microphone in the process of reciting the poem. She was presented as a powerful image as she raised her voice in the public forum. This NGO communicated the strength of young leaders and how these seek to challenge social norms, using hashtags such as #youthvoices and #youngleaders.

On 3 April 2019, Women Deliver uploaded a webinar (originally aired on 27 March 2019) on its YouTube channel entitled 'Gender Data: Why and How to Use Gender Statistics to Propel Your Advocacy'. It contained in-depth discussions on case studies of sex-disaggregated data used for successful policy advocacy across various regions. It further discussed various strategies to collect and leverage quantitative gender data for transforming policy. However, despite having a well-known panel of speakers, the video received only seven likes and 488 views, indicating the difficulties that organisations in the field have – be they from the North or the South – in transcending the 'bumble' of preaching only to the converted.

On 27 March 2019, ASAP posted a short one-minute video recorded by one of its 'youth champions', Asmita Ghosh. It featured a group of young people singing a song titled 'The #Abortionsong', which advocated for the right to bodily autonomy. The lyrics explored women's rights over their own bodies, featuring diverse women and transgender groups from across India to convey the message that people across genders and sexualities have the right to bodily autonomy. The lyrics of the song combined the categories of 'emotion' and 'reason' to get its message across, drawing attention to the fact that the worldwide practice of unsafe abortions is a leading cause of women's death. Different individuals with powerful expressions looked into the camera to reclaim agency through their voice, striving to undermine the anti-abortion discourse and to do so by uniting around collective action and movement building.[10]

The coordinator of ASAP described its videos on YouTube as a concerted strategy to ensure visibility for marginalised voices:[11]

> A lot of our youth champions have made short videos …
> For example, our youth champion for Bangladesh made a film on unsafe abortion in Bangladesh. It's literally the only film on unsafe abortion in Bangladesh. We just couldn't find any other. So, we thought it's very important for these films to be out there. There is someone from the Philippines who has made a film on

unsafe abortion there. Again, the only one that is available, in Sri Lanka, it's the only thing available. These are topics which are very taboo in these countries, no one talks about them. So, we've been trying to give space to these voices, and as I said, have more representation, more testimonies from the countries in Asia to say that these are our stories, we're not just numbers.

ASAP also had a unique component to its social media communications: the use of humour, internet *memes*, and *slang* with the objective of sharing information for advocacy purposes. One of the posts had a popular meme with the picture of a *Lord of the Rings* character, including the text: 'I need to gain weight. Oh look ... contraception pills.' The post aimed to debunk the myth that birth control pills can cause weight gain. Another attempted to deconstruct misinformation about safe abortion practice, underscoring how women 'are just going to start throwing themselves down the stairs again ... You are only getting rid of safe, medically supervised ones.' This post clearly tries to underscore the fact that abortions will not cease to occur if they are made illegal, as many women will ultimately have to resort to unsafe procedures. In a direct reference to the well-known English expression 'Keep calm and carry on', ASAP made use of the popular and catchy phrase 'keep calm and take the #abortion pill'.[12]

Such posts demonstrated ASAP's innovation and creativity as they appropriated popularly used internet artefacts to defend safe abortions. This is a clear indication of ASAP's ability to target young audiences by adapting its media messages to popular culture as well as to the overall *media logic*. ASAP thus mingled the categories of 'emotion' and 'reason' in order to increase engagement rather than simply resorting to the traditional advocacy practices of focusing solely on hard facts around SRHR. Additionally, the use of humour managed to convey rights-based messaging in a light and approachable tone as opposed to the assertive discourse used by most of the other material.

For *mobilisation* and *engagement* with the communities' categories, South Asian NGOs made further efforts to promote events. The focus of their communications varied, with some highlighting their presence at key international conferences and others stressing speeches. The Asia Pacific Alliance (APA) promoted the 52nd Commission on Population and Development (CPD) across all its social media handles using the hashtag #CPD52, with posts largely focused on establishing the organisation's role at the CPD, a critical international forum for advocacy of SRHR. One of its posts on Facebook placed APA's CEO in the spotlight, while at the same time promoting universal access to SRHR and the elimination of violence against marginalised communities. This text on Facebook posted on 5 April 2019 was accompanied by pictures of the CEO 'in action' at the CPD. This enabled APA to successfully demonstrate its active involvement in global advocacy efforts, further underlining its engagement with the communities 'on the ground.'[13]

Some NGOs promoted events they were organizing to increase engagement. CREA promoted Reconference 2019, a major conference it organizes annually. Almost all its posts in the period under study were about Reconference 2019, with the hashtag #recon2019. CREA hosted tweetchats aimed at producing debate on Twitter, with several well-known activists from India and the Global South being involved.[14] Conversations examined issues in SRHR, including the stigma attached to sexuality and pleasure. These debates provided the activists with a space to showcase their thinking around these topics and functioned to amplify their work. It was also considered one of the most successful communication strategies by the NGOs in this region, having generated significant engagement rates.

Various NGOs ran consistent campaigns during the period studied. This was the case for the Centre for Catalyzing Change, which publicised its 'YouthBolPoll' on 25 March on Twitter and included a poll of young individuals' opinions on sexual and reproductive health through extensive social media messaging. All eleven tweets posted by C3 during this period were about this poll. These were further accompanied by specific hashtags intended to mobilise younger users, such as #YouthVoicesCount.[15] This could be seen as an attempt to encourage youth to increase its participation in SRHR issues.

On 3 April 2019, the Population Foundation of India (PFI) showcased on Twitter the use of innovative tools to disseminate information through social media. It developed an AI-powered chatbot for information sharing, operated through its social media. The function of the chatbot was to engage with users' queries in both Hindi and English. The connection with users was established by giving the chatbot the avatar of the protagonist of the television show produced by PFI, called *Main Kuch Bhi Kar Sakti Hoon* (I can do anything).[16] Interviewed for this research, the communications manager at PFI defended the use of social media as a space for presenting SRHR advocacy in a freer manner than was possible elsewhere,[17] in a way that could transcend the self-censorship engaged in by the mainstream media around topics deemed too sensitive. She also spoke about the effectiveness of this strategy in reaching its target user base:

> SRHR for young people is something that needs to be focused on but would not be allowed on the state-run television because that is meant for 'family-viewing', and people would not be comfortable with it. So, to overcome that and to be able to reach out to adolescents and young people, we developed a chatbot which is based on the protagonist of the show [*Main Kuch Bhi Kar Sakti Hoon*] ... We've had more than a million conversations, and thirty-two thousand users regularly engaging in a month of the chatbot being live. This is an innovation because the chatbot uses entertainment content rather than text. It has been designed for people who are first-generation digital media users. We have embedded it on Facebook because we know a lot of people do not have access to personal devices, and the chatbot maintains confidentiality, so we have all those safeguards. The idea is to be able to reach out on a personalised level, but on aggregating you get a larger picture of what young people want.

PFI thus showed that it catered largely to users in rural geographies and to the urban poor through this chatbot, and it did so by embedding audio-visual content in the latter's responses. This addressed the low level of digital literacy in this audience, which often consisted of first-generation users with mobile phones who consume video content on social media and chat apps. PFI integrated the knowledge from the research done with sectors of the community to develop the chatbot. The senior manager of Knowledge Management and Partnerships at PFI described the innovation in the chatbot and its participatory focus,[18] noting how people from the community are invited to participate:

> It [the chatbot] uses the persona of Dr Sneha, the lead character of the series, and the chatbot is meant to answer questions around SRH. We have not even started promoting the chatbot, but we have seen extremely good subscription rates, of 60 percent. Even when we were designing the content, we have included the voices from the community. So, we did these pilots

and voice tests in Madhya Pradesh, Bihar, and Mewad. To get the voices of the community, what were they comfortable with, what were they not comfortable with, what terms they did not understand, what questions they had, the language that they're using, to make it more community friendly.

I thus conclude this chapter with a section on the topics the NGOs explored concerning reproductive health.

TOPICS ON SRHR COVERED BY THE SOUTH ASIAN NGOS

The results of the CDA conducted here shows that gender-based violence, reproductive rights, and gender equality were among the most popular topics investigated by the NGOs. All the NGOs included in this research support women's rights to make decisions regarding their bodies. There was some focus on intersectional perspectives on gender equality, but gender was largely treated as a binary with the adoption of the language of sustainable development goals in reference to 'women and girls' and the achievement of gender equality. Common topics were gender-based violence, human rights violations, and discrimination against minorities. The focus on gender-based violence could reflect the effort of the South Asian organisations to bridge this gap and include it within the ambit of their work as an important determinant of SRHR. Moreover, rights-based language was clearly present throughout the advocacy communications material, with several references to the right of choice.

ASAP was one of the very few organisations that directly linked its advocacy work to grassroots feminist movements in SRHR, confirming what is discussed in previous chapters regarding the existence of a 'disconnect' between some of the gender experts working within the UN orbit and the more local feminist grassroots networks. In a Facebook post on 5 April 2019, ASAP referred to a protest in which women across twenty states in India challenged the incumbent government and its 'attacks on minorities'.[19] While ASAP does not explicitly link its work to this protest, by bringing such movements within the ambit of its communications it indicates a connection between grassroots struggles for women's equality and its work on SRHR. Moreover, in overall references to grassroots movements in the social media communications of most organisations are either absent or scarce.

This is different with regard to the Latin American organisations, which had various forms of engagement with feminist groups and connections to local grassroots movements.

Another organisation that specifically linked its work to a grassroots struggle was Women Deliver. In a post on 29 March 2019 it refers to a protest in which survivors of sexual assault walked across twenty-four states in India, covering ten thousand kilometres, as part of a 'Dignity March' to bring attention to gender-based violence in that country.[20] Some NGO posts critiqued the political economy of development both globally and in India. They highlighted two interlinked problems that NGOs have been facing in the recent past: (1) increasing government hostility towards organisations involved in rights-based work globally and (2) project-dependent funding cycles. In one such post, on 1 April 2019, APA retweeted Open Democracy to clearly critique power hierarchies in international development, specifically targeting short funding cycles as opposed to funding for the 'long haul.'[21] Another APA retweet on 2 April 2019 challenged top-down decision making by funders, particularly critiquing the Global Gag Rule.[22] By framing this in a manner that gave primacy to women's health, the post approached this issue from a public health stance as a means of avoiding controversies.

On 30 March 2019, the NGO White Ribbon Alliance shared on Twitter some statistics on obstetric violence. The post was accompanied by a statement from Brazilian writer and journalist Vanessa Barbara in which she spoke about the rights of pregnant women to make decisions about their own medical care.[23] In a tweet posted on 27 March, APA discussed the imposition of the death penalty for consensual same-sex relations in Brunei, reinforcing the feminist conception of gender equality demonstrated across its communication.[24] By condemning the 'inhuman and degrading' treatment of same-sex relations, the post aimed to raise public awareness of the violation of sexual rights in conservative societies as well as drawing attention to states as perpetrators of violence on the basis of gender identity.

Another strain of gender-based violence was discussed by the NGO CREA in one of its tweet chats, called 'interrogating consent and pleasure', which included the tweets in the chat to reimagine consent by focusing on 'choice, agency, and autonomy'. The discussion considered various aspects of consent, such as the situations under which it can be given as well as the populations that may be unable to give it in a meaningful way. The tweet chat managed to further capture the ambiguities in the process of giving and revoking consent, which CREA characterised as being a 'grey zone' that didn't allow for straightforward constructions of 'right' and 'wrong'. ASAP also participated in this discussion, questioning the imperative people may place on themselves to participate in sexual relationships with their romantic partners. Both organisations sought to unpack the complexities of giving consent in dynamic and affirmative ways.

Many of the NGOs had several posts that advocated for marginalised groups, sexual minorities, and sex workers. These posts significantly broadened the scope of the discussion of SRHR issues by advocating for specific vulnerable groups, including women with disabilities and sexual minorities. On 29 March 2019, on Twitter CREA directed a lot of its posts towards supporting women with disabilities, stating that they are not given the space to raise their voice when it comes to advocacy on sports.[25] The director for programmes and operations explicitly stated that the focus is on intersectional perspectives as well as on broadening the scope of discussions on sexuality and reproductive health in India:[26]

> We are working towards pushing the boundaries of who you consider 'feminist' and who you consider women, like trans women get left out or other groups like sex workers and disabled women. And also the faultline globally between disability rights movement globally and abortion – in some circles. How do you uphold the rights of women with disabilities – that's a big one globally.

The analysis of the social media communications of the South Asian NGOs indicates pervasive underinvestment as well as an overall lack of focus on communications strategies. Some NGOs stated that they are in the process of developing communications strategies and are transitioning to more structured plans. This seems to be a requirement for each of the organisations, except for CREA and Women Deliver. Interviewed for this research, the senior advisor in gender and governance at C3 admitted to the lack of a more structured approach to its communications work:[27]

> If you check out our website or Facebook page then it's nothing great. We now have our own team working on a communications strategy ... on our branding, how to present information so

that it has a recall value ... Till the past year, our work was thematically structured, and our communications would be around an event, or sharing results of our programme, if we've had evaluations. So communications has been theme-focused, but we felt the need to have a structured plan.

Most of the South Asian NGOs studied here had some gaps in their communications strategy, with an absence of regular and consistent messaging around particular themes. Two major gaps could be identified. First, the organisations did not have a concerted focus on the topics of communications, and very few organisations had any regular posts on selected issues. This detracted from clear and consistent messaging as audiences received scattered information, with no specific focal points, regarding different topics aligned with SRHR. Second, there was a lack of investment in the type of communications, including the timeliness of the content, as most organisations posted inconsistently and used largely text-based posts. The absence of audio-visual material, as well as the adaptation of communications material across platforms, was also noted. This resulted in the inability to leverage different social media platforms for targeted communications involving specific stakeholders.

Underinvestment is also reflected in the overwhelming reliance on reposting and sharing other organisations' posts, something that also occurred with some of the organisations in the US and Latin America. In contrast to what was found in the South Asian organisations, NGOs like CREA and Women Deliver stood out in that each of these had a concerted focus and made use of a large volume of posts, including images and other media resources and tools. CREA made great use of tweet chats to encourage debate among key feminist organisations, bringing visibility to its work through events such as Reconference. The NGO Women Deliver, on the other hand, focused on policy-making, with its use of academic and informational posts indicating the gaps and negative outcomes of policy-making globally.

It is to an examination of how some of these organisations can overcome some of these challenges, embedding them within a context in which they can work on new approaches to gender and development theory and practice – a context that is decolonialist and in solidarity with various groups of women throughout the world – that I turn in the final chapter of this book.

13

Gender Development, Women's Reproductive Health, and Sexual Rights in Challenging Times

Communication Strategies Discussed and Concluding Remarks

This book highlights the numerous challenges faced by fifty-two feminist and health organisations and networks when it comes to advocacy communications on sexual and reproductive health, from those located in the North to those in the South, despite the differences in resources and funding, geographical location and culture, as well as in understandings and approaches to SRHR. This is particularly so when it comes to communicating with the wider public on matters concerning SRHR, including making full use of communications tools for social change and advancement on policies on gender equality and reproductive health. These organisations and grassroots networks have been working in an unfavourable environment that is affected not just by the dicta of a highly competitive and marketized global development industry, with its demands for cost-effective programmes and projects and with few funds to support causes, but also by a highly politicised (global) and increasingly conservative climate intent on turning back the clock on many of the policy advancements in the area of gender and minority rights throughout much of the world.

The problem has been exacerbated by the COVID-19 pandemic. The challenges posed by the coronavirus pandemic, particularly from March 2020 onwards, should not be taken lightly as they present another layer of difficulty for those working to improve access to quality health systems and to sexual and reproductive health services for more vulnerable women across many developing countries of the

Global South. The UN's specialised agency in the field, UNFPA, stated in March 2021 that nearly 12 million women in 115 countries lost access to family planning services, something that led to 1.4 million unintended pregnancies over the last year.[1] Various scholars in the field of public health have underlined the risk of inequalities in sexual and reproductive health being entrenched due to the coronavirus pandemic. Riley et al. (2020, 73–5) argue that failure to act in the post-COVID context would lead to this, particularly among the more disadvantaged and LGBT groups, reversing the advances made in the past decades.

Making use of data from the 2019 *Adding It Up* study on SRHR care provision, in 132 low and middle-income countries in Africa, Asia, Eastern and Southern Europe, Latin America, and the Caribbean, which accounts for a total of 1.6 billion women of reproductive age, Riley at al. (2020) indicate that a 10 per cent decline in the use of contraceptive methods in these countries due to reduced access to services would result in an additional 49 million women with an unmet need for contraception and another 15 million unintended pregnancies over the course of the year. There would be a further 28,000 maternal deaths, another 168,000 deaths of new-borns, and a likely further 3.3 million unsafe abortions. The authors make a series of recommendations, including facilitating access to services and making contraceptives available without prescriptions. They also underline the role that the US, as the largest donor for SRHR globally, could have in providing additional funding for global maternal health and family planning programmes to address the needs of marginalised groups. They conclude by emphasising the need for 'clear information on the functioning of sexual and reproductive health services as essential for understanding the impact of the pandemic on abortion'.

As I have stressed, before the pandemic, work and advocacy on gender equality and sexual and reproductive health was already taking place within an increasingly hostile, oppositional political environment. The attack on the 'gender agenda' by various conservative groups throughout the world was already ongoing and had intensified over the last decade, with various groups feeling empowered by the rise of populist and far-right movements and more at ease in lashing out against an ill-defined 'gender ideology' – an ideology that was supposedly propagated by feminists, policy-makers, and advocates of minority and equality rights, and even by governments seeking to implement gender policies as a means of boosting economic growth and productivity. The growth of this conservative opposition, which in the last years has become more vocal, had its roots in the 1980s and 1990s, following from the successes of the transnational feminist movements and the UN-led conferences on various women's rights.

Policies have ranged from the ratification of legislation on the elimination of all forms of gender discrimination to the embedding of sexuality and reproductive health within a human rights framework (Parker 2009; Lottes 2013; Butler 2019; Harcourt 2009, 2017). These led the way for the relaxing of certain legislations pertaining to SRHR, contributing to the expansion of sexuality education in schools and to reviewing abortion laws in various countries, including the wider recognition that women's rights are embedded in human rights frameworks and are aligned to the democratisation of societies everywhere.

This book has thus examined how feminism as a political movement and force has seen a significant revival throughout the world while at the same, paradoxically, being the subject of much scrutiny and attack from across the political spectrum, including from sectors of the left. The latter are concerned with the limits of the inclusivity of Western mainstream feminism ('white feminism' [Jonsson 2021] and the fact that the movement has largely benefitted small privileged groups of women (Fraser 2013) at the expense of working-class, racialised, and minoritized women in the North as well as in the global South. Making use of 'feminisms' in the plural (Alvarez 2014), I argue that feminism as a political, social justice movement has the potential to be truly transformative and to recapture the 'golden years' of transnational feminist networking, organising, and lobbying. Many health and feminist NGOs and organisations who operate in the field of sexuality and reproductive health can re-engage in new forms of transnational solidarity, empathy, and compassion around the pursuit of genuine change regarding gender justice both globally and locally (Fraser 2013).

The search for a way to strengthen feminism that is embedded in anti-colonialist practice and thinking (McLaren 2017) has yet to be achieved. However, it is a growing necessity, particularly within a world in which colonial relationships will continue to adversely affect the progress of various marginalised women and minority groups from various countries of the Global South. McLaren (2017) argues that feminist theory must address the historical legacy of colonialism, as well as postcolonialism and decoloniality, something that continues to be an unfinished project. If anything, the pandemic exposed numerous structural and deep-rooted inequalities (e.g., race inequalities through the #BlackLivesMatter movement) that, although visible before, had been downplayed or not fully addressed.

The inequalities of access to vaccinations for COVID-19 between countries of the North and those of the South – which, in the UK, culminated in the Global Justice Now! movement's attempt to get the government to suspend vaccine patents – is another example of the continuation of neocolonialist practices between the developed and the less-developed countries. The current intellectual debates around the decolonisation process that is taking place within institutions and academia in the UK, as well as throughout much of the West, is a further testament to the fact that – like the taken-for-granted assumptions that 'gender equality has been achieved' – issues of race, ethnicity, and nationality, and the inequalities that they continue to reproduce on a local and global scale, are far from over. If anything, both the New Right and the more participatory left have exposed the 'myths' and limits of the Western democratic consensus and of neoliberalism, particularly regarding its inclusivity and capacity to provide equal opportunities, prosperity, and wealth for wider groups across developed and developing countries alike. Even the rise of global far-right and populist movements, and the disenfranchisement of various citizens in many of the countries of the North, indicates that, for many, the Western democratic project has yet to deliver on its promise of wider equality, inclusion, and opportunities for all groups (including a more genuine political commitment to combatting structural social and economic inequalities).

Despite the current pessimism and the recognition of the numerous challenges and barriers to further advancements, many of the gender experts at the NGOs interviewed here shared a sense of purpose and momentum. They highlighted a widespread sense that concerns with women's bodily autonomy and health are topics destined to grow in importance, particularly in a post-COVID-19 context. The discussions around the Global Gag Rule, and how this had affected access to SRHR services and funding for NGOs across the world, were already providing people with more opportunities for in-depth debate on the quality of access to SRHR services before the Biden administration dropped the rule in 2021. As mentioned, the 2018 report of the Guttmacher-Lancet Commission defended a more holistic approach to SRHR, including the need to tackle neglected issues, from adolescent sexuality to gender-based violence, abortion, and diversity in sexual orientations and gender identities. It states that the gains of the past decades have been inequitable between and within countries, with services having fallen in quality and with people having insufficient access to SRHR services. As the document 'Accelerate Progress: Sexual and Reproductive Health Rights for All', further states:

> Progress in SRHR requires confrontation of the barriers embedded in laws, policies, the economy and in social norms and values ... that prevent people from achieving sexual and reproductive health. Improvement of people's well-being depends on individuals' being able to make decisions ... the right to control one's own body, define one's sexuality ... and receive confidential and high-quality services.

Thus within the context of the 'revival' of the feminist movement there has been an increasing growth of more in-depth debate on a range of issues concerning SRHR in the public sphere, from the decriminalization of abortion to the teaching of sexuality in schools, to respect to sexual identities, debates on male infertility, and the need for states to guarantee access to SRHR services for more vulnerable groups. The results of this study underline that, despite a lot of creativity shown in many of the communication campaigns and strategies of NGOs advocating for SRHR, there is still much more room to work on health communication messages and campaigns across different media outlets and social media platforms.

Messages for health advocacy for SRHR can take a variety of approaches, from a more entertainment-education format to digital storytelling and human interest stories. There can also be more strategic communications of both more 'hard evidence-based reports and facts' on reproductive health, from the impact of COVID-19 on maternal health services to the public health risks posed by unsafe abortion practices. How messages can be more engagingly framed is key here. As I have shown, new technologies offer opportunities for feminist mobilisation (Young 2015), but they can also be difficult to be heard in a crowded space (Thrall, Stecula, and Sweet 2014; McPherson 2015). Some NGOs with more resources for instance can thus afford focus groups to assess the impact of messages, or have advocacy and communications departments work together, as is the case with CARE UK and Family Planning.

NGOs, however, can do more to get their messages across, to move beyond elite publics or 'preaching to the converted', and have their content connect more to people's needs, aspirations, and cultural backgrounds and concerns on matters of sexuality and women's health. More personalized accounts of suffering and hardships, and of people's lived experiences, can function to create more compassion, empathy, and awareness around SRHR, as was found with the fund-raising campaigns of other NGOs working on humanitarian issues and development (Ascough 2018; Powers 2014) thus striving to encourage more in-depth discussion.

The use of digital communications for advocacy communications on SRHR has both limits and potential and can be a double-edged sword when it comes to feminist activism. Online networks are among many forms of communication use whereby media can be utilised to raise awareness, to mobilise, or to enact social change. Organisations should utilise all forms of communication channels in their advocacy efforts as no one model of communications fits all. Communications on SRHR needs to move beyond messages that seek to change individual behaviour (providing merely individual solutions while side-lining deep-seated structural gender inequalities) or simply to mimic traditional social marketing health campaigns (Waisbord and Obregon 2012b). Messages need to be sensitive to cultural contexts and to consider the needs of communities in order to understand *why* there is resistance. As I show, SRHR advocacy communications is inserted within a range of complex social and political issues. It is also very different from other forms of communications and social media used by other civic organisations (Thrall, Stecula, and Sweet 2014; Powers 2017) to advocate for causes such as climate change (although one could argue that the latter is equally challenging).

The findings of this research reveal how organisations are waking up to the need for better communicating, seeing communications as a tool for potential advocacy, even though some have yet to include communications in their strategic plans. The results further show diversity in the sharing capabilities of these organisations and that the larger ones and those with more resources have more and better means of advancing their messages. That said, the findings also highlight the need to know more about how specific publics, from the media to the 'general public', process content on SRHR. This needs to be combined with a more critical understanding of the development praxis, and of its roots in neoliberal economics, as well as how it continues to depict women as bodies lacking in agency (Wilkins 2016; Harcourt 2009). This is a first step towards the process of deconstructing the weak role of women within development, particularly women from the Global South and from developing countries, and to start moving towards the construction of a new agenda on women's rights, one that is capable of being truly inclusive and attentive to the needs of diverse groups of women across different locations and life experiences. As has been shown, stereotypical gendered discourses of 'women' are still being reproduced through development discourse and practice, including in the rhetoric and discussions of SRHR within international development.

Organisations need to utilise all forms of communication and channels, from television to social media, for advocacy. SRHR communication campaigns need to move beyond messages that seek to change attitudes and individual behaviour, as has traditionally been the case of social marketing messages on global health interventions in developing countries (Waisbord and Obregon 2012b). SRHR messages should take into consideration the specific cultural needs and differences of certain communities as well as their political and religious views. NGOs should also engage with communications from a more holistic and critical perspective, seeking to understand it as being more than just 'information sharing' for the sole purpose of behavioural change. There is more to be done than simply sharing the odd tweet on social media pertaining to SRHR during a project or a mainstream news report. However, that said, money and lack of resources is a problem, and there is only so much that can be done with limited funds.

NGOs working in the field can do more to get their messages across, moving beyond 'preaching to the converted' or the inner circles of UN-led debates as well as their professional networks and grassroots activists. They can make their content more widely known, working to connect to people's needs, interests, and feelings. This is something that is beginning to unite NGO advocates and others working in the field. Prior to COVID-19, in 2018, Share-Net International, a knowledge platform based in the Netherlands that aims to harness local knowledge to a network of experts and organisations as a means of promoting the development of SRHR policies, organised a series of workshops at The Hague on the theme 'effective SRHR messaging in changing times'. The intention was to examine SRHR advocacy and communications at a time when it is being challenged by groups that oppose it. On its institutional website, Share-Net International stated that its aim was to improve 'information and greater freedom of choice for young people about their sexuality.'[2] The report on the workshop stated that anti-SRHR messages were reaching out to wider publics and influencing them and that it was necessary to rethink how to communicate about sexuality and reproductive health by doing more than simply 'stating the facts'; rather, it was necessary to seek ways to resonate more with segments of the public so as to avoid the current 'disconnect' between the communities and how the issue is perceived by them.

Most of the organisations interviewed are waking up to this reality and are beginning to include more communications in their future strategic plans. The results of this research, from the interview with the gender experts of the organisations and the communication leads, underscores the urgent need to change messaging to better suit the current cultural, religious, economic, and geopolitical challenges under which the media content is produced and distributed. The importance of knowing the public better means that communications can be used to target diverse groups, many of which have different interests and media consumption habits and do not necessarily have access to social media or even enjoy it. With regard to the latter, communications through traditional media formats, such as posters, pamphlets, or radio, would be more appropriate. This was the case with the entertainment-education-led Feminina HIP citizen media project in Tanzania (Tufte 2020). Here civil society-driven media platforms – such as print media – made use of entertainment-education practices to tell 'real life' stories whose aim was to empower young people to make informed choices on sexuality and healthy lifestyles and so reduce the impact of HIV/AIDS.[3]

A decade ago Waisbord and Obregon (2012a, 643) underscored the existence of a 'paucity of studies about the linkage between communication, mobilisation and health policy in international settings'. They made the case for the need to adopt a wider perspective on health communications, one capable of constructing a convergence between public health and communication practices, including the need for the development of a critical mass of health communication professionals. As Waisbord and Obregon (2012a) point out, it is important to know how policies are communicated and how communications can shape them: for communications is more than information – it includes dialogue and participation, and messaging platforms as well as strategy and activism (643–5).

This research seeks to contribute to some of these theoretical perspectives through the empirical study of fifty-two health and feminist NGOs and their communications work, assessing how they seek to shape policy and debate in the public sphere relating to SRHR issues. It goes without saying that improvements in communications are closely interwoven with advancements in the political, social, and economic spheres. It is arguably not enough to strengthen communications advocacy strategies and practices in SRHR if the current geopolitical climate remains challenging, and if debate in the public sphere is skewed towards the interests of specific conservative groups or dictated by market imperatives and the specific needs of donors. We thus need to emphasise broader approaches to women's equality and health. As several NGOs have reported in their advocacy communications efforts, the greater use and adoption of entertainment-education formats to publicise and create deeper and more meaningful engagement with SRHR can be a way out of the current impasse. Workshops such as the one that was given in The Hague (see above) are already gathering professionals who work in the field to begin to articulate a new discourse and way of thinking about SRHR and its media messaging in the digital age.

I also show how frequently advocacy communications mingles 'objective' facts, statistics, scientific reports, and medical discourses around SRHR with more subjective and emotional stances, often blurring the boundaries between the 'hard facts' and human interest stories. The use of emotions in advocacy for various causes, including in the field of reproductive health, has been acknowledged by various scholars (Servaes 2008; Hemer and Tufte 2016; McPherson 2015; Britt Coe and Schnabel 2011). Advocacy communications, through the use of testimonials and storytelling, has the capacity to arouse 'powerful emotions' (Servaes 2008). Storytelling can make private experiences of suffering, hardship, or anxiety become public and can elicit empathy in the receiver, contributing to raising greater awareness and leading to potential engagement with the cause.

The findings also show that there needs to be wider engagement with and mobilisation of communities in a manner that enables people to feel more connected to the media health messages relating to SRHR. This includes the younger generation, who are beginning to discuss issues of reproductive health, as well as the wider public: who also need accurate information and communications on SRHR through targeted and meaningful health communication campaigns, as they both need to be able to make informed decisions in order to gain access to quality public (and private) health services.

More research on how targeted publics, from the media to policy-makers and the 'general public', process the content, information, and messages relating to SRHR would be welcome. This could be juxtaposed with a more critical and wider understanding of discourses on gender in development, both in terms of how, traditionally, development has understood 'women' within the literature and how it has depicted women's bodies in development practice. There is an urgent need for more in-depth and meaningful dialogue with the targeted publics and with those affected by both policy-making and health messages. More qualitative ethnographic research with sectors of the public in order to find out more about how people's attitudes towards abortion and gender equality are formed would also be beneficial. This includes assessing the ways in which discourses on SRHR that are circulating in the mediated global public sphere are shaping views on women's sexuality and reproductive health and are causing setbacks to women's rights in many countries across the world.

My current work in partnership with the NGO Reprolatina, which emerged from the GCRF project, looks at how targeted SRHR publics in Brazil consume media content within SRHR health communication campaigns. In July 2021, I conducted focus groups with the Brazilian NGO Reprolatina. Two of these were conducted with women from lower socio-economic income groups living in the state of Sao Paulo (these groups were separated by age – nineteen to twenty-nine years and twenty-nine to thirty-nine years). The results will be published in a future journal article.

An important finding that emerged from these focus groups was that the participants wanted better-quality information on reproductive health, including communication material that is more direct, that uses 'simple language' in entertaining ways, and that is capable of connecting personal, testimonial, and human interest stories on suffering and hardships to the 'hard facts' of inequalities in reproductive health and development without depoliticizing these structural problems (we are also developing an advocacy communications plan for NGOs working in the field). I intend to pursue research into the practices of evangelical and other religious groups and networks in Brazil as well as throughout Latin America and the US, including the discourses and narratives that these groups have been articulating in the mediated public sphere on 'gender ideology myths' regarding sexuality and reproductive health.

Funded by two separate small GCRF grants, this large-scale project started before the pandemic and was affected by it as, due to my teaching and childcare responsibilities, along with limited funds and time constraints, I could not further advance my research. Thus I believe that further research that engages quantitatively with the online communication practices of the NGOs on social media would be useful. More mixed methods studies, including quantitative methodology to assess the frequency and impact of SRHR messages combined with more ethnographic and qualitative studies on how sectors of the targeted communities understand SRHR and the ways in which they use the media to obtain information (including navigating online communication spaces), would produce useful insights into how they consume SRHR. This is what I have already started to work on with the NGO Reprolatina and the two focus groups. My purpose here is to understand more the types of engagement with media messages and health communication campaigns on reproductive health. Further quantitative and digital ethnography studies could also thus assist in measuring the impact of the social media and online communications tools used by the NGOs working in the field of gender and health, showing how this affects the discourses articulated in the mediated global public sphere. This includes the impact on decision making and policy interventions in SRHR not only in the Global South but also in other parts of the world.

Market dynamics and donor demands place a series of constraints on NGOs working in the health and gender sector which are the result of the imposition on these organisations of market dynamics and the demands of donors (Gideon and Porter 2016). Gideon and Porter (2016, 793) further argue that people experience health through *racialised* and *gendered* assumptions, and a growing body of evidence shows how the embedding of business norms within health funding, as well as the shift towards more scientific discourses, resulted in NGOs failing to challenge structural inequalities in the field. As Gideon and Porter (2016) maintain, because of this NGOs end up endorsing a limited understanding of gender inequalities – an understanding that does not address the social determinants of health. Arguably, the changing funding landscape over the last decades, with the increasing marketisation of development industry and practice (Wilkins 2016), has resulted in NGOs having to shift their work on health programmes, leading to the 'instrumentalisation' of understandings around maternal and reproductive health and rights (Gideon and Porter 2016, 786).[4] This has limited the type of projects that these organisations are able to promote, resulting in their often 'failing to give voice to the women they claim to be supporting'.

NGOs need to address priority areas stipulated by donors, and this is frequently tied to evaluation processes that are often dictated by measurements of efficiency that are not necessarily gender constrained. Thus organisations can be limited in how they engage with broader understandings of women's health, with certain concerns around sexuality and reproductive health often being neglected (Gideon and Porter 2016, 791). Gideon and Porter (2016) also note how stereotypes around African men's sexuality continue to exist, citing the example of the 'donor's prioritization of male circumcision' as an initiative promoted to combat AIDS, despite lack of medical evidence. In essence, this proposition simply endorses tired racialised stereotypes around African males' sexuality (and the view that they are the owners of a 'voracious sexual appetite' that cannot be controlled). This is similar to the discussions of women's bodies, although in the former case we also see connections being made between males' bodies and the control of reproduction and sexual desire. Gideon and Porter (2016) further underline how the Lancet Commission points to the existence of a 'democratic deficit' within the health sector globally, with a lack of representatives of civil society and other marginalised groups (including health experts) to engage in influencing policy, and with the field having become increasingly dominated by the corporate sector. They argue for a wider role for NGOs in shaping debate within the field, which is precisely what my research seeks to contribute towards.

Some interviewees, including the women's human rights programme manager at Amnesty International UK, talked about the need to improve the mainstream media's reporting of difficult issues such as SRHR. She and members of other NGOs acknowledge that there has been a revival of transnational feminist movements as well as of NGOs working in the field of reproductive health. She also underlined the growing mobilisation around SRHR in the last few years, albeit within a challenging global climate of 'push back' on the rights obtained by women over the last decades:[5]

> In 2018 we saw a positive conclusion in Ireland, of a struggle around safe ... abortion, which has been going on for at least thirty years. We have seen a lot of new mobilisations in response to new drugs, in ... Poland, Brazil ... in contexts where the restrictions in abortion already existed, and there was a

danger of them becoming more severe, and which is seen in ... movement building. To make sure ... not only that we keep the gains that we have made, but if possible we go further, in the wake of a huge backlash ... and also like real radical attempts, for example, the Polish Parliament to basically ban abortion ... It is a time I feel ... of resurgent activism, but also [a] resurgent attempt to curb women's rights and women's autonomy ... So these are worrying developments, from an advocate's perspective. What we find very worrying is that ... we have the blueprint of women's rights through Beijing, Cairo, of course, UN Security Council resolutions ... but the reality shows that if we had to renegotiate them ... we would get weaker agreements.

Focusing on Latin America as a case study, and comparing it with the case of other regions of the world, I would attempt to examine the impact on the public sphere of the communications and discourses of religious groups around sexuality and reproductive health. In the case of Latin America, for instance, research shows that Roman Catholicism, the traditional non-indigenous religion of the continent, has been in decline in the last decade, paving the way for the growth of Protestantism in its 'popular' form, mainly through the expansion of evangelicalism. Authors like Silva (2019) argue that the latter is gaining more power throughout the continent and is beginning to compete in the public sphere for influence and privileges through the State structures.[6] It is further seeking to impose on segments of the population its own private understanding of morality not only around sexuality but also around family values and the role of women in both the public and private spheres.

As has been examined here, SRHR issues within international development are complex but which still remain relatively 'behind the scenes', discussed either by informed players or manipulated by oppositional groups in the public sphere. Discussion needs to include multiple groups, engaging with and bringing into the debate segments of the younger generation (who are the most affected by SRHR), as well as LGBT and other sexual identity groups. More men need to be brought into the equation as well as population and family planning advocate representatives. It is clear from this research that the mere presentation of 'facts and statistics' on SRHR to support public health arguments is far from enough. Because this does not sufficiently mobilise various groups around the cause it is necessary to better 'frame' the narratives on SRHR (Friedman 2003). This would be similar to what other NGOs did within the context of the UN conferences of the 1980s and 1990s, particularly those engaged in the shift away from the old 'population' discourse and towards the notion of women's rights and reproductive health within a human rights framework (Friedman 2003; Harcourt 2017).

The question that I ask here is thus: How can development practitioners and academics working alongside various players in the development industry, from multilateral agencies to NGOs working with SRHR, ensure that development can work better for women 'on the ground' in an increasing challenging post-pandemic context? I believe that a key concern is to speak to those who are resisting in order to better understand how people form their values and political attitudes, what it is about 'gender equality' that scares them, and, in particular, how they connect to discussions of women's bodies and sexuality as well as to wider issues of reproductive health. Arguably, this may lead to uncomfortable discussions; however, what exists at present is discussions that are highly emotional, misinformed, and ideological. That said, a totally 'rational narrative' is not necessarily persuasive or fully workable. Thus talking and engaging with 'the other' – moving beyond the online/offline 'echo chambers' – is key here. We need to ask how it is possible to better communicate with these publics and to 'frame' issues in a way that is more meaningful, less 'threatening', and more relevant to people. In other words, we must speak directly to their lived experiences and to their hardships. In this situation 'facts' may be more effective if equipped with subjectivity and compassion.

Messages need to be made more relevant to the communities affected, and there should be more concern with religious and cultural norms, and how best to go about tackling these Thus there is a need to *reassess* language as well as to examine how we engage with certain concepts that are controversial and problematic for some people, and can cause alienation and disengagement in some publics (e.g., the focus on slogans and terms such as 'anti-choice' and 'my body'). I thus believe that both more education in gender literacy and more in-depth discussion and communications on these topics are crucial if we are to begin to break down the barriers that stand in the way of advancing progressive policies in the field.

As this research shows, in the last years human interest testimonials as well as storytelling have become more popular devices used in international development (Ascough 2018) and have started to be more widely adopted by various organisations working with SRHR. Evidently this communication format is capable of connecting to people; however, this is not enough if it fails to politicise these problems and if it disengages from the wider structural inequalities that have adversely affected the lives of millions of women. As we have seen, evidence-based research and the use of facts supported by public health arguments around SRHR are important, but they are not enough to actually mobilise people to engage in a way that enables more transformative social change in the field, particularly when it comes to sexual and reproductive health 'on the ground', and mostly also if the intention is to transform the lives of girls and women in more disadvantaged communities.

This research shows how the feminist and health NGOs located in countries in both the Global South and the Global North, from the US to Europe and Latin America, made strategic use of communications. It attempts to examine how they combined their offline media and communication activities with digital communications, assessing how they saw the effectiveness of the latter as a form of complementing traditional communications. As I show here, all the organisations that participated in this research made use of social media platforms as well as other online tools, including the wide use of Twitter and Facebook. There were, however, variations between the organisations, including regarding their use of YouTube videos, blogs, and other online communications. According to the survey-style questionnaire, most of the organisations started to make use of online media in the last five to ten years, having indicated that they would like to see more investments made in communications for SRHR advocacy. Out of the fifty-two organisations that took part in this research, only UNFPA and another twelve had clear strategic plans available on their websites (ready to download) during the period of analysis.[7] A few referred specifically to communications strategies, but many affirmed during the interviews that they intended to do more to embed communication activities in their advocacy communications on SRHR in the future. This was, for example, the case with Change and Family Planning 2020.

The head of digital communications of IPPF underlined how NGOs working in the field need to catch up, stating clearly that the 'opposition' is further ahead in mobilizing and using communications for reproductive health advocacy, both online and offline. She admitted that her organisation had not fully wakened to the importance of digital communications, emphasising the need to tap into the 'emotional side of our audiences':

> The opposition are years ahead of us and will continue to be until there is a sector-wide understanding of how to digitally transform us as a movement. We also need to understand our audience, yes policy-makers are important, so are other NGOs, but if we do not speak to the public ... we will lose ground ... Organisations need to stop relying on being seen as the 'good guys' ... Our comms needs to tap into the emotional side of our audiences, we needs to start creating real change from the ground up. The only successful movements in my eyes are the ones which started at a grassroots level – not bound by bureaucracy and fear of being called out ... If NGOs do not embrace becoming digital first – then it will make us redundant and ineffective ... Charities relying heavily on public donations are being forced to look at their business model ... millennials are more likely to support a local or grassroots organisation than one that has a one-hundred-year old history ... The digital natives ... are far more concerned about specific causes – especially on climate change, so an SRHR like ours may not appeal to them, though SRHR is interlinked with not only their personal development but the climate crisis issue (providing care to pregnant women during natural disasters) ... Larger NGOs really need to start thinking twenty years ahead, and what their audience landscape and supporter landscape will look like, and they must start developing the groundwork for attracting them now.

The foregoing interviewee, along with other gender experts who participated in this research, states what I have been arguing – mainly, that there is a need to rethink communications around SRHR for the twenty-first century. All the organisations acknowledged the many challenges in engaging with advocacy communications for SRHR, underlining the need to rethink the discourses used and moving away from one-way flows of communications (which, to some extent, still continue). Many said that they are seeking to combine the presentation of facts with human interest stories, mingling 'reason' with 'emotion' as well as resorting to popular communication devices such as digital storytelling. They are further seeking to design communication campaigns and strategies that are connected to some of the premises of entertainment-education formats and how they are used in health communication campaigns (Dutta 2011; Tufte 2012; Lewis and Lewis 2015). A key aim is to think more deeply about communications as well as to assess how different forms of media and communications – including offline and online tools (e.g., radio and social media) – can be used differently in order to target diverse publics. Organisations can also work to strengthen their relationships not only with their partners but also with the media and with journalists, including with NGO advocates and other civil society players both nationally and internationally.

If this current and unfavourable hostile climate, exacerbated by COVID-19, has posed a series of new challenges to advocacy communication strategies and practices for NGOs working in the field, it has also provided the sector with new opportunities for engaging with communications for social change and for sustainable development on gender equality and reproductive health. This includes, among other things, the need for an increase in the use of online communication tools and platforms that can assist in strengthening transnational feminist solidarity and activism at a time when the decolonising feminist project remains incomplete. The hope is that this would increase the future likelihood of (more equitable) partnerships between civil society players, organisations, and institutions from the North and from the South around the main challenges of our time. If anything, the COVID-19 pandemic has shown much of the world the limits of neoliberalism and of austerity, and the vital need for further investments in public health and political and economic equality – something that the West has taken too much for granted in the last decades. Sexuality and reproductive health is thus very much part of the women's rights agenda since it is interwoven with the social and health inequalities present in societies across both the developing and the developed world.

The use of online communications by NGOs working in the field seems thus destined to increase in the post-COVID-19 context, not just for advocacy but also for other activities, including research. Without a doubt, the shift towards online work during the pandemic has significantly increased the use of digital platforms for communications by NGOs as a means of targeting their publics. Inevitably, this process has accelerated the need for organisations to invest more in digital communications for advocacy on reproductive health, not just for mobilizing and fundraising activities. There has been more use of webinars for workshop events as well as for engagement with stakeholders, policy-makers, and other professional networks. This research shows that there needs to be more in-depth debate on sexual and reproductive health issues as these are closely connected to discussions of poverty and inequalities as well as to the quality and delivery of health systems. This should not occur just among those 'publics in the know', from NGO advocates to public health professionals and feminists working in the field; rather, it should also seek to engage the targeted publics, from members of the community to politicians and decision-making elites, as well as the general population.

NGOs should also seek to develop a proper advocacy communications plan, containing a rationale with aims, objectives, and targets and with details on how to go about developing communication campaigns, addressing both internal and external communications in order to make the most of different communication tools for SRHR advocacy. The advocacy communications plan should seek to include a rationale, with a few paragraphs outlining the principles of the organisation, its mission statement, what it stands for, how this translates into its policy work, and how it will appropriate communications to facilitate this work (Picketts 2012 in Lewis and Lewis 2015; Servaes 2008). A section on 'strategies for advocacy communications and its main aims and objectives' could also be included here, indicating the public health targets and what the organisation seeks to achieve.

It would also be wise to distinguish between the different target groups of the organisation (e.g., the media, policy-makers) and situate how different media could be used for each. A list of names of journalists in the mainstream media and of other partners could also be included. Policies and strategies for social media use may differ according to the platform: Twitter, Facebook, or YouTube. Twitter is more heavily associated with debate and with the formation of 'public opinion' in the Habermasian sense, particularly in many of the countries of the Global North, such as in the UK, whereas Facebook is more image-focused and provides more space for human interest stories. In line with the particularities of each platform, this could include a checklist with the 'do's' and 'don'ts' for each, including what language should be used in what situation and for what media (e.g., using digital storytelling on social media platforms to reach out to the younger population).

'Action campaigns' could be included here, such as a summary of their results or bullet points on what they have achieved. What exactly made these campaigns successful? This could be followed by information on 'how to prepare a communications campaign', starting from the research stage and going to the creation of a movement around the cause. This would include bringing in more support from mainstream media as well as from other civil society groups and mobilising these through online networks. It is also crucial to build the capacity of internal NGO staff to work with communications, or at least to have some understanding of communications in order to support the professionals working on this..

However, it goes without saying that no communications campaign will do the trick if other political and social inequalities within gender and international development are not tackled head on. As Serveas (2008) argues, each health issue requires a different communications response.[8] And, as I have discussed here, I am concerned with how these different forms of communications, from 'mass' to 'participatory', can make use of advocacy strategies – and media tools – to communicate their messages. Frequently, discussions on health do involve emotional responses (Serveas 2008), and it is precisely because of this that I make a distinction – as well as point out the blurring of the boundaries – between the categories of 'emotion' and 'reason' in the analysis of media content regarding SRHR.

Entertainment-education formats for health communication messages have, as we have seen, shown themselves to be useful communication approaches that can make scientific medical discourses more appealing to targeted publics. The combination of 'reason' and 'emotion' emerges as an interesting formula that is beginning to be more utilized by NGOs working with reproductive health advocacy (e.g., from Promsex to the chatbot used by PFI for information sharing that generated more than a million conversations). A key issue is how to construct creative health communication campaigns that can address various SRHR themes and engage larger segments of the population in order to shape policy and deepen discussions in the public sphere, thus further undermining religious and/or political opposition. These health communication campaigns for SRHR, regardless of whether they are articulated by organisations in the Global South or in the Global North, should be attentive to the persistence of discourses and representations within the development industry that continue to essentialise the experiences of women from developing countries or from more vulnerable communities, particularly when it comes to images of female bodies in family planning programmes (Wilkins 2016; Harcourt 2017).

It is thus not enough that these narratives are discourses that are considered to be inaccurate and old-fashioned representations that reinforce power relations and dynamics: they also contribute to alienating publics (Choularaki 2006; Ascough 2018) both in the Global North and in the Global South. They provide little incentive to promote wider in-depth debate and understanding on sexual and reproductive health issues within international development (Cornwall et al. 2008) and therefore do not contribute to a more holistic understanding of SRHR's connection with inequality as well as with the stigmatisation of sexual identities and of other vulnerable groups (including the link with philosophical and moral debates around the family and women's sexuality). Such communication campaigns thus cease to promote wider compassion and empathy between transnational feminist groups and NGOs working in the field, and this at a time when there is urgent need to unite them in global partnerships to advance gender justice and SRHR rights under challenging circumstances – circumstances that are determined by socio-economic factors and that are thus political.

In her introduction to McLaren's edited collection of work on decolonizing feminism, Mohanty (2017) stresses the difficulties of operationalising a vision of feminism for the 99 per cent that can connect to the material reality of gendered and racialised communities of women from around the world and from different backgrounds. This is particularly so under the current geopolitical circumstances of globalization, economic recession, and persistent inequalities. Mohanty and I come from the same epistemological standpoint – one that sees dialogue as crucial to enabling transformative change. Quoting Mohanty, McLaren (2017, 4) underscores how she 'articulates a vision of a world that is pro-sex and pro-women', a world where 'women and men are free to lead creative lives, in security and with bodily health and integrity', being free to choose their romantic relationships and who they want to spend time with. This also needs to be equated with *quality of life* and human dignity for all people, granting them everything from economic stability and racial equality to wider wealth redistribution, and thus guaranteeing their well-being irrespective of their country of birth or socio-economic background.

As the McClaren further notes (2017, 8), to decolonise should not be restricted only to the 'theoretical and epistemological level' but, rather, it should be part of an 'active, ongoing struggle for social justice' in every sphere, ranging from the economic and the political to the cultural. As Fraser (2013) puts it, it should combine cultural recognition with redistribution. It is thus a mistake to assume that the struggle for economic justice should be prioritized and dissociated from the impact of identity and culture on one's life chances and propensity either to be discriminated against or to be included within economic prosperity. Such a vision opens up the possibilities of engaging in new and innovative approaches to contemporary global challenges (McLaren 2017, 8) and to the intersections of gender (as well as race and class) and reproductive health with inequalities.

Identifying cultures as 'open systems', Fultner (2017, 203–30) also makes the case for the construction of *meaningful dialogue* that can cut across borders, coming from an epistemological standpoint that sees dialogue as *enabling transformative practice*. This is very much in line with communications as a *dialogical* process, one that is embedded within a participatory and human rights framework (Manyozo 2012a; Tufte 2012; Wilkins 2016). When interviewed for this research, the head of SRHR from Global Fund for Women said that she sees room for building bridges between the North and the South, with the voices of women from the South having a crucial role to play in the process of creating meaningful dialogue in order to construct solidarity and compassion, and, in so doing, to bring about transformative change through feminist transnational activism. They should thus be able to engage with some of the most challenging political issues of our time, from the elimination of poverty to climate change, gender equality, and advancement in sexuality and reproductive health and rights, in a way that gives voice to all those concerned and who seek to be heard irrespective of differences.[9]

The Sustainable Development Goals already emphasise the centrality of global partnerships for development in many areas, including in gender and reproductive health. These can be further strengthened and better explored under the principles of equal opportunities and with the commitment to delivering a global agenda of gender justice for a postcolonial – and even 'post-neoliberal' – digital age. The failures of development 'on the ground' have become all the more pressing in the face of the global recession caused by the COVID-19 pandemic and the threats to our planet from climate change, not to mention the rise of extremist governments and far-right populist politics/movements as well as wars in the Global North (e.g., Russia and Ukraine). There is also the problem of the persistence of the kind of thinking around development that continues to uphold, albeit indirectly or implicitly, the legacy of the North/South divide, thus continuing to affect, even after decades of independence, the decisions of former colonies and of other less powerful countries. Such issues need to be fully overcome if we are to construct a sustainable, equitable, fair, and just world for women and girls across the world, if not for humanity itself.

APPENDICES

APPENDIX A

List of Organisations

Acoes Afirmativas em Direito e Saude (AADS) (former Ipas Brasil) – http://www.aads.org.br

Akahata – http://www.akahataorg.org

Amnesty International UK – https://www.amnesty.org.uk

ANIS – http://www.anis.org.br

ASAP – http://asap-asia.org

Asia Pacific Alliance – http://www.asiapacificalliance.org

CARE International UK – https://www.careinternational.org.uk

Catolicas pelo Direito de Decidir (Catholics for the Right to Decide) – http://www.catolicasonline.org.br

Center for Catalyzing Change in India – http://www.c3india.org

Center for Health and Gender Equity (Change) – http://www.genderhealth.org

Center for Reproductive Rights – https://www.reproductiverights.org

Centro de Estudos de Estado y Sociedade de Argentina – http://www.cedes.org

CEPIA (Cidadania, Estudo, Pesquisa, Informacao e Acao) (Citizenship, Study, Research, Information and Action) – https://cepia.org.br/pt

Cfemea (Centro Feminista de Estudos e Assessoria) (Feminist Centre of Studies and Consultancy) – https://www.cfemea.org.br

Colectivo de Salud Feminista (Argentina) – http://comohacerseunaborto.com/es/inicio

Coletivo Feminino Plural – http://femininoplural.org.br

Consorcio latino-americano contra el aborto inseguro – http://clacai.org

CREA India – https://creaworld.org

Family Planning 2020 – https://www.familyplanning2020.org

Fundacion Desafio – https://www.fundaciondesafio-ec.org

Global Fund for Women – https://www.globalfundforwomen.org

Guttmacher Institute – https://www.guttmacher.org

Human Rights Law Network - https://www.inclo.net/members/hrln

IAW (International Alliance of Women) – https://womenalliance.org

Ibis Reproductive Health – https://ibisreproductivehealth.org

Inspire Euro NGOs – https://inspire-partnership.org/home.html

International Planned Parenthood Federation – https://www.ippf.org

Latin American and Caribbean Committee for the Defence of Women's Rights – https://cladem.org

La Mesa por la vida de las mujeres – http://www.despenalizaciondelaborto.org.co/la-mesa

Movimento Nacional das Cidadas Posithivas (National Movement of Positive Citizens) – no website, Facebook page: https://www.facebook.com/cidadasposithivas

Mujer y Salud Uruguay – http://www.mysu.org.uy

Population Foundation of India – https://www.populationfoundation.in

Promsex – Centro de Promocion y Defensa de los Derechos Sexuales y Reprodutivos (Centre for the Promotion and Defense of Sexual and Reproductive Rights) – http://promsex.org

Realizing Sexual and Reproductive Justice (RESURJ) – http://resurj.org

Rede Feminista de Saude, Direitos Sexuais e Reprodutivos – http://redesaude.org.br/home

Reproductive Health Supplies Coalition – https://www.rhsupplies.org

Reprolatina – https://reprolatina.org.br

Safe Abortion Women's Rights – http://www.safeabortionwomensright.org

Sexual and Reproductive Health Matters (formerly RHM) – http://www.srhm.org

Sexual Policy Watch – https://sxpolitics.org

Sexual Rights Initiative (SRI) – https://www.sexualrightsinitiative.com

SheDecides – https://www.shedecides.com

SOS Corpo – http://soscorpo.org

Swasti – http://swasti.org

United Nations Population Fund – https://www.unfpa.org

Universal Access Project – http://universalaccessproject.org

White Ribbon Alliance India – https://www.whiteribbonalliance.org

Women Deliver – https://womendeliver.org

Women's Global Networking for Reproductive Rights – http://beta.wgnrr.org

Women's Learning Partnership – https://learningpartnership.org

Women's Link Worldwide – https://www.womenslinkworldwide.org

YouAct – http://youact.org

Youth Coalition – http://www.youthcoalition.org

APPENDIX B

NGOs by Region

Asia	9
Europe	11
International	3
Latin America	20
USA	9
Total	52

APPENDIX C

Budget Information for Twenty-Two NGOs

NGO budget (GBP)	Period	Total income	Total expenditure	Yearly surplus/ deficit
Akahatá	1 January– 31 December 2018	364,278.11	-403,225.39	-38,947.28
Amnesty International UK	1 January– 31 December 2018	20,122,00.00	-20,004,000.00	118,000.00
Asia Pacific Alliance	1 January– 31 December 2018	140,689.27	-116,020.52	24,668.74
Care International UK	1 July 2018– 30 June 2019	65,079,000.00	-66,882,000.00	-1,803,000.00
Center for Catalyzing Change India	1 April 2017– 31 March 2018	1,602,868.77	-1,523,302.12	79,566.65
Center for Health and Gender Equity	1 July 2018– 30 June 2019	2,113,660.51	-1,852,825.05	260,835.46
Center for Reproductive Rights	1 July 2018– 30 June 2019	26,337,046.04	-25,866,442.05	510,603.99
Crea India	1 April 2018– 31 March 2019	1,080,399.78	-1,026,341,53	54,058.25
Global Fund for Women	1 July 2018– 30 June 2019	14,197,774.39	-14,165,575.04	32,199.35
Guttmacher Institute	1 January– 31 December 2018	7,614,748.60	-21,478,243.54	-13,863,494.94
IAW	1 January– 31 December 2018	7,264.71	-5,510.95	1,753.76
Ibis Reproductive Health	1 July 2018– 30 June 2019	3,102,580.62	-5,009,772.65	-1,907,192.03
International Planned Parenthood Federation	1 January–3 1 December 2016	97,812,547.87	-92,903,579.00	4,908,968.51

NGO budget (GBP)	Period	Total income	Total expenditure	Yearly surplus/ deficit
Population Foundation of India	1 April 2017– 31 March 2018	3,236,807.95	-2,656,567.36	580,240.59
Promsex	2018	1,521,166.90	-1,251,848.00	269,319.20
Realizing Sexual and Reproductive Justice	2017	255,050.32	-254,397.69	652.63
Sexual and Reproductive Health Matters	2018	458,479.21	-442,047.21	16,431.99
Swasti	2018–19	1,994,648.96	-2,069,215.28	-74,566.32
White Ribbon Alliance India	1 January– 31 December 2018	5,692,049.51	-3,003,539.33	2,688,510.18
Women Deliver	1 January– 31 December 2018	10,235,368.88	-6,582,738.49	3,652,630.39
Women's Learning Partnership	1 July 2015– 30 June 2016	1,533,398.53	-1,528,674.85	4,723.68
You Act	1 August 2017– 31 July 2018	13,632.74	-15,448.38	-1,815.64

APPENDIX D

NGOs and Type of Communications (Sample)

	Ações Afirmativas em Direito e Saúde (AADS)*	Akahatá	Amnesty International UK	Anis	ASAP	Asia Pacific Alliance	Care International UK	Católicas pelo Direito de Decidir	Center for Catalyzing Change India
INFORMATION									
a) Policy reports	0	1	0	1	1	1	1	1	0
b) Press releases	0	0	1	0	0	0	1	1	1
c) Media articles	0	0	1	1	0	1	1	1	1
d) Publications	0	1	1	1	0	1	1	1	1
e) Facts and figures	0	1	0	1	1	1	1	1	1
f) CEO speeches	0	0	0	1	1	0	0	1	0
g) Archives	0	1	1	1	1	1	0	1	1
ADVOCACY									
a) Information (emotion)	1	1	1	1	1	0	1	1	1
b) Campaigns	1	1	1	0	1	1	1	1	1
c) Events	0	1	1	0	1	0	1	1	0
d) Discussion forums	0	0	1	1	0	0	0	1	0
e) Membership	0	0	1	0	0	1	0	0	0
f) Volunteering	0	0	1	0	0	0	1	0	1
g) Newsletter	0	0	1	0	1	1	1	0	0

	Ações Afirmativas em Direito e Saúde (AADS)*	Akahatá	Amnesty International UK	Anis	ASAP	Asia Pacific Alliance	Care International UK	Católicas pelo Direito de Decidir	Center for Catalyzing Change India
COMMUNITY ENGAGEMENT									
a) Emails	0	1	1	1	1	1	1	1	0
b) Discussion forums	0	0	1	1	0	0	0	0	0
c) Contact organisation	0	1	1	1	1	1	1	1	1
d) Member profiles	0	0	1	0	1	1	0	0	0
e) Local events	1	1	1	0	1	0	1	1	0
f) Workshops and training	0	1	1	1	1	0	0	1	1
g) International agenda	0	1	1	0	0	1	1	1	0
FUNDRAISING AND RESOURCES									
a) Donations	0	1	1	1	0	0	1	1	0
b) Funding	0	0	1	0	1	1	1	0	1
c) Partners	0	0	1	0	0	0	1	1	0
d) Lobbying politicians	0	1	1	1	0	0	1	1	0
MOBILIZATION									
a) Online petitions	0	0	1	0	0	0	1	1	0
b) Action alerts	1	0	1	0	1	1	1	1	1
c) Protests	1	0	1	0	0	0	1	1	0
d) Organization of campaigns	1	0	1	0	1	1	1	1	1

	Center for Health and Gender Equality (Change)	Centre for Reproductive Rights	Centro de Estudios de Estado y Sociedad de Argentina	Cepia	Cfemea	Colectivo de Salud Feminista	Coletivo Feminismo Plural	Consorcio latino-americano contra el aborto inseguro (CLACAI)	Crea India
INFORMATION									
a) Policy reports	1	1	1	1	1	0	0	1	1
b) Press releases	1	1	0	0	0	1	0	1	0
c) Media articles	1	1	0	0	1	0	0	1	1
d) Publications	1	1	1	1	1	1	1	1	1
e) Facts and figures	1	1	1	1	1	0	0	1	1
f) CEO speeches	1	1	1	1	0	0	0	1	0
g) Archives	1	1	1	1	1	1	1	1	1
ADVOCACY									
a) Information (emotion)	1	1	1	1	1	1	1	1	1
b) Campaigns	1	1	0	1	1	1	0	1	1
c) Events	1	1	1	1	1	0	1	1	1
d) Discussion forums	1	1	1	1	1	0	1	1	0
e) Membership	1	0	0	0	1	0	0	0	0
f) Volunteering	1	0	0	0	0	0	1	0	0
g) Newsletter	1	1	1	0	0	0	0	1	0

COMMUNITY ENGAGEMENT						
a) Emails	1	1	1	1	0	0
b) Discussion forums	1	0	1	1	0	0
c) Contact organisation	1	1	1	1	1	1
d) Member profiles	0	0	0	0	1	0
e) Local events	1	1	1	1	1	1
f) Workshops and training	1	1	1	1	1	1
g) International agenda	1	1	1	1	0	1
FUNDRAISING AND RESOURCES						
a) Donations	1	0	0	0	1	0
b) Funding	1	1	1	1	0	1
c) Partners	1	1	1	1	0	1
d) Lobbying politicians	0	0	0	1	1	0
MOBILIZATION						
a) Online petitions	0	1	0	0	0	1
b) Action alerts	1	0	0	0	1	1
c) Protests	1	0	1	1	1	0
d) Organization of campaigns	1	1	1	1	1	1

	Family Planning 2020	Fundacion Desafio	Global Fund for Women	Guttmacher Institute	IAW (International Alliance of Women)	Ibis Reproductive Health	Inspire Euro NGOS	International Planned Parenthood Federation	La Mesa por la vida de las mujeres
INFORMATION									
a) Policy reports	1	1	0	1	1	1	1	1	1
b) Press releases	1	1	1	1	1	1	1	1	1
c) Media articles	1	1	1	1	0	0	0	1	1
d) Publications	1	1	0	1	1	1	1	1	1
e) Facts and figures	1	1	1	1	1	1	0	1	0
f) CEO speeches	0	1	1	0	1	1	0	0	0
g) Archives	1	1	0	1	1	1	1	1	1
ADVOCACY									
a) Information (emotion)	1	1	1	1	1	1	1	1	1
b) Campaigns	1	1	1	1	1	0	0	1	1
c) Events	1	1	0	1	0	0	1	1	0
d) Discussion forums	1	0	0	0	0	0	1	1	0
e) Membership	1	0	1	0	1	0	1	1	0
f) Volunteering	0	0	1	0	0	0	0	1	0
g) Newsletter	1	0	1	1	1	1	1	1	0

COMMUNITY ENGAGEMENT								
a) Emails	1	1	1	1	0	1	1	1
b) Discussion forums	1	1	0	0	0	1	1	0
c) Contact organisation	1	1	1	1	1	1	1	1
d) Member profiles	1	0	1	0	1	1	1	0
e) Local events	1	1	1	0	1	0	1	1
f) Workshops and training	1	1	0	0	0	1	1	1
g) International agenda	1	0	1	1	1	1	1	1
FUNDRAISING AND RESOURCES								
a) Donations	0	1	1	1	1	0	1	0
b) Funding	1	1	1	1	1	0	0	1
c) Partners	1	0	1	1	1	1	0	0
d) Lobbying politicians	0	0	1	1	0	0	0	0
MOBILIZATION								
a) Online petitions	0	0	1	0	0	0	1	0
b) Action alerts	0	0	1	1	0	0	1	1
c) Protests	0	0	1	0	1	0	1	1
d) Organization of campaigns	0	1	1	0	1	0	1	1

	Latin American and Caribbean Committee for the Defense of Women's Rights (CLADEM)	Movimento Nacional das Cidadãs Posithivas*	Mujer y Salud Uruguay	Population Foundation of India	Promsex - Centro de Promocion y Defensa de los Derechos Sexuales y reprodutivos	Realizing Sexual and Reproductive Justice (RESURJ)	Rede Feminista de Saúde, Direitos Sexuais e Reprodutivos	Reproductive health supplies coalition	Reprolatina
INFORMATION									
a) Policy reports	1	1	1	1	1	1	1	1	1
b) Press releases	1	0	1	0	1	1	1	1	0
c) Media articles	0	1	1	1	0	0	0	1	0
d) Publications	1	1	1	1	1	1	1	1	1
e) Facts and figures	1	1	1	1	1	1	1	1	1
f) CEO speeches	0	0	0	1	1	0	0	0	1
g) Archives	1	1	1	1	1	1	1	1	1
ADVOCACY									
a) Information (emotion)	1	1	1	1	1	1	1	0	0
b) Campaigns	1	1	0	0	1	0	1	0	1
c) Events	1	1	0	0	0	0	1	1	1
d) Discussion forums	0	1	0	0	0	0	0	0	0
e) Membership	0	1	0	0	0	1	0	1	0
f) Volunteering	0	0	0	0	0	1	0	0	0
g) Newsletter	0	0	0	0	1	1	1	1	0

COMMUNITY ENGAGEMENT								
a) Emails	0	1	1	0	1	1	1	0
b) Discussion forums	0	1	0	0	0	0	1	0
c) Contact organisation	1	1	1	1	1	1	1	1
d) Member profiles	0	0	1	0	1	0	1	1
e) Local events	1	1	0	0	0	1	0	1
f) Workshops and training	0	0	1	1	0	1	1	1
g) International agenda	1	1	0	0	1	0	1	0
FUNDRAISING AND RESOURCES								
a) Donations	1	0	0	0	0	0	1	1
b) Funding	0	0	1	1	0	0	1	1
c) Partners	1	1	1	1	1	1	1	0
d) Lobbying politicians	0	0	1	0	0	0	0	0
MOBILIZATION								
a) Online petitions	0	1	0	0	0	0	0	0
b) Action alerts	0	1	0	0	0	1	1	0
c) Protests	0	1	0	0	0	1	0	0
d) Organization of campaigns	1	1	0	1	0	1	0	1

	Safe Abortion Women's Rights	Sexual and Reproductive Health Matters (RHM)	Sexual Policy Watch	Sexual Rights Initiative (SRI)	SheDecides	SOS Corpo	Swasti	United Nations Population Fund	Universal Access Project
INFORMATION									
a) Policy reports	1	1	1	1	0	1	1	1	1
b) Press releases	1	1	1	0	0	1	0	1	1
c) Media articles	1	0	1	0	0	0	0	1	1
d) Publications	1	1	1	1	0	1	1	1	1
e) Facts and figures	1	1	1	1	1	1	1	1	1
f) CEO speeches	1	0	0	0	0	0	0	1	0
g) Archives	1	1	1	1	0	1	1	1	1
ADVOCACY									
a) Information (emotion)	1	0	1	0	1	1	1	1	0
b) Campaigns	1	0	0	0	1	1	0	0	1
c) Events	1	1	1	0	0	1	0	1	0
d) Discussion forums	0	0	0	0	0	0	0	0	0
e) Membership	1	0	0	0	0	0	0	0	0
f) Volunteering	1	0	0	0	0	0	0	0	0
g) Newsletter	1	1	1	1	0	0	0	1	0

COMMUNITY ENGAGEMENT							
a) Emails	1	1	1	0	0	1	0
b) Discussion forums	0	0	0	0	0	1	0
c) Contact organisation	1	1	1	1	1	0	1
d) Member profiles	0	1	1	0	0	0	0
e) Local events	1	1	0	1	0	1	0
f) Workshops and training	1	0	0	0	1	1	1
g) International agenda	1	1	1	1	0	1	1
FUNDRAISING AND RESOURCES							
a) Donations	1	0	0	0	0	1	1
b) Funding	1	0	0	0	1	1	0
c) Partners	1	1	1	1	1	1	0
d) Lobbying politicians	0	0	0	1	0	0	1
MOBILIZATION							
a) Online petitions	1	0	0	1	0	0	0
b) Action alerts	1	0	0	1	1	0	1
c) Protests	1	0	0	1	1	0	1
d) Organization of campaigns	1	0	0	1	0	1	1

	White Ribbon Alliance India	Women Deliver	Women's Global Network for Reproductive Rights	Women's Learning Partnership	Women's Link Worldwide	You Act	Youth Coalition for Sexual and Reproductive Rights
INFORMATION							
a) Policy reports	1	1	1	0	0	1	0
b) Press releases	1	1	1	1	0	1	0
c) Media articles	1	1	0	0	1	0	0
d) Publications	1	1	1	1	1	1	1
e) Facts and figures	0	1	1	1	1	1	1
f) CEO speeches	0	0	0	1	0	0	1
g) Archives	1	1	1	1	1	1	0
ADVOCACY							
a) Information (emotion)	1	1	1	1	1	1	0
b) Campaigns	0	0	1	1	0	0	1
c) Events	0	1	1	1	0	0	0
d) Discussion forums	0	0	1	0	0	0	0
e) Membership	1	0	1	0	1	1	1
f) Volunteering	1	0	1	0	1	1	1
g) Newsletter	1	1	1	0	1	1	1

COMMUNITY ENGAGEMENT							
a) Emails	1	1	0	1	1	0	0
b) Discussion forums	0	0	1	0	0	0	0
c) Contact organisation	1	1	1	1	1	1	1
d) Member profiles	1	0	1	1	1	1	1
e) Local events	0	0	0	1	0	1	0
f) Workshops and training	0	0	0	1	0	0	1
g) International agenda	1	1	1	1	0	1	1
FUNDRAISING AND RESOURCES							
a) Donations	1	1	1	1	1	0	0
b) Funding	1	1	1	1	0	1	1
c) Partners	1	1	1	1	1	1	1
d) Lobbying politicians	0	0	0	0	0	0	0
MOBILIZATION							
a) Online petitions	0	0	0	0	0	0	0
b) Action alerts	1	1	0	0	0	0	0
c) Protests	0	0	1	0	0	0	0
d) Organization of campaigns	0	1	1	0	1	0	1

APPENDIX E

Tables and References from the NGOs' Blogs

DATES OF THE CDA OF THE NGOS' BLOG POSTS

NGO	Posts in time frame	Next blog date (after time frame)	Blog used for DA	In time frame
Amnesty International UK	4	8 April 2019	'The Women Risking Their Lives to Save the Planet'	No: 30 April 2019
Asia Safe Abortion Partnership (ASAP)	1	17 April 2019	'Keep Calm and Take the Medical Abortion Pill'	Yes: 26 March 2019
Asia Pacific Alliance (APA)	0	30 April 2019	'Population, Development, Governments and YOU!'	No: 0 April 2019
CARE International UK (CARE)	6	9 April 2019	'Cyclone Idai: Women and Girls Face Risk of Abuse in Camps'	Yes: 28 March 2019
Centre for Catalysing Change India (C3)	0	2 March 2020	'"Thappad", Not a Movie But a Page from Every Woman's Life in India'	No: 2 March 2020
Centre for Health and Gender Equity (CHANGE)	0	8 April 2019	'New Documentary: The Global Gag Rule – The "Prolife" Death Warrant'	No: 8 April 2019
Family Planning 2020 (FP2020)	5	1 May 2019	'Finding Reproductive Healthcare In The World's Biggest Refugee Camp'	Yes: 1 April 2019
International Campaign for Women's Right to Safe Abortion (Campaign)	0	17 July 2019	'South Africa: Need for National Traction on Reproductive Justice in South Africa following Elections'	No: 17 July 2019

NGO	Posts in time frame	Next blog date (after time frame)	Blog used for DA	In time frame
International Planned Parenthood Federation (IPPF)	2	29 April 2019	'I Decide: A Global Campaign to Break Down Barriers for Safe Abortion Access'	Yes: 26 March 2019
Realizing Sexual and Reproductive Justice (RESURJ)	0	18 April 2019	'The FAWE Girls' Scholarship Case: Three Critical Aspects to Learn – Opinion'	No: 18 April 2019
Sexual and Reproductive Health Matters (SRHM)	1	18 April 2019	'Fecundity in Art'	Yes: 1 April 2019
Swasti	0	6 September 2019	'Chapter 4: Without Gender Equity, Universal Health Coverage Is a Pipe Dream'	No: 10 September 2019
Women Deliver	0	n.d., 10 July 2019	'From Syria to Sudan, Women Rights Defenders Need More Than Likes'	No: 10 July 2019
Women's Learning Partnership (WLP)	2	20 November 2019	'Women from Across the Middle East and Africa Gather for Peace, Security, and Equality – Nigeria'	Yes: 31 March 2019
YouAct	0	9 May 2019 (recruitment call)	'Advocacy Toolkit: The European Parliament Our Ally'	No: 22 May 2019

BLOG POST REFERENCES

Alkanawati, L. 2019. 'From Syria to Sudan, Women Rights Defenders Need More Than Likes', *The New Humanitarian*, 10 July 2019, https://womendeliver.org/2019/from-syria-to-sudan-women-rights-defenders-need-more-than-likes.

CARE. 2019. 'Cyclone Idai: Women and Girls Face Risk of Abuse in Camps.' 28 March 2019. https://www.careinternational.org.uk/stories/cyclone-idai-women-and-girls-face-risk-abuse-camps.

Chadband, E. 2019. 'Finding Reproductive Healthcare in the World's Biggest Refugee Camp'. *Family Planning 2020*, 1 April 2019. https://medium.com/@FP2020Global_20685/finding-reproductive-healthcare-in-the-worlds-biggest-refugee-camp-5c8b7dbab8of.

Dalvie, S. 2019. 'Keep Calm and Take the Medical Abortion Pill'. ASAP, 26 March 2019. http://asap-asia.org/blog/keep-calm-and-take-the-medical-abortion-pill/#sthash.r8mNTjHA.dpbs.

Fauveau, V. 2019. 'Fecundity in Art'. SRHM, 1 April 2019. http://www.srhm.org/news/fecundity-in-art.

IPPF. 2019. 'I Decide: A Global Campaign to Break Down Barriers for Safe Abortion Access'. 26 March 2019. https://www.ippf.org/blogs/i-decide-global-campaign-break-down-barriers-safe-abortion-access.

Minter, G. 2019. 'The Women Risking Their Lives to Save the Planet'. *Amnesty International UK*, 30 April 2019. https://www.amnesty.org.uk/blogs/ether/women-saving-planet.

Narang, V. '"Thappad", Not a Movie But a Page from Every Woman's Life in India'. *Center for Catalyzing Change*, 2 March 2020. http://www.c3india.org/blogs/thappad-not-a-movie-but-a-page-from-every-woman-s-life-in-india.

Nolan, N. 2019. 'New Documentary: The Global Gag Rule – The "Prolife" Death Warrant'. SRHR, 8 April 2019. https://srhrforall.org/new-documentary-the-global-gag-rule-the-prolife-death-warrant.

Nunag, J.M. 2019. 'Population, Development, Governments and YOU!' *Asia Pacific Alliance*, 30 April 2019. https://www.asiapacificalliance.org/our-work/blog/population-development-governments-and-you.

Stevens, M. 2019. 'South Africa: Need for National Traction on Reproductive Justice in South Africa Following Elections'. *International Campaign for Women's Right to Safe Abortion*, 17 July 2019. https://www.safeabortionwomensright.org/south-africa-need-for-national-traction-on-reproductive-justice-in-south-africa-following-elections.

Swasti. 2019. 'Chapter 4: Without Gender Equity, Universal Health Coverage is a Pipe Dream.' 10 September 2019. https://swasti.org/without-gender-equity-universal-health-coverage-is-a-pipe-dream.

Umuhoza, C. 2019. 'The FAWE Girls' Scholarship Case: Three Critical Aspects to Learn – Opinion'. RESURJ, 18 April 2019. http://resurj.org/post/fawe-girls-scholarship-case-three-critical-aspects-learn-opinion.

WLP Team. 2019. 'Women from Across the Middle East and Africa Gather for Peace, Security, and Equality – Nigeria'. *Women's Learning Partnership*, 31 March 2019. https://learningpartnership.org/blog/

women-from-across-middle-east-and-africa-gather-for-peace-security-and-equality-nigeria.

YouAct. 2019. 'Advocacy Toolkit: The European Parliament our Ally'. 22 May 2019, http://youact.org/2019/05/22/advocacy-toolkit-the-european-parliament-our-ally.

APPENDIX F

South Asian NGOs' Social Media Engagement Figures

NGO	Facebook	Twitter	Blog
ASAP	10	18	1
APA	6	58	2
C3	7	13	0
CREA	48	165	0
PFI	2	5	0
Swasti	0	14	0
White Ribbon Alliance	6	30	0
Women Deliver	24	50	0
Women's Global Network for Reproductive Rights	1	7	0

Notes

INTRODUCTION

1 This fund supports research that addresses the challenges faced by developing countries. It is a £1.5 billion fund that forms part of the UK's Official Development Assistance (ODA) commitment. It is administered by a number of delivery partners, including the four UK funding bodies, the research councils, the four national academies, and other research-active universities across the UK.
2 See the November 2020 edition of the journal *Feminist Media Studies* here (*https://0-www-tandfonline-com.wam.city.ac.uk/doi/full/10.1080/14680777.2020.1841813*).
3 See LIDC's YouTube platform: https://www.youtube.com/watch?v=7Ia7jnTP4ko.

CHAPTER ONE

1 See King's College website for more details: https://www.kcl.ac.uk/news/half-a-billion-people-could-be-pushed-into-poverty-by-covid-19.
2 See "The World's Abortion Laws" and the full statistics here: https://maps.reproductiverights.org/worldabortionlaws.
3 In June 2022 the US Supreme Court overturned *Roe v. Wade*, which recognised women's constitutional right to abortion, a decision condemned by US president Joe Biden. In a five to four vote, the court upheld a Mississippi law that banned abortions after fifteen weeks of pregnancy. States now have the power to ban abortion, making the United States an exception among other developed nations with regard to protecting reproductive rights, according to the US president. For more, see https://

www.reuters.com/world/us/us-supreme-court-overturns-abortion-rights-landmark-2022-06-24.

4 I do not intend to provide factual information on all the activities of these conservative groups throughout the world (e.g., Trump in the US, Bolsonaro in Brazil), particularly as these activities are highly complex, fragmented, and contradictory and have, in fact, been taking place since before the last decade and had already started to emerge during the 1980s and 1990s in the UN-led conferences on women's rights (Friedman 2003). However, I do mention some of these actions within the context of specific case studies of Latin America and South Asia.

5 The last decades have also seen a growth of writing and critique within the Western feminist movement on the continuation of the practices of reproduction of inequalities and exclusions of women of colour from some strands of the movement. For recent writings on this see the work of authors such as Jonsson (2016, 2021) and Beck (2021), among other feminist postcolonial scholars (Mohanty 2000; Yuval-Davis 2010; McLaren 2017).

6 The campaign #NiUnaaMenos (Not One Less) was organised in solidarity with women fighting against discrimination and violence and took place in various countries, from Argentina to Italy. Like other Latin American countries, the anti-abortion movement is strong in Italy due to the influence of the Roman Catholic Church. Under law 194, women have the right to an abortion in the first ninety days of pregnancy for health reasons. Italy has been criticised by the UN and the Council of Europe for its various obstacles to access to safe abortion. Between the twelfth and the twentieth week, a foetal abnormality must be present and pose a risk to a woman's mental or physical health, and be life-threatening, to terminate the pregnancy. The law also permits medical professionals to refuse abortion on the grounds of conscientious objection, a practice that also occurs in countries like Brazil and is considered highly controversial.

7 Cornwall, Correa, and Jolly (2008, 5) also define 'sexuality' as being about 'the social rules, economic and structures, political battles and religious ideologies that surround psychical expressions of intimacy and the relationship with which such intimacy takes place'.

8 These are the 1994 International Conference on Population and Development (ICPD), held in Cairo, Egypt, and the 1995 Fourth World Conference on Women, held in Beijing.

9 Signed interview consent form on 18 November 2019.

10 Interviewed on the 14 May 2019.

11 The Global Gag Rule is a Republican policy that was reinstated by Donald Trump during his first day in office and that states that if an

international organisation receives American funding it cannot provide abortion services or advocate for the abortion law. This rule had an impact on public health funds, costing $9 billion in foreign aid in a year. NGOs were not able to receive money for sanitation or HIV/AIDS programming if they offered abortion services. This had implications for women's health organisations in various regions of the Global South, including in countries like India. The Global Gag Rule was repealed by the new Biden administration (2021–24).

12 In an article in the magazine *New Statesman America* published in 2019, Butler criticised the backlash, underscoring how gender theory should not be considered 'indoctrinating'. Instead, she argues that the discipline seeks to be a 'form of political freedom', one that is necessary to 'live in a more equitable and liveable world'. See Judith Butler, 'The Backlash against "Gender Ideology" Must Stop,' *New Statesman America*, 21 January 2019.

13 Interviewed for this research in March 2019.

14 Agenda Europe is an extremist Christian network committed to 'pro-life' and family values. For more, see N. Datta, 'Agenda Europe: An Extremist Network in the Heart of Europe', Heinrich Boll Stiftung Gunda Werner Institute: Feminism and Gender Democracy, 2019, https://www.gwi-boell.de/en/2019/04/29/agenda-europe-extremist-christian-network-heart-europe.

15 The organisations that participated in this seminar included Rutgers, Amref Flying Doctors, AFEW, and Doortje Braeken, https://share-netinternational.org/resources/report-thematic-meeting-effective-srhr-messaging-in-changing-times.

16 The Republic of Ireland voted to overturn its abortion ban in a national referendum held in May 2018. This saw 66.4 per cent of the votes in favour as opposed to 33.6 per cent against. The previous law had allowed abortion only when a woman's life was at risk, but not in cases of rape or fatal foetal abnormality. The 8th Amendment thus granted the equal right to life to the mother and the unborn.

17 Interviewed on 15 March 2019.

18 See 'India Has Achieved Ground-Breaking Success in Reducing Maternal Mortality', World Health Organisation, Southeast Asia, 2019, http://www.searo.who.int/mediacentre/features/2018/india-groundbreaking-sucess-reducing-maternal-mortality-rate/en.

19 See 'India Is What Happens When Rich People Do Nothing,' *Atlantic*, 27 April 2021.

20 Interviewed for this research on the 22 April 2019.

21 Interviewed for this research on the 19 June 2020.

22 See Gary Younge, 'Streets on Fire: How a Decade of Protest Shaped the World', *Guardian*, 23 November 2019.
23 See list of organisations in the appendices.
24 See appendices F (South Asian NGOs) and E (tables and graphs from the NGOs' blogs).
25 See appendices A and B for full list of organisations as well as the NGOs by region.
26 For more information, see the website https://polioeradication.org.
27 These were: Alessandra Brigo (IESP UERJ/New York University, March-August 2019); Aline Carvalho (UFRJ Brazil, March-May 2019); Tatiane Leal (UFRJ/Fiocruz, April-July 2019); Ambika Tandon (CIS India, March-August 2019); Sarah Molisso (City, University of London, UK, April-August 2020); and Jamile Dalpiaz (independent early career research, UK, May-August 2021).

CHAPTER TWO

1 Rappaport (1987) describes 'empowerment' as being a psychological sense of personal control as well as concern with social influence, political power, and rights. Melkote (in Moday and Gudykunst 2003) provides a good definition of empowerment as manifesting itself as social power from the individual to the organisation levels of analysis.
2 See full report: *Accelerate Progress: Sexual and Reproductive Health Rights for All*, Guttmacher-*Lancet* Commission 391 (June 2018): 2642–92, https://www.thelancet.com/pdfs/journals/lancet/PIIS0140-6736(18)30293-9.pdf.

CHAPTER THREE

1 Answered the in-depth interview question sheet on 2 March 2019.
2 Interviewed for this research on 18 April 2019.
3 Interviewed for this research on 15 March 2019.
4 Interviewed on 12 March 2019.
5 Interviewed for this research on the 19 March 2019.
6 Interviewed for this research on 18 March 2019.
7 Interviewed for this research on the 20 March 2019.
8 Interviewed for this research in May 2019.
9 Interviewed for this research together with the director of policy research on 12 March 2019.
10 Interviewed on the 15 March 2019.

CHAPTER FOUR

1 Sternbach et al. (1992, 400) point out that Argentina was an exception, having seen feminist movements formed largely by professional women. The authors quote the late Brazilian scholar Paul Singer, who made a distinction between 'feminine' and 'feminist'; "The struggles against the rising cost of living or for schools, day-care centres etc. ... It is possible to consider them *feminine* revindications. But they are not feminist to the extent that they do not question the way women are inserted into the social context" ('O feminismo e o feminino', in Sao Paulo, O *povo em movimento*, ed. P. Singer and V.C. Brant, 116–17 [Petropolis: Vozes, 1980] in Sternbach et al. 1992, 401). However, the plurality of the diverse forms of contemporary Latin American feminisms might blur these distinctions even further. Demands made by women's groups regarding maternity policies or day care could also be seen as early manifestations of feminist thinking – something that could later give rise to more mature, active, and self-conscious forms of engagement with women's issues in the pursuit of change.
2 Interviewed via email in June 2019.
3 Chile is still seen as the reference for more institutionalised and organised feminist NGOs. Contemporary feminist movements in Brazil, on the other hand, include those from the various 'Marchas' movements, such as the Marcha das Vadias (Marches of the Sluts), including Marcha Mundial das Mulheres (World March of Women), Marcha das Mulheres Negras (March of Black Women) as well as NGO networks and organisations like SOF, SOS Corpo, and Articulacao de Mulheres Brasileiras.
4 Most nations allow abortions in exceptional circumstances, such as when the pregnancy is a threat to a woman's life, while others ban it altogether (Kulezycki 2011). In nations like El Salvador, Honduras, Haiti, Nicaragua, Dominican Republic, and Suriname, abortion is forbidden, whereas countries like Uruguay, Cuba, and Guyana allow women to interrupt their pregnancy up until the twelfth week. Brazil, Panama, and Chile permit abortion in exceptional circumstances, such as to save lives in cases of rape.
5 For more, see "Open Data about Femicide in Brazil" in the Open Government Partnership https://www.opengovpartnership.org/stories/open-data-about-femicide-in-brazil.
6 Interviewed for this research on 10 April 2019.
7 See 'Brasil se abstem em voto sobre saude sexual e reprodutiva na ONU' (Brazil abstains in vote on sexual and reproductive health at the UN), 26 June 2019, https://jamilchade.blogosfera.uol.com.br/2019/06/26/brasil-se-abstem-em-voto-sobre-saude-sexual-e-reprodutiva-na-onu.

As the journalist Igor Mello notes in the piece, the ten-page document provided by the Brazilian government made no mention of LGBT rights, which were included under the generic term 'vulnerable groups'. It stated that Brazil would 'combat violence and discrimination' but did not mention actions to guarantee the inclusion of LGBT communities or reproductive rights. However, it did assume a commitment to combat violence against women and feminicide. In March 2019, Brazil also opposed a document elaborated by the Commission on the Status of Women (CSW), criticising the guarantee of 'access to universal services of sexual and reproductive health'.

8 Interviewed for this research on the 26 November 2019.
9 Interviewed for this research on 25 March 2019.
10 Interviewed for this research on 9 May 2019.
11 The research was conducted by the Global Advisor online platform between 25 June and 9 July 2021. For more, see https://www.ipsos.com/en/global-views-abortion-2021.

CHAPTER FIVE

1 See 'India's Failure to Include Enough Women in Politics', *Interpreter*, 21 April 2021, https://www.lowyinstitute.org/the-interpreter/india-s-failure-include-enough-women-politics.
2 For more, see UNICEF *India* (https://www.unicef.org/india/what-we-do/gender-equality).
3 India is known for having a gender population gap. According to the 2011 census, girls account for 48 per cent of the population, and, out of 12.15 million married children, 8.9 million are girls, numbers that are likely to be even higher following the COVID-19 pandemic. See 'Gender Inequality Continues to Affect the Lives of Many Girls in India', https://www.cry.org/blog/gender-inequality (put out by CRY, an Indian charity that specialises in children's rights).
4 See 'As India Advances, Women's Workforce Participation Plummets', *Strategy and Business*, 15 May 2020.
5 See *Status of Human Rights in the Context of Sexual Health and Reproductive Health Rights in India*, https://nhrc.nic.in/sites/default/files/sexual_health_reproductive_health_rights_SAMA_PLD_2018_01012019_1.pdf.
6 The grounds include the risk to the physical or mental health of a woman when contraceptive methods have failed or on humanitarian grounds, such as risks posed to the foetus (e.g., deformities) (Hirve 2004).

7 Interviewed on 3 April 2019.
8 Interviewed for this research in May 2019.
9 See *Partnering for a Better Future for India's Women and Children: India*, 17 July 2019, https://2017-2020.usaid.gov/india/health-partnerships.
10 See World Bank, 2003, 'India- Improving Reproductive and Child Health (English)', in *Results Profile*, Washington, DC: World Bank Group, http://documents.worldbank.org/curated/en/867551468257075769/India-Improving-reproductive-and-child-health.
11 Interviewed for this research on the 10 April 2019.
12 Interviewed for this research on the 25 March 2019.
13 Interviewed for this research on the 29 May 2019.

CHAPTER SEVEN

1 See http://www.who.int/topics/millennium_development_goals/about/en/index.html.
2 Interviewed for this research on 8 May 2019.
3 See https://amnistia.org.ar/esiya.
4 Responded to the questionnaire on 28 May 2019.
5 See campaign here (http://mujeresimparables.co) and here: http://www.despenalizaciondelaborto.org.co/2018/09/27/el-arte-alza-su-voz-por-el-aborto-legal-en-colombia.
6 Responded to the gender question sheet and the communications survey on 1 April 2019.
7 For an example, see https://www.facebook.com/promsex/videos/10156165537804127.

CHAPTER EIGHT

1 The Argentinian NiUnaMenos (Not One Less) was a grassroots feminist movement that began in 2015 in the streets of Buenos Aires, later spreading throughout other Latin American countries and having an impact on global feminism. The campaign was organised by female journalists, artists, and academics and was known for having been a 'collective scream against *machista* violence'. The popular hashtag on social media, #NiUnaMenos, was posted following mass demonstrations held in Buenos Aires in June 2015, following the murder of a fourteen-year-old girl, Chiara Paez, who was found buried in her boyfriend's house and who had been beaten by him after he found out that she was pregnant and wanted to keep the baby. Since then, there have been

various protests against femicide throughout Argentina as well as in Uruguay, Chile, and Brazil. These have influenced other protests in the US, such as the International Women's Strike in 2017. In December 2020, Argentina legalised abortion during the first trimester, with the NiUnaMenos campaign being seen as having been crucial in paving the way for change.
2. Interviewed for this research on 1 May 2019.
3. The term 'ICTs' (information and communication technologies) can include any form of communication device or application, from radio, TV, mobile phones to computers, hardware and software networks, as well as satellite systems (Kleine and Unwin 2009).
4. This includes some of the 'quirky' types of radical and creative forms of feminist protesting and activism that have become popular in the 'new' young feminist movements, such as the different SlutWalk editions and the use women in these protests make of their own bodies – including demonstrating without their shirts or wearing 'sexy clothes' – to call out bodily control and sexual repression. This is also true of campaigns that advocate for the liberalisation of abortion.
5. Family Planning 2020 works with sixty-nine countries, including in Africa and Southeast Asia and a few other nations in Latin America.
6. Interviewed on 2 April 2019.
7. Interviewed for this research on 18 March 2019.

CHAPTER NINE

1. Only a few networks and NGOs had a strategic plan that could be accessed through their website. These are: (1) Akahata; (2) Amnesty International; (3) CARE International; (4) UNFPA 2018–21; (5) International Alliance of Women; (6) Ibis; (7) Promsex; (8) RESURJ; (9) Consorcio Latin American Contra el Aborto Inseguro (2020–24); (10) Women Deliver; and (11) White Ribbon Alliance.
2. Interviewed on 13 May 2019.
3. Interviewed on 13 May 2019.
4. Interviewed on 18 March 2019.
5. Responded to the communications questionnaire in June 2019.
6. There were links provided for each, which were: https://amnistia.org.ar; https://amnistia.org.ar/todas-las-ciberacciones; https://amnistia.org.ar/participa; https://amnistia.org.ar/sumate; and https://amnistia.org.ar/areas-tematicas/educacion-en-derechos-humanos-y-jovenes.

7   Responded to the communications questionnaire on 28 May 2019.
8   Responded to the questionnaire on 20 March 2019.
9   For further information, see https://www.fundaciondesafio-ec.org.
10 Responded to the communications questionnaire on 14 May 2019.
11 For more, see the website: www.freethepill.org.
12 For more here, see the website: https://www.mmoho.org.
13 Responded to the questionnaire on 23 May 2019.
14 Responded to the communications survey on 30 April 2019.
15 Responded to the questionnaire on the 4 April 2019.
16 The communications lead responded to the communications questionnaire on the 13 May 2019.
17 Interviewed for this research on 11 April 2019.

CHAPTER TEN

1   See the videos of the campaigns here: https://www.facebook.com/promsex/videos/10156165537804127; https://www.facebook.com/promsex/videos/10155010543609127 and https://www.facebook.com/promsex/videos/10155912033194127.
2   Responded to the communications questionnaire on the 12 March 2019.
3   Both responded to the communications questionnaire on the 10 April 2019.
4   See https://www.mysu.org.uy/web.
5   See http://www.mysu.org.uy/haceclick.
6   See https://www.mysu.org.uy/web.
7   These are www.reprolatina.org.br; www.adolescencia.org.br; and www.anticoncepcao.org.br.
8   Interviewed and responded to the questionnaire on the 18 March 2019.
9   An example of a successful campaign cited by the CEO is the 'Fazer Valer' (Make It Worth It) of the Youth for Integral Education in Sexuality project. Here an advocacy campaign was carried out using social media with the aim of joining allies who were in favour of the delivery of full-time sexuality education in schools. Some results listed here included having had seventy people sign a letter of support for this goal.
10 Both were interviewed on 26 April 2019.
11 See https://fpvoices.tumblr.com.
12 See the post at https://www.facebook.com/UNFPA/photos/a.762970977068554/2362886100070108/?type=3&theater.
13 Interviewed for this research on 18 June 2020.
14 Responded to the communications questionnaire on 21 May 2020.

CHAPTER ELEVEN

1. Six posts in this time frame were related to the core themes of SRHR, GBV, and CSE.
2. See full list of blog posts and references in appendix E.
3. A total of thirty-five posts were collected from the following organisations: Amnesty International (2), ASAP (1), CARE UK (4), IPPF (9), RESURJ (6), Campaign (1), SRHM (3), Swasti (8), and WLP (1). Examples included: CARE, 'COVID-19: How CARE Is Responding to an Unprecedented Global Crisis', 6 April 2020, https://www.careinternational.org.uk/stories/covid-19-how-care-responding-unprecedented-global-crisis; IPPF, 'What You Need to Know about Sex and COVID-19', 27 March 2020, https://www.ippf.org/blogs/what-you-need-know-about-sex-and-covid-19; and WLP Team, 'The WLP Partnership Is Empowering Vulnerable Populations during the Coronavirus Crisis', *Women's Learning Partnership*, 7 April 2020, https://learningpartnership.org/index.php/blog/wlp-partnership-empowering-vulnerable-populations-during-coronavirus-crisis.
4. See appendix E.
5. Ibid.
6. As of 4 August 2020.
7. S. Dalvie, "Keep Calm and Take the Medical Abortion Pill', *that which I am*, 17 June 2019, https://thatwhichiam.wordpress.com/2019/06/17/keep-calm-and-take-the-medical-abortion-pill.
8. UNFPA, 'Finding Reproductive Healthcare un the World's Biggest Refugee Camp', *Reliefweb*, 5 April 2019, https://reliefweb.int/report/bangladesh/finding-reproductive-healthcare-world-s-biggest-refugee-camp.
9. UNFPA Bangladesh, 'Finding Reproductive Healthcare in the World's Biggest Refugee Camp', 4 April 2019, https://bangladesh.unfpa.org/en/news/finding-reproductive-healthcare-worlds-biggest-refugee-camp.
10. L. Alkanawati, 'From Syria to Sudan, Women Rights Defenders Need More Than Likes', *The New Humanitarian*, 10 July 2019, https://www.thenewhumanitarian.org/opinion/2019/07/10/syria-sudan-women-rights-defenders-need-more-likes.
11. See https://twitter.com/CRCMSUDAN/status/1148926116419162113.
12. See https://www.facebook.com/womendeliver/posts/10157734733031844.
13. These included: UNFPA (2018), *International Technical Guidance on Sexuality Education: An Evidence-Informed Approach*; UNESCO, UNAIDS, UNFPA, UNICEF, UN Women, and WHO; UNFPA ESARO (2016), *How Effective Is Comprehensive Sexuality Education in Preventing HIV?*; UNFPA, ESARO, BZgA (Federal Centre for Health Education) and

IPPF EN (International Planned Parenthood Federation – European Network), *Sexuality Education in Europe and Central Asia: State of the Art and Recent Developments: An Overview of 25 Countries* (Cologne: BZgA, 2017).

14 See J. Nilsson and S.M. Spencer, '1965: The Birth Control Revolution', *Saturday Evening Post*, 31 December 2015, https://www.saturdayeveningpost.com/2015/12/50-years-ago-the-birth-control-revolution.

15 Global Gag Rule, 'The Global Gag Rule: The "Prolife" Death Warrant', YouTube, 9 March 2019, https://www.youtube.com/watch?v=D7Jm9ZDQIW4.

16 These included: L. Carmody and M. Stevens, 'Reproductive Justice: The Missing Issue in Party Manifestos for 2019 Election', *Daily Maverick*, 5 May 2019, https://www.dailymaverick.co.za/article/2019-05-05-reproductive-justice-the-missing-issue-in-party-manifestos-for-2019-election; and P. Pilane, '"Top Three Parties" Position on Sexual and Reproductive Justice', *Health-E News*, 18 March 2019, https://health-e.org.za/2019/03/18/top-three-parties-position-on-sexual-reproductive-justice.

17 See IPPF's post '#IDECIDE What happens to My Body Pledge Your Voice', https://www.ippf.org/idecide/pledgeyourvoice.html, no longer available, viewed 6 August 2020.

18 Mehta, S., B.S, Mehta, and A. Kumar 'Addressing Domestic Violence: A Forgotten Agenda While Locking India Down', *Observer Research Foundation*, 8 April 2020, https://www.orfonline.org/expert-speak/addressing-domestic-violence-a-forgotten-agenda-while-locking-india-down-64301.

19 Amnesty International, 'Ecuador: They Will Not Stop Us – Justice and Protection For Amazonian Women, Defenders of the Land, Territory and Environment', 30 April 2019, https://www.amnesty.org/en/documents/amr28/0039/2019/en.

20 For further information see blog references in the appendices.

CHAPTER TWELVE

1 See https://twitter.com/WRAglobal/status/1111995267853811712.
2 See https://twitter.com/gogiinc/status/1113331971222962176.
3 See https://twitter.com/Youthbolpoll/status/1110058878371356672.
4 See https://twitter.com/c3_india/status/1113373821766176774.
5 See https://twitter.com/WomenDeliver/status/1114180143499575298.
6 See https://www.facebook.com/CREAworld.org.
7 Interviewed for this research on 8 April 2019.

8 See N. Palshetkar, 'Unsafe Abortions and Third Leading Cause of Maternal Deaths', *DNA India*, 8 March 2019, https://www.dnaindia.com/analysis/column-unsafe-abortions-are-third-leading-cause-of-maternal-deaths-2727362.

9 See A. Hardon, C. Pell, E. Taqueban, and N. Narasimhan, 'Sexual and Reproductive Self-Care among Women and Girls: Rights from Ethnographic Studies', *BMJ* 365 (2019): 1333, https://www.bmj.com/content/365/bmj.l1333.

10 See https://www.youtube.com/watch?v=qBbpED2GfP0.

11 Interviewed for this research in May 2019.

12 See S. Dalvie, 'Keep Calm and Take the Medical Abortion Pill', *ASAP Blog*, 26 March 2019, https://asap-asia.org/blog/keep-calm-and-take-the-medical-abortion-pill.

13 See https://www.facebook.com/pg/AsiaPacAlliance/posts/?ref=page_internal.

14 See https://twitter.com/ThinkCREA.

15 See https://twitter.com/Youthbolpoll/status/1110058878371356672.

16 See https://twitter.com/gogiinc/status/1113331971222962176.

17 Interviewed for this research on 4 June 2019.

18 Interviewed for this research on 12 April 2019.

19 See 'Hundreds of Women March across India For Their Right: All about the Growing Movement You Haven't Heard of', *QRIUS*, 5 April 2019, https://qrius.com/hundreds-of-women-march-across-india-for-their-rights-all-about-the-growing-movement-you-havent-heard-of.

20 See https://twitter.com/WomenDeliver/status/1111639149335986176.

21 See https://twitter.com/FundHumanRights/status/1112729006581972993.

22 See tweets at http://ow.ly/qPPQ30oiiyH and @*AJENews* at https://twitter.com/pai_org/status/1113101356343156736.

23 See https://twitter.com/WRAglobal/status/1111705064886976518.

24 See https://twitter.com/AsiaPacAlliance/status/1113628901698203648.

25 See https://twitter.com/ThinkCREA/status/1111635233194037248.

26 Interviewed for this research on 30 March 2019.

27 Interviewed on 10 April 2019.

CHAPTER THIRTEEN

1 For further information, see the UNFPA website at https://www.unfpa.org/press/new-unfpa-data-reveals-nearly-12-million-women-lost-access-contraception-due-disruptions.

2 See Share's website at https://share-netinternational.org.
3 This case study was delivered by Thomas Tufte in a guest lecture to the postgraduate students in the Master's programme in International Communications and Development at the Department of Sociology, City, University of London, on 10 November 2020.
4 Development assistance has tended to target maternal health with the aim of reducing maternal mortality as well as increasing access to contraception for women. Gideon et al. (2016, 792) argue that the priorities of certain players in the field have influenced the shifts. This was the case with programmes such as Safe Motherhood Initiative and the 2021 Gates Foundation Family Planning, which shifted towards more technical concerns.
5 Interviewed for this research on 1 May 2019.
6 According to the official statistics of the Brazilian Institute for Geography and Statistics, there are 22 million evangelicals in Brazil (or 22 per cent of the total) as opposed to 125 million Catholics, or 64 per cent of the total.
7 These included Akahata, Amnesty International, CARE International UK, IAW Action Programme, Ibis Reproductive Health, Promsex, RESURJ, Reproductive Health Supplies Coalition, Women Deliver, the Latin American Consortium Against Unsafe Abortion (CLACAI), Women's Global Network for Reproductive Rights, and the White Ribbon Alliance.
8 Serveas (2008, 45) outlines the shift in development from the focus on results to empowerment processes, including the example of the campaign 'Abstinence – Be Faithful and Use a Condom ABC' model in HIV prevention to Panos's (2006) document (in Serveas 2008) on how communication can help HIV social movements to enact social change. In the latter cases, the expected outcome is a process of empowerment. A focus on communities as units of analysis emerged as critical to understanding the effectiveness of interventions in health promotion campaigns (Omoto 2005 and Papa, Singhal, and Papa 2006, both in Servaes 2008, 45).
9 Fultner (2017, 205) goes on to note that transnational feminists argue that women's issues vary according to geographical locations, with Peggy Antrobus (2016) noting how Nigerian women are frequently less interested in equality with men but nonetheless want to affirm their reproductive and property rights and consider themselves feminists.

References

Aasen, B. 2006. 'Lessons from Evaluations of Women and Gender Equality in Development Cooperation'. Report from the Norwegian Institute for Urban and Regional Research (NIBR). https://www.oecd.org/derec/norway/37880765.pdf.

Airhihenbuwa, Collins, and Mohna J. Dutta. 2012. 'New Perspectives on Global Health Communication: Affirming Spaces for Rights, Equity and Voices'. In *The Handbook of Global Health Communication*, ed. Rafael Obregon and Silvio Waisbord, 34–51. Chichester: Wiley-Blackwell.

Alvarez, S. 1998. 'Latin American Feminisms Go Global: Trends of the 1990s and Challenges for the New Millennium.' In *Culture of Politics, Politics of Cultures: Re-Visioning Latin American Social Movements*, ed. S.A. Alvarez, E. Dagnino, and A. Escobar, 293–317. New York: Routledge.

– 2009. 'Beyond NGO-ization? Reflections from Latin America'. *Development* 52, no. 2: 175–84.

– 2014. 'Para além da sociedade civil: Reflexões sobre o campo feminista'. *Cadernos Pagu* 43 (January-June): 13–56.

Antrobus, P. 2016. 'Feminism as Transformational Politics: Towards Possibilities for Another World'. In *The Palgrave Handbook of Gender and Development: Critical Engagement in Feminist Theory and Practice*, ed. Wendy Harcourt, 583–93. London: Palgrave.

Arnaudo, D. 2017. 'Computational Propaganda in Brazil: Social Bots during the Elections'. Report of the Computational Propaganda Research Project, University of Oxford. https://ora.ox.ac.uk/objects/uuid:e88de32c-baaa-4835-bb76-e00473457f46.

Ascough, Hannah. 2018. 'Once upon a Time: Using the Hero's Journey in Development Stories'. *Canadian Journal of Development Studies* 39, no. 4: 533–49.

Auger, G. 2013. 'Fostering Democracy through Social Media: Evaluating Diametrically Opposed Non-Profit Advocacy Organisation's Use of Facebook, Twitter and Youtube'. *Public Relations Review* 39: 369–76.

Babugura, A. 2016. 'Gender Equality in Combatting Climate Change.' In *Policy Briefing – Women, Power and Policy-making*, report from the Centre for International Governance Innovation and South African Institute of International Affairs. https://www.africaportal.org/documents/19278/Babugura__Gender_equality_in_combatting_climate_change.pdf.

Baltiwala, S. 2007. 'Taking the Power Out of Empowerment: An Experiential Account'. *Development in Practice* 17, nos. 4–5: 557–65.

Bandura, A. 1977. 'Social Learning Theory.' Englewood Cliffs, NJ: Prentice Hall.

Banet-Weiser, S., and K.M. Miltner. 2016. 'Masculinity so Fragile: Culture, Structure and Networked Misogyny'. *Feminist Media Studies* 16, no. 1: 171–4.

Baru, R. 2006. 'Privatisation of Health Care in India: A Comparative Analysis of Orissa, Karnataka and Maharashtra States.' In *The Indian Institute of Public Administration, Centre for Multi-Disciplinary Development Research, and United Nations Development Programme*, India. https://www.iipa.org.in/common/pdf/PAPER%204_Privatisation%20of%20Health%20Care.pdf.

Bebbington, A., S. Hickey, and D. Mitlin. 2008. 'Introduction: Can NGOs Make a Difference? The Challenge of Development Alternatives'. In *Can NGOs Make a Difference? The Challenge of Development Alternatives*, ed. Anthony Bebbington, Samuel Hickey, and Diana C. Mitlin, 3–55. London: Zed Books.

Bordo, S. 1992. 'The Body and the Reproduction of Femininity: A Feminist Appropriation of Foucault'. In *Gender/Body/Knowledge: Feminist Reconstructions of Being and Knowing*, ed. Alison M. Jaggar and Susan Bordo, 13–34. New Jersey: Rutgers University Press.

Britt Coe, A., and A. Schnabel. 2011. 'Emotions Matter After All: How Reproductive Rights Advocates Orchestrate Emotions to Influence Policies in Peru'. *Sociological Perspectives* 54, no. 4: 665–88.

Butler, J. 1993. 'Bodies That Matter'. In *Bodies That Matter: On the Discursive Limits of 'Sex'*, 27–57, New York: Routledge.

– 2017. 'The Phantom of Gender: Reflections on Freedom and Violence', *Folha de Sao Paulo*, 21 November 2017. https://www1.folha.uol.com.br/internacional/en/culture/2017/11/1936921-the-phantom-of-gender-reflections-on-freedom-and-violence.shtml.

– 2019. 'Anti-gender Ideology and Mahmood's Critique of the Secular Age'. *Journal of the American Academy of Religion* 87, no. 4: 955–67.

Cardoso, F. 1972. 'Dependency and Development in Latin America'. In *The Globalization and Development Reader*, ed. Amy Hite and J. Timmons Roberts, 85–95. London: Blackwell.

Carpenter, R.C. 2007. 'Setting the Advocacy Agenda: Theorizing Issue Emergence and Non-Emergence in Transnational Advocacy Networks.' *International Studies Quarterly* 51, no. 1: 99–120.

Centre for Reproductive Rights and the Inter-American Dialogue. 2015. 'Abortion and Reproductive Rights in Latin America: Implications for Democracy.' Report. https://www.reproductiverights.org/sites/crr.civicactions.net/files/documents/IAD9794%20Repro%20Rights_web.pdf.

Chadwick, A. 2006. *Internet Politics: States, Citizens and New Communication Technologies*. New York: Oxford University Press.

Chambers, R. 2005. *Ideas for Development*. London: Earthscan.

Chant, S. 2011. 'The "Feminization of Poverty" and the "Feminization" of Anti-Poverty Programs: Room for Revision?' In *The Women, Gender and Development Reader*, ed. Nalini Visvanathan and Lynn Duggan, 174–97. London: Zed Books.

Chant, S., and Craske, N. 2003. 'Feminisms in Latin Americ.a.' In *Gender in Latin America*, 162–91. London: Latin America Bureau.

Chenou, J.M., and C. Cepeda-Masmeda. 2019. '#NiUnaMenos Data Activism: From the Global South'. *Television and New Media* 20, no. 4: 396–411.

Chouliaraki, L. 2006. *The Spectatorship of Suffering*. London: Sage.

Chowdhry, G. 1995. 'Engendering Development? Women in Development (WID) in International Development Regimes'. In *Feminism/Postmodernism/Development*, ed. Marianne Marchand and Jane L. Parpart, 26–42, Oxon: Routledge.

Chua, P., K.K. Bhaunani, and J. Foran. 2000. 'Women, Culture and Development: A New Paradigm for Development Studies?' *Ethnic and Racial Studies* 23, no. 5: 820–41.

Colle, R.D. 2008. 'Threads of Development Communication'. In *Communication for Development and Social Change*, ed. Jan Servaes, 96–158, Los Angeles: Sage.

Cornwall, A., S. Correa, and S. Jolly. 2008. 'Development with a Body: Making the Connections between Sexuality, Human Rights and Development'. In *Development with a Body: Sexuality, Human Rights and Development*, ed. Andrea Cornwall, Sonia Correa, and Susie Jolly, 1–22, London: Zed Books

Cornwall, A., and C. Nyamu-Musembi 2006. 'Putting the "Rights-Based Approach" to Development into Perspective'. *Third World Quarterly* 25, no. 8: 1415–37.

Cornwall, A., and A. Rivas. 2015. 'From Gender Equality and Women's Empowerment to Global Justice: Reclaiming a Transformative Agenda for Gender and Development'. *Third World Quarterly* 30, no 2: 396–415.

Correa, S., A. Germain, and R. Petchesky. 2005. 'Thinking beyond ICPD + 10: Where Should Our Movement Be Going?' *Reproductive Health Matters* 13, no. 25: 109–19.

Correa, S., and S. Jolly. 2008. 'Development's Encounter with Sexuality: Essentialism and Beyond.' In *Development with a Body: Sexuality, Human Rights and Development*, ed. Andrea Cornwall, Sonia Correa, and Susie Jolly, 22–45. London: Zed Books.

Correa, S., and R. Petchesky. 1994. 'Reproductive and Sexual Rights: A Feminist Perspective'. In *Population Policies Reconsidered: Health, Empowerment and Rights*, ed. Gita Sen, Adrienne Germain, and Lincoln C. Chen, 107–26, Boston: Harvard University Press

Crane, B.B., and J. DusenberryJ. 2004. 'Power and Politics in International Funding for Reproductive Health: The US Global Gag Rule'. *Reproductive Health Matters* 12, no. 24: 128–37.

Dahlgren, P. 2009. *Media and Political Engagement: Citizens, Communication and Democracy*. Cambridge: Cambridge University Press.

Daniels, J. 2009. 'Rethinking Cyberfeminism(s): Race, Gender, and Embodiment.' *Women's Studies Quarterly* 37, nos. 1 and 2: 101–24.

Datta, B., and G. Misra. 2000. 'Advocacy for Sexual and Reproductive Health: The Challenge in India'. *Reproductive Health Matters* 8, no. 16: 24–34.

Dean, J., and K. Aune 2015. 'Feminism Resurgent? Mapping Contemporary Feminist Activisms in Europe'. *Social Movement Studies* 14, no. 4: 375–95.

Della Porta, D. 2012. 'Communication in Movement: Social Movements as Agents of Participatory Democracy'. In *Social Media and Democracy: Innovations in Participatory Politics*, ed. Brian Loader and Dan Mercea, 39–55, London: Routledge.

Desai, V., and R.B. Potter. 2014. *The Companion to Development Studies*. Oxford: Oxford University Press.

Diniz, D., and M. Medeiros. 2010. 'Aborto no Brasil: Uma pesquisa domiciliar com técnica de urna.' In *Anis – Instituto de Biotécnica, Direitos Humanos e gênero*. Brasilia: DF.

Dinz, D., M. Medeiros, and A, Madeiro 2017 'Pesquisa Nacional de Aborto 2016.' *Ciência Sociais Saúde Coletiva* 22, no 2: 653–60.

Dutta, M.J. 2006. 'Theoretical Approaches to Entertainment-Education'. *Health Communications* 20, no. 3: 221–31.

– 2011. 'Theorizing Social Change Communication'. In *Communicating Social Change*, 29–65. New York and London: Routledge.

Earl, J., and K. Kimport. 2013. *Digital Enabled Social Change: Activism in the Internet Age*. Cambridge, MA: MIT Press.

Enghel, F., and J. Noske-Turner. 2018. 'Introduction: Communication in International Development – Towards Theorizing across Hybrid Practices'. In *Communication in International Development: Doing Good and Looking Good?*, ed. Florencia Enghel and Jessica Noske-Turner, 1–19. London: Routledge.

Fairclough, N. 1998. *Discourse and Social Change*. Cambridge: Polity.

Ferreira, C. Branco de Castro. 2015. 'Feminisms on the Web: Lines and Forms of Action in Contemporary Feminist Debate'. *Cadernos Pagu* 44 (January-June): 199–228.

Foot, K.A., and S.M. Schneider. 2006. *Web Campaigning*. Cambridge, MA: MIT Press.

Foucault, M. 1972. *The Archaeology of Knowledge*. London: Routledge

– 1980. *The History of Sexuality*. Vol. 2, *The Use of Pleasure*. London: Penguin.

Frank, A. Gunder. 1969. 'The Development of Underdevelopment'. In *The Globalization and Development Reader*, ed. Amy Hite and J. Timmons Roberts, 76–85. London: Blackwell.

Fraser, N. 2013. *Fortunes of Feminism: From State-Managed Capitalism to Neoliberal Crisis*. London: Verso

Freedman, L.P., and S.I. Isaacs. 1993. 'Human Rights and Reproductive Choice'. *Studies in Family Planning* 24, no. 1: 18–30.

Freire, P. 1970. *The Pedagogy of the Oppressed*. London: Penguin.

Friedman, E.J. 2003.'Gendering the Agenda: The Impact of Transnational Women's Rights Movement at the UN Conferences of the 1990s'. *Women's Studies International Forum* 26, no. 4: 313–31.

– 2005. 'The Politics of Information and Communication Technology Use among Latin American Gender Equality Organisations'. *Knowledge, Technology and Policy* 18, no. 2: 30–40.

Fotopoulou, A. 2016a. 'Digital and Networked by Default/Women's Organisations and the Social Imaginary of Networked Feminism'. *New Media and Society* 18, no. 6: 989–1005.

– 2016b. *Feminist Activism and Digital Networks*. London: Palgrave Studies in Communication for Social Change.

Fuchs, C. 2003. 'Structuration Theory and Self-Organisation'. *Systemic Practice and Action Research* 16, no. 2: 133–67.

Fultner, B. 2017. 'The Dynamics of Transnational Feminist Solidarity Dialogue'. In *Decolonizing Feminism: Transnational Feminism and Globalization*, ed. Margaret A. McLaren, 203–31. Maryland: Rowman and Littlefield.

Gajjala, R. 2003. 'South Asian Digital Diasporas and Cyberfeminist Webs: Negotiating Globalization, Gender and Information Technology Design'. *Contemporary South Asia* 12, no. 1: 41–56.

Gajjala, R., and A. Mamidipudi. 1999. 'Cyberfeminism, Technology and International Development'. *Gender and Development* 7, no. 2: 8–16.

Garita, A. 2015. 'Moving towards Sexual and Reproductive Justice: A Transnational and Multigenerational Feminist Remix'. In *The Oxford Handbook of Transnational Feminist Movements*, ed. Wendy Harcourt and Rawwida Baksh, 271–91, Oxford: Oxford University Press.

George, A. 2009. 'Quantitative and Qualitative Approaches to Content Analysis'. In *The Content Analysis Reader*, ed. Klaus Krippendorff and Mary Bock, 144–55. London: Sage.

Germain, A. 2004. 'Reproductive Health and Human Rights'. *Lancet* 363: 65–6.

Ghosh, M. 2018. 'Gender Equality, Growth and Human Development in India'. In *Asian Development Perspectives* 9, no. 1: 68–87.

Giddens, A. 1991. *Modernity and Self-Identity*. Los Angeles: Stanford University Press.

Gideon, J. 2020. 'Introduction to Covid-19 in Latin America and the Caribbean'. *Bulletin of Latin American Research* 39, no. S1: 4–6.

Gideon, J., and F. Porter. 2016. 'Challenging Gendered Inequalities in Global Health: Dilemmas for NGOs'. *Development and Change* 47, no. 4: 782–97.

Gill, R. 2000. 'Discourse Analysis.' In *Qualitative Researching with Text, Image and Sound*, ed. Martin W. Bauer and George Gaskell, 173–90, London: Sage.

- 2007a. *Gender and the Media.* Cambridge: Polity. 16-44.
- 2007b. 'Postfeminist Media Culture: Elements of a Sensibility'. In *European Journal of Cultural Studies* 10, no. 2: 142–66.
- 2018. 'Discourse Analysis in Media and Communication Research'. In *The Craft of Criticism: Critical Media Studies in Practice*, ed. Michael Kackman and Mary C. Kearney, 23–35. London: Routledge.

Gomes, C., and B. Sorj. 2014. 'Corpo, geracao e identidade: A Marcha das Vadias no Brasil'. *Sociedade e Estado* 29, no. 2: 433–42.

Gonzaga, P., R. Bacellar, and L.M.B. de Aras. 2015. 'Mulheres latino-americanas e a luta por direitos reprodutivos: o panorama da conjuntura politica e legal do aborto nos paises da America Latina'. *Revista de Estudos e Pesquisa sobre as Americas* 9, no. 2: 1–31.

Graham, P. 2018. 'Ethics in Critical Discourse Analysis'. *Critical Discourse Analysis* 15, no. 2: 186–203.

Green, M. 2002. 'Social Development Issues and Approaches.' In *Development theory and Practice: Critical Perspectives*, ed. Uma Kothari and Martin Minogue, 52–71. Basingstoke: Palgrave.

Grewal, I. 1999. 'Women's Rights as Human Rights: Feminist Practices, Global Feminism and Human Rights Regimes In Transnationality'. *Citizenship Studies* 3, no. 3: 337–59.

Grewal, I., and C. Kaplan 2009. 'Postcolonial Scholarship'. In *A Companion to Gender Studies*, ed. Philomena Essed, David Theo Goldberg, and Audrey L. Kobayashi, 51–9. Oxford: Wiley-Blackwell.

Grint, K., and R. Gill. 1995. *The Gender-Technology Relation: Contemporary Theory and Research*, 1–28. London: Taylor and Francis.

Habermas, J. 1992. *The Structural Transformation of the Public Sphere.* Cambridge: Polity.

Haraway, D. 1991. 'Situated Knowledges: The Science Question in Feminism and the Privilege of Partial Perspective'. In *Simians, Cyborgs and Women: The Reinvention of Nature*, 183–201. London: Free Association.
- 2000. 'A Cyborg Manifesto: Science, Technology and Socialist Feminism in the Late 20th Century'. In *The Cyberculture Reader*, ed. David Bell and Barbara M. Kennedy, 291–324. London: Routledge.

Harcourt, W. 1994. 'Negotiating Positions in the Sustainable Development Debate: Situating the Feminist Perspective.' In *Feminist Perspectives on Sustainable Development*, 11–26. London: Zed Books.
- 1999. 'Reproductive Health and Rights and the Quest For Social Justice'. *Development* 3, no. 42 (1 March): 7–10.

- 2009. 'Reproductive Bodies'. In *Body Politics in Development: Critical Alternatives in Gender and Development*, 38–65. London: Zed Books.
- 2013. 'Transnational Feminist Engagement with 2010 Plus Activisms'. *Development and Change* 44 (May): 621–37.
- 2017. 'The Development Industry and the Co-Optation of Body Politics'. In *Bodies in Resistance: Gender Politics in the Age of Neoliberalism*, 19–213. London: Palgrave Macmillan.

Harding, S. 1993. 'Rethinking Standpoint Epistemology: What Is "Strong Objectivity"?' *Centennial Review* 36, no. 3 (1992): 437–70.

Hawkesworth, M.E. 2006. *Globalization and Feminist Activism*. Maryland: Rowman and Littlefield.

Hemer, O., and T. Tufte. 2016. 'Introduction: Why Voice and Matter Matter'. In *Communication, Development and the Cultural Return*, ed. Oscar Hemer and Thomas Tufte, 11–25. Nordicom: University of Gothenburg.

Heriot, J. 1996. 'Fetal Rights versus the Female Body: Contested Domains'. *Medical Anthropology Quarterly* 10, no. 2: 176–94.

Hirve, S.S. 2004. 'Abortion Law, Policy and Services in India: A Critical Review'. *Reproductive Health Matters* 12, no. 24: 114–21.

Huesca, R. 2003. 'Participatory Approaches to Communication for Development'. In *International Development Communication: A 21st Century Perspective*, ed. Bella Mody and William B. Gudykunst, 209–27. London: Sage.

- 2008. 'Tracing the History of Participatory Communication Approaches to Development: A Critical Appraisal'. In *Communication for Development and Social Change*, ed. Jan Serveas, 180–98. Sage Publications India.

Iosifidis, P. 2011. 'The Public Sphere, Social Networks and Public Service Media'. *Information, Communication and Society* 14, no. 5: 619–37.

Jain, D. 2005. *Women, Development and the UN – A Sixty-Year Quest for Equality and Justice*. Bloomington and Indianapolis: Indiana University Press.

Jaworski, A., and N. Coupland. 2014. 'Power, Ideology and Control'. In *The Discourse Reader*, ed. A. Jaworski and N. Coupland, 408–28. London: Routledge.

Jonsson, T. 2021. *Innocent Subjects: Feminism and Whiteness*. London: Pluto Press.

Jorgensen, M., and L. Philips. 2002. *Discourse Analysis as Theory and Method*. London: Sage.

Kabeer, N. 2015. 'Gender, Poverty and Inequality: A Brief History of Feminist Contributions in the Field of International Development'. *Gender and Development* 23, no. 2: 189–205.

Kaplan, C. 1997. 'The Politics of Location as Transnational Feminist Critical Practice.' In *Scattered Hegemonies: Postmodernity and Transnational Feminist Critical Practice*, ed. Inderpal Grewal and Caren Kaplan, 137–53. Minneapolis, MN: University of Minneapolis Press.

Kapoor, P. 2003. 'Gendered Sites of Conflict: Internet Activism in Reproductive Health'. *Feminist Media Studies* 3, no. 3: 368–71.

Kavada, A. 2014. 'Transnational Civil Society and Social Movements'. In *The Handbook of Development and Social Change*, ed. Karin G. Wilkins, Thomas Tufte, and Rafael Obregon, 351–69. Chichester, West Sussex: Wiley-Blackwell.

Keck, M.E., and K. Sikkink. 1998. *Activists beyond Borders: Advocacy Networks in International Politics*. Ithaca, NY: Cornell University Press

Khamis, S. 2015. 'Gendering the Arab Spring: Arab Women Journalists/ Activists, Cyber-Feminism and the Socio-Political Revolution.' In *The Routledge Companion to Media and Gender*, ed. Cynthia Carter, Linda Steiner, and Lisa McLaughlin, 565–75. London: Routledge.

Kindornay, S., J. Ron, and R.C. Carpenter. 2012. 'Rights-Based Approaches to Development: Implications for NGOs'. *Human Rights Quarterly* 34, no. 2: 472–506.

Kingston, L.N., and K.R. Stam. 2013. 'Online Advocacy: Analysis of Human Rights NGO Websites'. *Journal of Human Rights Practice* 5, no. 1: 75–95.

Kismodi, E., and L. Ferguson. 2018. 'Celebrating the 70th Anniversary of the UDHR, Celebrating Sexual and Reproductive Rights.' In *Reproductive Health Matters* 26, no. 52: 1–5.

Kleine, D., and T. Unwin. 2009. 'Technological Revolution, Evolution and New Dependencies: What's New about ICT4D?' *Third World Quarterly* 30, no. 5: 1045–67.

Kothari, U. 2002. 'Feminist and Postcolonial Challenges to Development'. In *Development Theory and Practice: Critical Perspectives*, ed. Uma Kothari and Martin Minogue, 35–52. Basingstoke: Palgrave.

Kothari, U., and M. Minogue. 2002. 'Critical Perspectives on Development: An Introduction'. In *Development Theory and Practice: Critical Perspectives*, ed. Uma Kothari and Martin Minogue, 1–16. Basingstoke: Palgrave.

Krippendorff, K., and M.A. Bock. 2009. *The Content Analysis Reader*. London: Sage.

Kulezycki, A. 2011. 'Abortion in Latin America: Changes in Practice, Growing Conflict and Recent Policy Development'. *Studies in Family Planning* 42, no. 3: 199–220.

Lazar, M. 2007. 'Feminist Critical Discourse Analysis: Articulating a Feminist Discourse Praxis 1'. *Critical Discourse Studies* 4, no. 2: 141–64.

Lebon, N. 2010. 'Women Building Plural Democracy in Latin America and the Caribbean'. In *Women's Activism in Latin America and the Caribbean – Engendering Social Justice, Democratizing Citizenship*, ed. Elizabeth Maier and Nathalie Lebon, 3–26. New Brunswick: Rutgers University Press.

Lee, M. 2006. 'What's Missing in Feminist Research in New Information and Communication Technologies?' *Feminist Media Studies* 6, no. 2: 191–210.

Lerner, D., and W. Schramm 1967. *Communication and Change in Developing Countries*. Honolulu: East-West Centre Press.

Lewis, B., and J. Lewis. 2015. *Health Communications: A Media and Cultural Studies Approach*. London: Palgrave Macmillan.

Lindekilde, L. 2014. 'Discourse and Frame Analysis: In-Depth Analysis of Qualitative Data in Social Movements Research'. In *Methodological Practices in Social Movement Research*, ed. Donatella Della Porta, 1–35. Oxford: Oxford Scholarship.

Lottes, I.L. 2013. 'Sexual Rights: Meanings, Controversies, and Sexual Health Promotion'. *Journal of Sex Research* 50, nos. 3–4: 367–91.

Lovejoy, K., and G.D. Saxton. 2012. 'Information, Community and Action: How Nonprofit Organisations Use Social Media'. *Journal of Computer-Mediated Communication*, 17: 337–53.

Lugones, M. 2016. 'The Coloniality of Gender'. In *The Palgrave Handbook of Gender and Development: Critical Engagement in Feminist Theory and Practice*, ed. Wendy Harcourt, 13–34. London: Palgrave.

Machado, M., R. de Assis, and Maciel, D. Alves. 2017. 'The Battle over Abortion Rights in Brazil's State Arena's, 1995–2006.' *Health and Human Rights* 19, no. 1: 119–32.

Machado, M. das D.C. 2018. 'O discurso cristão sobre a "ideologia de gênero"'. *Revista Estudos Feministas* 26, no. 2: 1–18.

Maier, E., and N. Lebon, eds. 2010. *Women's Activism in Latin American and the Caribbean: Engendering Social Justice, Democratizing Citizenship*. New Brunswick: Rutgers University Press.

Makkar, S. 2019. 'Marital Rape: A Non-Criminalized Crime in India.' *Harvard Human Rights Journal* 35 (Spring). https://harvardhrj.com/2019/01/marital-rape-a-non-criminalized-crime-in-india.

Mansell, R. 2014. 'Power and Interests in Information and Communication and Development: Exogenous and Endogenous Discourses in Contention'. *Journal of International Development* 26, no. 1: 109–27.

Mansell, R., and U. When, eds. 1998. *Knowledge Societies: Information Technology for Sustainable Development*. New York: Oxford.

Manyozo, L. 2012a. 'Community Media, Health Communication and Engagement: A Theoretical Matrix'. In *The Handbook of Global Health Communications*, ed. Rafael Obregon and Silvio Waisbord, 233–51. Chichester, West Sussex: Wiley-Blackwell.

– 2012b. 'Media, Communication and Development: School of Thoughts and Approaches'. In *Media, Communication and Development*, 1–53. London: Sage.

– 2017. *Communicating Development with Communities*. Abingdon, Oxon: Routledge

Marchand, M. 1995. 'Latin American Women Speak on Development – Are We Listening Yet?' In *Feminism, Postmodernism, Development*, ed. Marianne Marchand and Jane L. Parpart, 56–71. London: Routledge

Martin, E. 1987. 'Science as a Cultural System – Medical Metaphors of Women's Bodies: Menstruation and Menopause.' In *The Woman in the Body: A Cultural Analysis of Reproduction*, 25–69. Milton Keynes: Open University Press.

Matos, C. 2012. *Media and Politics in Latin America: Globalization, Democracy and Identity*. London: I.B. Tauris.

– 2016. *Globalization, Gender Politics and the Media*. Maryland: Lexington Books

– 2017. 'New Brazilian Feminisms and Online Networks: Cyberfeminism, Protest and the Female "Arab Spring"'. *International Sociology* 32, no. 3: 417–34. – 2022. 'NGOs and Advocacy Communications on Sexual and Reproductive Health and Rights: From the North to the South'. *Feminist Media Studies* 22, no. 2: 183–204.

McCann, H., and I. Nicholas. 2019. 'Gender Troubles: Is "Gender Ideology" Really a Danger to Feminism?' *Inside Story*, 18 February 2019, https://insidestory.org.au/gender-troubles.

McLaren, M. 2017. 'Introduction: Decolonizing Feminism.' In *Decolonizing Feminism: Transnational Feminism and Globalization*, ed. Margaret McLaren, 1–19. Maryland: Rowman and Littlefield.

McMillan, S. J. 2009. 'The Challenge of Applying Content Analysis to the World Wide Web'. In *The Content Analysis Reader*, ed. Klaus Krippendorff and Mary Bock, 60–7. London: Sage.

McPhail, T.L. 2009. 'The Roles of Non-Governmental Organisations (NGOs)'. In *Development Communications: Reframing the Role of the Media*, 67–83. West Sussex: Wiley-Blackwell.

McPherson, E. 2015. 'Advocacy Organisations' Evaluation of Social Media Information for NGO Journalism: The Evidence and Engagement Models'. *American Behavioral Scientist* 59, no. 1: 124–48.

– 2017. 'Social Media and Human Rights Advocacy'. In *The Routledge Companion to Media and Human Rights*, ed. Howard Tumber and Silvio Waisbord, 279–88. London and New York: Routledge.

McRobbie, A. 2009. *The Aftermath of Feminism: Gender, Culture and Social Change*. London: Sage.

Melkote, S. 2003. 'Theories of Development Communication'. *International and Development Communication: A 21st Century Perspective*, ed. Bella Mody and William B. Gudykunst, 129–47. London: Sage.

Melkote, S., and A. Singhal, eds. 2021. *The Handbook of Communication and Development*. Cheltenham: Edward Elgar.

Melkote, S.R, and L.H. Steeves. 2001. *Communication for Development in the Third World: Theory and Practice for Empowerment*. London: Sage.

Mendes, K., J. Ringrose, and J. Keller. 2019. *Digital Feminist Activism: Girls and Women Fight Back against Rape Culture*. New York: Oxford University Press.

Michailidou, M. 2018. 'Feminist Methodologies for the Study of Digital Worlds.' *International Journal of Media and Cultural Politics* 14, no. 1: 19–33.

Miguel, L.F., F. Biroli, R. Mariano. 2017. 'O direito ao aborto no debate legislativo brasileiro: A ofensiva conservadora na Câmara dos Deputados'. *Opinião Pública* 23, no 1: 230–60.

Miller, A.M., and Roseman, M. J. 2011. 'Sexual and reproductive rights at the United Nations: frustration and fulfilment?' In *Reproductive Health Matters* 19, no. 38: 102–18.

Miller, T. 2005. 'Conclusions and Reflections: Making Sense of Motherhood'. In *Making Sense of Motherhood: A Narrative Approach*, 138–61. Cambridge: Cambridge University Press.

Miskolci, R., and M. Campana. 2017. '"Ideologia de gênero": Notas para a genealogia de um pânico moral contemporâneo'. *Sociedade e Estado* 32, no. 3: 725–48.

Mitra, A. 2011. 'Feminist Organizing in India: A Study of Women in NGOs'. *Women's Studies International Forum* 34, no. 1: 66–75.

Mody, B., and W.B. Gudykunst. 2003. *International and Development Communication: A 21st Century Perspective*. London: Sage.

Mohanty, C.T. 2017. 'Toward a Decolonial Framing for the 99 Percent'. In *Decolonizing Feminism: Transnational Feminism and Globalization*, ed. Margaret McLaren, vii–1. Maryland: Rowman and Littlefield.

– 2000. 'Under Western Eyes: Feminist Scholarship and Colonial Discourses'. In *Feminist Theory: A Reader,* ed. Wendy K. Kolmer and Frances Kouski, 372–439. New York: McGraw Hill.

Morgan, L.M., and E. Roberts. 2012. 'Reproductive Governance in America'. *Anthropology and Medicine* 19, no. 2: 241–54.

Morgan, R. 2016. 'Sexual and Reproductive Health and Rights'. In *The Palgrave Handbook of International Development*, ed. Jean Grugel and Daniel Hammett, 471–85, London: Palgrave Macmillan.

Nah, S., and G.D. Saxton. 2012. 'Modelling the Adoption and Use of Social Media by Non-Profit Organisations'. *New Media and Society* 15, no. 2: 294–313.

Narayanaswamy, L. 2014. 'NGOs and Feminisms in Development: Interrogating the "Southern Women's NGO"'. *Geography Compass* 8, no. 8: 576–89.

– 2017. *Gender, Power and Knowledge For Development*. New York: Routledge.

Natansohn, G. 2013. 'Introdução: o que tem a ver as tecnologias digitais com o gênero?' In *Internet em código feminino: Teorias e práticas*, ed. Graciela Natansohn, 15–38. Buenos Aires: La Crujía.

Nederveen Pieterse, J. 2010. *Development Theory*. London: Sage.

Newsom, V.A., and L. Lengel. 2012. 'Arab Women, Social Media and the Arab Spring: Applying the Framework of Digital Reflexivity to Analyze Gender and Online Activism'. *Journal of International Women's Studies* 13, no. 5: 31–45.

Noske-Turner, J. 2017. *Rethinking Media Development through Evaluation: Beyond Freedom*. Melbourne: Palgrave Macmillan.

Obregon, R., and T. Tufte. 2017. 'Communication, Social Movements, and Collective Action: Toward a New Research Agenda in Communication for Development and Social Change'. *Journal of Communications* 67, no. 5: 635–45.

Obregon, R., and S. Waisbord. 2012. 'Capacity Building (and Strengthening) in Health Communication: The Missing Link'. In

The Handbook of Global Health Communications, ed. Rafael Obregon and Silvio Waisbord, 559–82. Chichester, West Sussex: Wiley-Blackwell.

O'Donnell, A., and C. Sweetman. 2018. 'Introduction: Gender, Development and ICTs'. *Gender and Development* 26, no. 2: 217–29.

Parker, R. 2009. 'Sexuality, Culture and Society: Shifting Paradigms in Sexuality Research'. *Culture, Health and Sexuality* 11, no. 3: 251–66.

Parpart, J., P. Connelly, and E.V. Barriteau. 2000. *Theoretical Perspectives on Gender and Development*. Canada, International Development Research Centre. ix–xiii.

Partners for Law in Development and SAMA Resource Group for Women and Health (PLD and SAMA). 2018. *Status of Human Rights in the Context of Sexual Health and Reproductive Rights in India*. April 2018. https://nhrc.nic.in/sites/default/files/sexual_health_reproductive_health_rights_SAMA_PLD_2018_01012019_1.pdf.

Petchesky, R.P. 2003. *Global Prescriptions: Gendering Health and Human Rights*. Switzerland: Zed Books.

Philips, L., and M.W. Jorgensen. 2002. 'Critical Discourse Analysis'. In *Discourse Analysis as Theory and Method*, 60–96. London: Sage.

Pieck, S.K. 2013. 'Transnational Activist Networks: Mobilisation between Emotion and Bureaucracy'. *Social Movement Studies: Journal of Social, Cultural and Political Protest* 12, no. 2: 121–37.

Plant, S. 1995. 'The Future Looms: Weaving Women and Cybernetics'. In *Body and Society*, 45–64. London: Sage

Provost, C., and N. Archer. 2020. 'Revealed: $280 Million "Dark Money" Spent by US Christian Right Groups Globally'. Open Democracy, 27 October 2020. https://www.opendemocracy.net/en/5050/trump-us-christian-spending-global-revealed.

Powers, M. 2014. 'The Structural Organisation of NGO Publicity Work: Explaining Divergent Strategies at Humanitarian and Human Rights Organisations'. *International Journal of Communication* 8: 90–107.

– 2017. 'Civic Organisations, Human Rights and the News'. In *The Routledge Companion to Media and Human Rights*, ed. Howard Tumber and Silvio Waisbord, 248–57. London and New York: Routledge.

Radcliffe, S.A. 2015. 'Gender and Post-colonialism'. In *The Routledge Handbook of Gender and Development*, ed. Ann Coles, Leslie Gray, and Janet Momsen, 35–47. London: Routledge.

Rai, S.M. 2011. 'Gender and Development: Theoretical Perspectives'. In *The Women, Gender and Development Reader*, ed. Nalini Visvanathan, Lynn Duggan, Nan Wiegersma, and Laurie Nisonoff, 28–38. London: Zed Books.

Reimeryte, E., and L. Ferreira. 2021. 'What Is Crisis Pregnancy?' Open Democracy, 8 December 2021. https://www.opendemocracy.net/en/5050/explainer-crisis-pregnancy.

Richardson, E., and A. Birn. 2011. 'Sexual and Reproductive Health and Rights in Latin America: An Analysis of Trends, Commitments and Achievements'. *Reproductive Health Matters* 19, no. 38: 183–96.

Ridgeway, C., and L. Smith-Lovin. 1999. 'The Gender System and Interaction'. *Annual Review of Sociology* 25, no. 1: 191–216.

Ridgeway, C., and S.J. Correll. 2004. 'Unpacking the Gender System: A Theoretical Perspective on Gender Beliefs and Social Relations'. *Gender and Society* 18, no. 4: 510–31.

Riley, T., E. Sully, Z. Ahmed, and A. Biddlecom. 2020. 'Estimates of the Potential Impact of the Covid-19 Pandemic on Sexual and Reproductive Health in Low and Middle-Income Countries'. *International Perspectives on Social and Reproductive Health* (Guttmacher Institute) 46: 73–6.

Rimon, J.G. 2001. 'Behaviour Change Communication in Public Health: Beyond Dialogue – Moving towards Convergence'. Paper presented at the United Nations Roundtable on Development Communication, sponsored by the UNFPA and Panos Institute, Managua, Nicaragua.

Risman, B.J. 2004. 'Gender as a Social Structure, Theory Wrestling with Activism'. *Gender and Society* 18, no. 4: 429–50.

Rogers, E.M. 1976. 'Communication and Development: The Passing of the Dominant Paradigm'. In *Communication and Development: Critical Perspectives*, ed. Everett M. Rogers, 121–48. London: Sage.

Roth, R. 2014 (1998). 'Backlash and Continuity: The Political Trajectory of Fetal Rights.' In *The Politics of Women's Bodies: Sexuality, Appearance and Behaviour*, ed. Rosa Weitz and Samantha Kwan, 322–30. New York: Oxford University Press.

Sadah, S.A., M. Shahbazi, M.T. Wiley, and V. Hristidis. 2016. 'Demographic-Based Content Analysis of Web-Based Health-Related Social Media'. *Journal of Medical Internet Research* 18, no. 6: 1–13.

Sandoval, C. 2000. 'New Sciences – Cyborg Feminism and the Methodology of the Oppressed.' In *The Cyberculture Reader*, ed. David Bell and Barbara M. Kennedy, 374–85. London: Routledge.

Sardenberg, C.M. 2007. 'Back to Women? Translations, Resignations and Myths of Gender in Policy and Practice in Brazil'. In *Feminisms in Development: Contradictions, Contestations and Challenges*, ed. Andrea Cornwall, Elizabeth Harrison, and Ann Whitehead, 48–65. London: Zed Books.

Sarikakis, K. 2014. 'Arriving at a Crossroads: Political Priorities for a Socially Relevant Feminist Media Scholarship.' In *Current Perspectives in Feminist Media Studies*, ed. Lisa McLaughlin and Cynthia Carter, 105–111. London: Routledge.

Sassen, S. 2002. 'Towards a Sociology of Information Technology'. *Current Sociology* 50, no. 3: 365–85.

Schramm, W. 1964. *Mass Media and National Development: The Role of Information in the Developing Countries*, 1–58. California: Stanford University Press.

Sebastian, M.P., M.E. Khan, and D. Sebastian. 2014. *Unintended Pregnancy and Abortion in India: Country Profile Report*. Population Council, New Dehli, 122. https://www.gov.uk/research-for-development-outputs/unintended-pregnancy-and-abortion-in-india-country-profile-report.

Sen, A. 1999. 'Women's Agency and Social Change'. In *Development as Freedom*, 189–203. Oxford: Oxford University Press

Sen, G., and A. Mukherjee. 2014. 'No Empowerment without Rights, No Rights without Politics: Gender Equality, MDGs and the Post-2015 Development Agenda'. *Journal of Human Development* 15, nos. 2–3.

Servaes, J. 2008. *Communication for Development and Social Change*. London: Sage.

– 2017. 'All Rights Are Local: The Resiliency of Social Change.' In *The Routledge Companion to Media and Human Rights*, ed. Howard Tumber and Silvio Waisbord, 136–47. London and New York: Routledge.

Servaes, J., and P. Malikhao. 2010. 'Advocacy Strategies for Health Communication'. *Public Relations Review* 36, no. 1: 42–9.

Sharma, A. 2008. *Logics of Empowerment: Development, Gender and Governance in Neoliberal India*. Minneapolis, MN: University of Minnesota Press.

Sharma, D. 2015. 'India Still Struggles with Rural Doctor Shortages'. *Lancet* World Report 386, no. 10011: 2381–82. https://www.thelancet.com/journals/lancet/article/PIIS0140-6736(15)01231-3/fulltext.

Silva, H. 2019. 'Os novos atores evangélicos e a conquista do espaço público na América Latina'. *Revista Reflexão* 43, no. 2: 243–63.

Simon-Kumar, R. 2006. *Marketing Reproduction: Political Rhetoric and Gender Policy in India*. New Delhi: Zubaan Books

Singh, S., R. Hussai, C. Shekhar, R. Archarya, A.M. Moore, M. Stillman, J.L. Frost, H. Sahoo, M. Alagarajan, A. Sundaram, S. Kalyanwala, and H. Ball. 2018. 'Abortion and Unintended Pregnancy in Six Indian

States: Findings and Implications for Policies and Programs'. In *Guttmacher Institute,* IPAS and Population Council of India, November 2018. https://www.guttmacher.org/sites/default/files/report_pdf/abortion-unintended-pregnancy-six-states-india.pdf.

Singhal, A. 2013. 'Introduction: Fairy Tales to Digital Games: The Rising Tide of Entertainment Education.' In *Critical Arts: A Journal of South-North Cultural and Media Studies* 27, no. 1: 1–8.

Singhal, A., and E. Rogers. 1999. *Entertainment Education: A Communication Strategy for Social Change.* London: Mahwah N.J.

Snyder, L.B. 2003. 'Development Communication Campaigns'. In *International and Development Communication: A 21st Century Perspective*, ed. Bella Mody and William B. Gudykunst, 167–89. London: Sage.

Sood, S., C. Shefner-Rogers, and J. Skinner. 2014. 'Health Communication Campaigns in Developing Countries'. *Journal of Creative Communications* 9, no. 1: 67–84.

Sotelo, M.V., and F. Arocena. 2021. 'Evangelicals in the Latin American Political Arena: The Cases of Brazil, Argentina and Uruguay'. *SN Social Sciences* 180: 1–26.

Sparks, C. 2007. *Globalization, Development and the Mass Media.* London: Sage.

Spivak, G. 1988. 'Can the Subaltern Speak?' In *Marxism and the Interpretation of Cultures*, ed. Cary Nelson and Lawrence Grossberg, 271–316. Basingstoke: Macmillan Education.

Starrs, A., A. Ezeh, G. Barker, A. Basu, J.T. Betrand, and R. Blum. 2018. 'Accelerate Progress: Sexual and Reproductive Health and Rights for All'. Report of the Guttmacher-*Lancet* Commission 391, 30 June 2018. https://www.thelancet.com/journals/lancet/article/PIIS0140-6736(18)30293-9/fulltext.

Steeves, H.L. 2003. 'Development Communication as Marketing, Collective Resistance and Spiritual Awakening.' In *International and Development Communication: A 21st Century Perspective*, ed. Bella Mody and William B. Gudykunst, 227–44. London: Sage

Stein, L. 2009. 'Social Movement Web Use in Theory and Practice: A Content Analysis of US Movement Websites'. *New Media and Society* 11, no. 5: 749–71.

Sternbach, N.S., M. Navarro-Aranguren, P. Chuchryk, and S. Alvarez. 1992. 'Feminisms in Latin America: From Bogota to San Bernardo'. *Signs* 17, no. 2 (1992): 393–434.

Stillman, M., J.J. Frost, S. Singh, A.M. Moore, and S. Kalyanwala. 2014. *Abortion in India: A Literature Review*, 12–14. New York: Guttmacher Institute.

Stroup, S., and A. Murdie. 2012. 'There's No Place Like Home: Explaining International NGO Advocacy'. *Review of International Organisations* 7, no. 4: 425–48.

Sumner, A., and M.A. Tribe. 2008. 'How Are Research and Practice Linked to Development Studies?' In *International Development Studies: Theories and Methods in Research and Practice*, 129–63. London: Sage.

Tacchi, J., and J. Lennie. 2014. 'A Participatory Framework for Researching and Evaluating Communication for Development and Social Change'. In *The Handbook of Development Communication and Social Change*, ed. Karin Wilkins, Thomas Tufte, and Rafael Obregon, 298–320. Chichester, West Sussex: Wiley-Blackwell.

Thrall, T., D. Stecula, and D. Sweet. 2014. 'May We Have Your Attention Please? Human-Rights NGOs and the Problem of Global Communications'. *International Journal of Press/Politics* 19, no. 2: 1–25.

Trevisan, F., B. Bello, M. Vaughan, and A. Vromen. 2020. 'Mobilizing Personal Narratives: The Rise of Digital "Story Banking": in US Grassroots Advocacy'. *Journal of Information Technology and Politics* 17, no. 2: 146–60.

Tufte, T. 2001. 'Entertainment-Education and Participation Assessing the Communication Strategy of Soul City'. *Journal of International Communication* 7, no. 2: 25–51.

– 2005. 'Entertainment-Education in Development Communication: Between Marketing and Empowering People'. In *Media and Glocal Change: Rethinking Communication for Development*, ed. Thomas Tufte and Oscar Hemer, 159–76. Goteborg: Nordicom.

– 2012. 'Communication and Public Health in a Glocalised Context: Achievements and Challenges'. In *The Handbook of Global Health Communications*, ed. Rafael Obregon and Silvio Waisbord, 608–23. Chichester, West Sussex: Wiley-Blackwell.

UNDP. 2009. 'Communications for Development: A Glimpse at UNDP's Practice'. Report of the United Nations Development Programme (UNDP). https://www.undp.org/publications/communication-development-glimpse-undps-practice.

UNFPA. 2020. 'Sexual and Reproductive Health and Rights, Maternal and Newborn Health and Covid-19'. Report of the United Nations Population Fund, March 2020. https://www.unfpa.org/resources/

sexual-and-reproductive-health-and-rights-maternal-and-newborn-health-covid-19-0.

Van Dijk, T.A. 2016. 'Critical Discourse Analysis: A Socio-Cognitive Approach'. In *Methods of Critical Discourse Studies*, ed. Ruth Wodak and Michael Meyer, 62–86. London: Sage.

Vargas, V. 2010. 'Constructing New Democratic Paradigms for Global Democracy: The Contributions of Feminisms.' In *Women's Activism in Latin American and the Caribbean: Engendering Social Justice, Democratizing Citizenship*, ed. Elizabeth Maier and Nathalie Lebon, 319–34. New Brunswick: Rutgers University Press.

– 2017. 'Some Thoughts on New Epistemologies in Latin American Feminism.' In *Bodies in Resistance – Gender Politics in the Age of Neoliberalism*, ed. Wendy Harcourt, 259–309. London: Routledge.

Vokes, R. 2018. 'ICT4D in New Media Worlds'. In *Media and Development*, 192–33. London: Routledge.

Wahl-Jorgensen, K., and T.R. Schmidt. 2019. 'News and Storytelling'. In *The Handbook of Journalism Studies*, ed. Karin Wahl-Jorgensen and Thomas Hanitzsch, 261–76. London: Routledge.

Waisbord, S. 2015. 'Three Challenges for Communication and Global Social Change'. *Communication Theory* 25, no. 2: 144–65.

– 2020. 'Family Tree of Theories, Methodologies and Strategies in Development Communication'. In *Handbook of Communication for Development and Social Change,* ed. Jan Serveas, 93-133 .Singapore: Springer Nature.

Waisbord, S., and R. Obregon. 2012a. 'Conclusions: Why Communication Matters in Global Health'. In *The Handbook of Global Health Communications*, ed. Rafael Obregon and Silvio Waisbord, 642–52. Chichester, West Sussex: Wiley-Blackwell.

– 2012b. 'Theoretical Divides and Convergence in Global Health Communication'. In *The Handbook of Global Health Communications*, ed. Rafael Obregon and Silvio Waisbord, 9–34. Chichester, West Sussex: Wiley-Blackwell.

Wajcman, J. 2000 (1991). *Feminism Confronts Technology*. London: Polity.

Walby, S. 2000. 'Gender, Globalization and Democracy'. *Gender and Development* 8, no. 1: 20–8.

Waylen, G. 1993. 'Women's Movements and Democratisation in Latin America'. *Third World Quarterly* 14, no. 3: 573–87.

– 1996. *Gender in Third World Politics*. Buckingham: Open University Press.

Wenham, C., J. Smith, and R. Morgan. 2020. 'Covid-19: The Gendered Impacts of the Outbreak'. *Lancet* 395: 846–8.

WHO. 2016. 'Action Plan for SRHR: Towards Achieving the 2030 Agenda for Sustainable Development in Europe – Leaving No One Behind'. World Health Organisation, Copenhagen, Denmark, 12–15 September. https://www.euro.who.int/__data/assets/pdf_file/0018/314532/66wd13e_SRHActionPlan_160524.pdf.

– 2017. *Strategic Communications Framework for Effective Communications*. Report of the World Health Organisation. https://www.who.int/docs/default-source/documents/communicating-for-health/communication-framework.pdf.

Wilkins, K.G. 2014. 'Advocacy Communications'. In *The Handbook of Development Communication and Social Change*, ed. Karin Wilkins, Thomas Tufte, and Rafael Obregon, 57–71, Chichester, West Sussex: Wiley-Blackwell.

– 2016. *Communicating Gender and Advocating Accountability in Global Development*. New York: Palgrave Macmillan

Wilkins, K.G., and B. Mody. 2001. 'Reshaping Development Communication: Developing Communication and Communicating Development'. *Communication Theory* 11, no. 4: 385–96.

Wilkins, K.G., T. Tufte, and R. Obregon. 2014. 'Developing Strategic Communication for Social Change'. In *The Handbook of Development Communications and Social Change*, ed. Karin Wilkins, Thomas Tufte, and Rafael Obregon, 145–329. Chichester, West Sussex: Wiley-Blackwell.

Williams, L.D., and G.A. Artzberger. 2019. 'Developing Women as ICT Users: A Miniature Scoping Review of Gender and ICTs for Development'. *Gender, Technology and Development* 23, no 3: 234–56.

Wilson, K. 2015. 'Towards a Radical Re-Appropriation: Gender Development and Neoliberal Feminism'. In *Development and Change* 46, no. 4: 803–32.

– 2018. 'For Reproductive Justice in an Era of Gates and Modi: The Violence of India's Population Policies'. *Feminist Review* 119, no. 1: 89–105.

Wodak, R., and M. Meyer, eds. 2016. 'Critical Discourse Analysis Studies: History, Agenda, Theory and Methodology'. In *Methods of Critical Discourse Analysis*, ed. Ruth Wodak and Michael Meyer, 1–33. London: Sage.

Yanacopulos, H. 2016. *International NGO Engagement, Advocacy, Activism: The Faces and Spaces of Change*. London: Palgrave Macmillan.

Yang, A., and A. Saffer. 2018. 'NGOs Advocacy in the 2015 Refugee Crisis: A Study of Agenda Building in the Digital Age'. *American Behavioural Scientist* 62, no. 4: 421–39.

Yokoe R., R. Rowe, S.S. Choudhury, A. Rani, F. Zahir, and M. Nair. 2019. 'Unsafe Abortion and Abortion-Related Death among 1.8 Million Women in India'. *BMJ Global Health* 4, no. 3: 1–13.

Youngs, G. 2002. 'Closing the Gaps: Women, Communications and Technologies'. *Development* 45, no. 4: 23–8.

– 2015. 'Digital Transformations of Transnational Feminism in Theory and Practice'. In *The Oxford Handbook of Transnational Feminist Movements*, ed. Rawwida Baksch and Wendy Harcourt, 857–66. Oxford: Oxford University Press.

Yuval-Davis, N. 2010 (1997). 'Theorising Gender and Nation'. In *Gender and Nation*, 1–25. London: Sage.

Index

abortion, 9–11, 13–14, 18–22, 30–2, 42, 50, 58, 71–4, 81–5, 87–8, 90, 93–6, 100–2, 121, 124, 128, 143, 145, 158, 160, 167, 171, 175, 180, 186, 192–5, 197–9, 202–7, 209–11, 217–18, 226–7, 229, 234, 236–7. *See also* anti–abortion

advocacy communication, 35, 37, 39–40, 50–1, 53, 121, 123, 128–9, 133–5, 138, 145, 152, 155, 163–4, 170, 179, 183–4, 189–91, 194–5, 200, 203, 209, 213–14, 221, 225, 230, 233–4, 239–40; advocacy around SRHR, 35, 66, 81, 117, 148; in health and feminist NGOs, 27, 34, 36, 40–1, 43, 54, 93, 101, 122, 129, 134, 227, 233; professional information led–type of, 44

Agenda Europe, 273

Akahata, 139, 145, 147, 176, 180

Alvarez, Sonia, 11, 16, 29, 35, 43–5, 64–5, 75–7, 79–80, 95, 103, 227

Amnesty International, 23–4, 42, 120–1, 124, 136, 145–9, 152, 156–8, 176–7, 180, 198, 200, 202–3, 207–8, 210–11, 236; Amnesty International Argentina, 120, 136, 156–7

anti-abortion, 14, 23, 217, 272. *See also* abortion

anti-colonialist, 4, 227

Arab Spring Uprising, 32

Argentina, 13, 23–4, 36, 77, 81, 83, 93, 120–1, 124, 136, 140, 145, 156–7

Australian National University, 8

Bangladesh, 31, 97, 102, 153, 201, 217

Bill Gates Foundation, 38, 100

body politics, 16, 60, 62

Bolsonaro, Jair, 5, 14, 21–2, 29, 87–9, 126, 193

Bolsonarismo political movement, 31

Brazil, 5, 12, 15, 18, 21–2, 29–32, 36–7, 40, 42, 68, 70, 74–5, 79–84, 86–91, 93–4, 126, 138, 147, 159, 182, 185, 188, 193–5, 222, 234, 236; catholic church in, 86; right

wing military dictatorship in, 31, 75. *See also* Bolsonaro, Jair; *Bolsonarismo* political movement
Butler, Judith, 22

Cairo Action Plan, 90
Care International UK, 42, 136, 139, 145–6, 148, 152–3, 162, 176
CDA's Moral And Ethical Dimensions, 50
Center for Catalyzing Change, 139, 214
Center for Reproductive Rights, 140, 146, 148–9, 177–8
Centre for Health and Gender Equity, 72, 130
Centro de Estudo, Pesquisa, Informacao e Acao (Centre of Studies and Research, Information and Action) (CEPIA), 18, 91, 140, 145, 148–9, 152, 176, 178
Centro de Promocion y Defensa de los Derechos Sexuales y Reprodutivos (Centre for the Promotion and Defence of Sexual and Reproductive Rights) (Promsex), 77, 121, 136, 142, 148, 150–1, 176–81
child mortality, 116
Chile, 23, 77, 84, 88, 93, 275, 278
Christian right groups (US), 14; and pro-life arguments, 11. *See also* Bolsonaro, Jair; Trump, Donald
civil society, 18, 23, 41–2, 64, 67, 71–2, 89, 97, 125, 213, 232, 236, 241, 243

climate change, 28, 32, 79, 230, 240, 245
colonialism, 60, 62, 75, 227
communications and new technologies, 27, 79, 81; communications for social change, 4, 26, 34, 105–6, 108, 241; digital divide, 30, 53, 126; internet users, 30; online and offline communications, 40
contraception, 43, 66, 68, 72, 91–2, 99, 152–3, 169, 190, 193, 195, 199, 204, 212, 216, 218, 226; sterilisation, 99. *See also* abortion; anti-abortion
Convention on the Elimination of all Forms of Discrimination Against Women (CEDAW), 24
Cornwall, Andrea, 10, 14–15, 28, 35, 41, 55–7, 59–61, 63, 66, 244, 272
Correa, Sonja, 10, 14–16, 18, 20, 28, 35, 55, 57, 59–63, 190, 272
COVID-19 pandemic, 8, 199, 225, 241, 245
Creating Resources for Empowerment in Action India (CREA India), 101, 141, 148–9, 151–2, 176–8, 180, 198
critical discourse analysis (CDA), 5, 36–7, 48, 104, 132, 135, 173–4, 197, 200, 213

development, 3–6, 8–11, 14–19, 23–30, 34–8, 40–5, 50–1, 55–70, 73, 76, 95–100, 105–13, 115–20, 122–3, 126–9, 132, 152, 161, 173, 181, 186, 206, 208, 211, 216, 218, 221–2, 224–5, 230–2, 234–5, 237–41,

243–6; and decolonisation, 4, 60, 228; industry, 6, 18, 56, 105, 126, 225, 235, 238, 243
digital storytelling, 5, 45, 120, 132, 174, 179, 191, 194–5, 198, 216, 229, 240, 242; communication and new technologies, 27, 126; deconstruction of language, discourses, and narratives, 6; fact checking in, 5, 45, 132, 190; narratives round sexual and reproductive health, 6, 54; sexuality (SRHR), 3, 5–6, 9, 11, 13, 15, 17–18, 20, 22–3, 25–8, 30–2, 34–51, 54, 58–9, 63, 66, 68–9, 71–5, 79, 81, 84, 86, 88, 92, 94–9, 101, 116–17, 120–2, 127–32, 134–8, 145, 147–8, 152–5, 157–8, 161–4, 166, 168–73, 175–6, 179–91, 193–5, 197–203, 205, 207, 209, 212–13, 215, 218–21, 223–40, 242–5; suffering and hardships, 230, 234
Donovan, Jack, 22

education, 4, 8, 10, 13, 19, 23, 27, 33, 43, 57, 58–9, 81, 84–5, 92, 95, 97–8, 107–8, 110–11, 113, 115, 118, 121–2, 161, 164, 169, 175, 179, 181, 186, 189, 192–3, 195, 199, 204, 227, 229, 232–3, 238, 241, 243
Ecuador, 84, 159–60, 208, 210
Egypt, 69, 95, 120
empowerment, 11, 16, 43–4, 56–5, 66, 71, 80, 97–8, 103, 105, 109, 123, 125, 145, 153, 193. *See also* development; gender ideology

European Parliamentary Forum Population and Development, 23

Family Planning 2020, 130, 135–6, 147–8, 152, 156, 168, 176–7, 179–80, 193, 239
far right, 5, 10, 13–14, 20, 31, 36, 226, 245; Trump, Donald, 4–5, 10, 14, 21–3, 73, 88, 193; Bolsonaro, Jair, 5, 14, 21–2, 29, 88–9, 126, 193; right-wing movements, 4
female bodies, 6, 61, 64, 74, 244; abortion, 9–11, 13–14, 16, 18–24, 30–2, 42, 50, 58, 68, 71–4, 81–5, 87–8, 90, 93–6, 100–2, 121, 124, 128, 143, 145, 158, 160, 167, 171, 175, 180, 182–6, 190, 192–5, 197–9, 202–7, 209–11, 215, 217–18, 223, 226–7, 229, 234, 236–7; decriminalization of abortion, 124, 175; *Roe v. Wade*, 9–10. *See also* abortion; anti-abortion; sexuality and reproductive health
female genital mutilation, 193
FEMEN, 124
feminism, 9, 11–13, 15, 20, 26–7, 29, 55, 57, 75–7, 79–80, 82, 121, 124, 125, 127, 189, 227, 244; Black, 15–16; and contemporary feminist activism, 12; and culture of death, 13, 30, 50; empowerment, 11, 16, 43–4, 56–7, 66, 71, 80, 97–8, 103, 105, 109, 123, 125, 145, 153, 193; feminist waves, 55; and global gender justice, 12, 29, 55, 74; intersectional, 46; and LGBT rights, 20–1, 73, 86, 191; liberal,

55; revival of, 9; and the 'Third World woman,' 56; and transgender rights, 12; transnational feminist advocacy, 11; white, 12, 26, 227
fertility, 11, 16–17, 50, 62, 68, 71, 81, 85, 95, 152, 195, 203, 209; sterilisation, 99. *See also* contraception

gender and development (GAD), 3, 6, 34, 50, 55, 57, 126, 224; 1994 International Conference for Population and Development (ICPD), 9, 16–17, 19, 39, 58, 71–2, 78, 97, 101–2, 201, 211; equality agenda, 13, 16, 21, 24, 76; sustainable development, 8, 24–25, 30, 58, 108, 114, 221, 241, 245; sustainable development goals (SDGS), 114, 221, 245; woman and development (WAD), 55; women in development (WID), 55. *See also* development; sexuality and reproductive health
gender-based violence, 12, 58, 82, 165, 194–5, 199, 207–8, 221–2, 229
gender equality, 3–4, 6, 8–9, 13, 16, 19, 24–5, 27–9, 34–5, 37, 41–4, 46, 60, 67, 74–6, 79, 82, 88, 95, 105, 112, 128–30, 139, 145, 153–4, 159, 180, 193, 195, 212, 221–2, 225–6, 228, 234, 238, 241, 245, 256. *See also* gender ideology; sexuality and reproductive health
gender ideology, 6, 13, 24, 33, 39, 49, 85–7, 92, 94, 137–8, 174, 188, 191, 226, 234; anti-gender ideology, 20; gender myths, 50
Global Challenges Research Fund, 3
Global Fund for Women, 11, 67, 136, 141, 146–9, 163–4, 170, 176–8, 180, 245
#GlobalGagRule, 190
Global Gender Gap Index, 95
globalisation, 9, 13–14, 38, 244
Global North, 3, 18, 24, 34, 36, 51, 74, 106, 120, 161, 239, 242, 243, 244–5
Global South, 3, 10, 12, 15, 17–18, 25–6, 29, 34–5, 38, 51, 56, 62–3, 65, 74, 77–8, 94, 101–2, 104, 106, 124, 126–7, 152, 171, 194, 216, 219, 226–7, 231, 235, 239, 243–4
Guttmacher and Lancet Commission, 31, 58, 228

Hague, The, 23, 231, 233
Haraway, Donna, 46, 61, 123, 125
health/healthcare, 3–6, 8–11, 13, 15–19, 21, 23–5, 27–32, 34–6, 38–44, 46, 48–51, 54–60, 63–4, 66–74, 76–7, 79–85, 87–96, 98–102, 104–5, 109–10, 112–24, 127–36, 138–9, 141, 143, 145–8, 150, 152–3, 155–6, 158–67, 171–6, 178–81, 183–4, 186–8, 190, 193, 195, 197, 199, 202, 204–16, 219, 221–3, 225–39, 241–2; HIV/Aids, 15, 27, 59, 90, 115–16, 118, 191, 232; National Health Service (NHS), 30; NGO and public health advocates, 13; Sistema Unico de Saude (SUS), 30
hidden pockets, 101, 215

HIV/Aids, 15, 27, 59, 90, 115–16, 118, 191, 232
human rights, 4, 15–17, 19, 27, 31, 32, 37, 39, 41–2, 50, 57, 59, 63, 66, 68–71, 88, 91, 107–9, 112, 124, 128–9, 132, 145, 158–9, 163, 173, 181, 193, 203, 208, 211, 221, 227, 236, 238, 245
Human Rights Law Network, 31
Hungary, 23

IESP UERJ, 23
imperial legacy, 17
India, 12–13, 24, 29–31, 36–7, 41, 71, 94–9, 102, 116, 126, 136, 138–9, 142, 145, 153, 156, 176, 204, 207, 214, 216–17, 219, 221–3; Modi, Narendra, 29
International Alliance of Women (IAW), 23, 66–7, 141
International Conference for Population and Development (ICPD), 9, 16–17, 19, 39, 58, 71–2, 78, 97, 101–2, 201, 211
International Planned Parenthood Federation (IPPF), 23, 31, 136, 141, 145–7, 156, 195
IPSOS, 93
Ireland, 13, 24, 121, 124, 195, 197, 206, 236

Jolly, Suzy, 10, 14–15, 28, 35, 55, 57, 59–61, 63

King's College London, UK, 8

Latin America, 4, 10, 13–14, 30, 35–6, 42, 68–9, 74–82, 84, 86–93, 95, 106, 124–6, 136, 159, 161, 166, 169, 171, 175, 179–82, 193, 215–16, 222, 224, 226, 234, 237, 239
Latin American and Caribbean Committee for the Defence of the Rights of Women (CLADEM), 92, 141
London International Development Centre (LIDC), 10. *See also* decolonisation; development

males, 236
Malthusian: agenda, 17; approach, 96; framework, 152; theory, 17
masculinity, 22. *See also* female bodies; feminism
media and communications, 4, 27, 36, 42, 44, 105–6, 128, 133, 241
Mesa por la Vida de Las Mujeres, La, 90, 120–1, 136, 141, 145, 156–7
#MeToo movement, 13, 24, 124, 194; sexual harassment, 11–12, 25, 194
modernisation theory, 15, 26–7, 105, 115. *See also* decolonisation; development
Mohanty, Chandra, 4, 12, 17, 55–7, 62, 73, 103, 120, 244
Mujer y Salud, 84, 131, 141, 148, 156, 185–7

neoliberalism, 22, 30–1, 33, 76–7, 101, 228, 241
New Right, 16, 228. See also, Bolsonaro, Jair; far right; Trump, Donald
NGO journalism, 5, 48; advocacy communication, 5, 35, 40, 42,

44–5, 48, 54, 112, 122, 129–31, 181, 191, 210, 214–15, 241
Non-profit organisations (NGO), 11, 13, 16, 18, 22–3, 27, 31, 37, 39, 42–3, 48, 64–8, 70–2, 77, 81, 84, 89–91, 97, 100–2, 117, 119–21, 124, 127, 130–1, 134–6, 145–7, 157, 159, 161, 163–4, 167, 171, 175–6, 179, 181, 184–5, 190–1, 193–4, 200–3, 206, 209–11, 214, 216–17, 222, 224, 231, 234–5, 241–3, 252–3, 266–7; health and feminist NGOs, 27, 34, 36, 40–1, 43, 54, 93, 101, 122, 129, 134, 227, 233; NGO activists, 11, 22, 23; professionalised non-profits, 103
Northern NGO, 65, 214

Open Democracy, 14, 222
Orban, Viktor, 17, 62
'Other', the, 17, 62; differences, 6, 9, 18, 25, 28–9, 38, 40, 44, 94, 128–9, 133, 152, 174–5, 183, 206, 225, 231, 245
Oxfam, 8

Peru, 36, 77, 87
pleasure, 11, 60, 62–3, 85, 160, 193, 219, 22. *See also* contraception; fertility; sexuality and reproductive health
'Politization of pregnancy', 10; culture of death, 13, 30, 50; fertility and childcare, 11; pro-life arguments, 11. *See also* abortion
population, 8–9, 16–17, 19, 23, 32, 34, 61, 63, 68–9, 89–90, 92, 95–7, 99, 106, 108–9, 115, 119–20, 122, 131, 136, 138, 142–3, 145–6, 159–61, 171, 184, 187–9, 211, 218–19, 222, 237–8, 242–3, 253, 260, 262; and family planning; 237; Malthusian theory, 17; population control, 16–17, 30, 63, 95–6. *See also* feminism; social movements
Population Foundation of India, 97, 136, 138, 142, 145, 146, 219
postcolonial scholars, 12, 15, 17, 26, 55, 120. *See also* development; imperial legacy
poverty, 8–9, 11, 15, 17, 27, 29–30, 45, 56–9, 63, 65, 73, 79, 88, 105, 109, 114, 129, 152, 242, 245; child deaths, 9; deprivation, 11; impact of COVID-19, 9, 229; reduction in the 'Third World', 17; reproduction of inequalities, 22; web of disadvantages, 15, 59
Pussy Riot, 124

Racism, 50, 60, 158, 194
Realisation of Sexual and Reproductive Health and Rights Justice (RSRJ), 101
reproductive bodies, 14, 56, 73
reproductive health, 3–6, 9–11, 13, 16–17, 19, 23–5, 28–32, 34–6, 38–42, 44, 48–51, 54–5, 58–60, 63–4, 66, 69, 71, 73–4, 76–7, 79, 81–4, 87–9, 92–6, 98–9, 101–2, 104, 112, 115–16, 118, 120, 123–4, 127–9, 134–6, 141, 143, 145–8, 150, 152, 155, 158, 159–61, 163–7, 172, 174–6,

178–80, 183–4, 186–7, 190, 193, 197, 199, 205, 208, 210–13, 215–16, 219, 221, 223, 225–7, 229, 232–9, 241–5
Reprolatina, 11, 70, 81, 91, 136, 143, 156, 159, 185, 188–9, 234–5

sexuality, 3–4, 6, 10–11, 13–17, 24–2, 28–30, 33–4, 38–40, 44, 49–50, 58–63, 69–70, 72–4, 77, 81–2, 84–9, 92, 94, 102, 104, 112, 118, 120, 127, 129, 134, 160, 164, 169, 172, 189, 192, 195, 199, 205, 208, 210, 213, 215–17, 219, 223, 227–30, 232, 234, 236–8, 241, 244–5, 272; and human rights, 4, 15–17, 19, 27, 31–2, 37, 39, 41–2, 48, 51, 57, 59, 63, 66, 68–71, 88, 91, 107–9, 112, 124, 128–9, 132, 145, 158–9, 163, 171, 181, 193, 203, 208, 211, 221, 227, 236, 238, 245; and motherhood and maternity, 28; and pleasure, 11, 60, 62–3, 65, 160, 193, 219, 222; transgender people, 15; of women, 28. *See also* poverty; sexuality and reproductive health
sexuality and reproductive health, 3–4, 6, 10–11, 13, 29–30, 39–40, 44, 50, 58, 60, 63, 69, 74, 82, 84, 87–8, 94, 104, 112, 118, 127, 134, 205, 213, 215–16, 223, 227, 232, 234, 236, 237, 241, 245; birth control, 17, 19, 68, 91, 152, 154, 162, 169, 204, 218; *deconstruction* of language,

discourses, and narratives, 6; 'Effective SRHR Messaging in Changing Times' (The Hague), 23, 231; entertainment-education, 119, 122, 137; mediated public sphere, 5, 50, 69, 182, 234; misinformation, 13, 32, 34, 38, 49–50, 54, 87, 136, 138, 163, 166, 181, 187, 189, 215–16, 218; public sphere, 5–6, 11, 13, 25, 27, 30, 33–4, 38, 50–1, 60, 64, 69, 71, 75, 80, 83, 92, 94, 182, 191, 210, 229, 233–5, 237, 243; safe abortion services, 20; social movements, 5, 12, 29, 38, 64, 81, 86, 95, 100, 110, 120, 123, 196, 283. *See also* Bolsonaro, Jair; far right; Trump, Donald; women's rights
Sexual Policy Watch, 143, 148, 150, 176, 178–80, 182
SheDecides, 20, 143, 193
SlutWalk, 124
social movements, 5, 12, 29, 38, 64, 81, 86, 95, 100, 110, 120, 123, 196
sustainable development, 8, 24–5, 30, 58, 108, 114, 172, 221, 241, 245–6

transformative social change, 4, 67, 239
transgender people, 12, 15, 18, 217

UN Conference on Environment and Development (1992), 15
United Kingdom (UK), 5, 12, 36–7, 41–2, 124, 136, 139, 145–6, 148–9, 152–3, 157–8, 162, 176–7, 183, 193, 195, 200,

202–3, 207–8, 210, 228–9, 236, 242
United Nations (UN), 8, 69, 109
United Nations Children's Fund (UNICEF), 38, 95
United Nations Children's Fund India (UNICEF India), 95
United Nations Population Fund (UNFPA), 8, 72, 161, 193, 201, 226, 239
United States of America (USA), 73, 271
Uruguay, 23, 36, 83–4, 132, 141, 185, 187, 275, 278
US Agency for International Development (USAID), 99
US Occupy Wall Street, 32

Vatican, 33

Western liberal democracy, ix, 9; SRHR advocacy, 27, 36–7, 40, 47, 135, 154, 158, 181, 185, 212–13, 219, 230–1, 239, 242; Western institution, 26, 56
White Ribbon Alliance, 157, 214, 222; White Ribbon Coalition, 100; White Ribbon Alliance India, 144, 146
World Bank, 99
World Conference on Human Rights (1993), 15
World Health Organisation (WHO), 19, 66, 70–1, 110, 114, 204
World Social Forum (WSF), 77

Youth Coalition for Sexual and Reproductive Rights (YCSRR), 169–70, 206
YouAct, 144